369 0246450

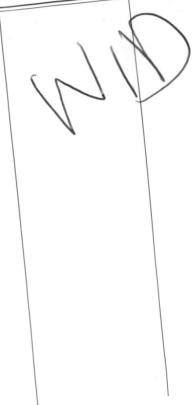

WD

D1471322

Notice

a LANGE medical book

THE ULTIMATE GUIDE TO
CHOOSING
A MEDICAL
SPECIALTY

THIRD EDITION

Brian S. Freeman, MD
Department of Anesthesiology
Georgetown University Medical Center
Washington, DC

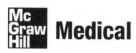 **Medical**

New York   Chicago   San Francisco   Lisbon   London
Madrid   Mexico City   Milan   New Delhi   San Juan
Seoul   Singapore   Sydney   Toronto

The Ultimate Guide to Choosing A Medical Specialty, Third Edition

1 2 3 4 5 6 7 8 9 0   DOC/DOC   17 16 15 14 13 12
ISBN 978-0-07-179027-7
MHID 0-07-179027-6
ISSN 1545-3626

This book was set in Electra by Aptara, Inc.
The editors were Catherine A. Johnson and Cindy Yoo.
The production supervisor was Jeffrey Herzich.
Project management was provided by Ruchira Gupta, Aptara, Inc.
The interior design was adapted from the original by Marsha Cohen/Parallelogram; the cover designer was Joanne Lee.
Cover image: Female surgeon anesthetizing a patient in an operating room. Credit: Glow Wellness.
RR Donnelley was printer and binder.

This book is printed on acid-free paper.

McGraw-Hill books are available at special quantity discounts to use as premiums and sales promotions, or for use in corporate training programs. To contact a representative please e-mail us at bulksales@mcgraw-hill.com.

For my wife, Rebecca:

Without you, this book would never have been conceived. You are my
inspiration—each and every day—for all that I do and all that
I hope to achieve. Thank you for your love, for your never-ending
support and devotion, and for always being there with a soft "pet"
whenever I need one. I am yours forever.

CONTENTS

CONTRIBUTORS

Vicki Anderson, MD, MBA
Assistant Professor of Physical Medicine and Rehabilitation
Spinal Cord Injury Medicine Fellowship Program Director
Medical College of Wisconsin
Milwaukee, Wisconsin
Physical Medicine and Rehabilitation

Kathleen Ang-Lee, MD
Clinical Instructor
Department of Psychiatry and Behavioral Sciences
University of Washington School of Medicine
Seattle, Washington
Psychiatry

Gregory H. Borschel, MD, FACS, FAAP
Assistant Professor
Department of Surgery
University of Toronto
Division of Plastic and Reconstructive Surgery
The Hospital for Sick Children
Toronto, Ontario, Canada
Plastic Surgery

Amy J. Derick, MD
Clinical Instructor
Department of Dermatology
Feinberg School of Medicine
Northwestern University
Chicago, Illinois
Dermatology

Kelly Oberia Elmore, MD
Obstetrician/Gynecologist
President, KOE Medical Consulting, Inc.
San Diego, California
Obstetrics and Gynecology

Derek L. Fimmen, MD
General Radiologist
Cape Radiology
Cape Girardeau, Missouri
Radiology

Brian S. Freeman, MD
Department of Anesthesiology
Georgetown University Medical Center
Washington, DC
Anesthesiology

Jeremy Graff, MD
Medical Director
Emergency Services
St. Rose Hospital
Hayward, California
Emergency Medicine

Arjun Joshi, MD, FACS, FRCSC
Assistant Professor
Division of Otolaryngology—Head and Neck Surgery
The George Washington University
Washington, DC
Otolaryngology

John C. Langland, MD
Orthopedic Surgeon
Steindler Orthopedic Clinic, P.L.C.
Iowa City, Iowa
Orthopedic Surgery

Jane M. Lewis, MD
Assistant Professor
Department of Urology
University of Minnesota Medical School
Minneapolis, Minnesota
Urology

Michael Mendoza, MD, MPH
Assistant Professor
Department of Family Medicine
University of Rochester School of Medicine and Dentistry
Medical Director
Highland Family Medicine
Rochester, New York
Family Medicine

Aaron J. Miller, MD, MPA
Assistant Professor of Clinical Pediatrics
Weill Cornell Medical College
Director, Lincoln Child Advocacy Center
Lincoln Medical & Mental Health Center
New York, New York
Pediatrics

Ashish Raju, MD
Vascular Fellow
Division of Vascular and Endovascular Surgery
Department of Cardiovascular and Thoracic Surgery
Montefiore Medical Center and Albert Einstein College of Medicine
Bronx, New York
General Surgery

Edmunds Z. Reineks, MD, PhD
Associate Staff
Pathology and Laboratory Medicine Institute
Cleveland, Ohio
Pathology

Andrew P. Schwartz, MD, FAAO
Clinical Instructor
Department of Ophthalmology
Mount Sinai School of Medicine
New York, New York
Ophthalmology

Kiarash Shahlaie, MD, PhD
Assistant Professor
Department of Neurological Surgery
University of California Davis School of Medicine
Sacramento, California
Neurosurgery

Neil Tanna, MD, MBA
Institute of Reconstructive Plastic Surgery
New York University
New York, New York
Otolaryngology

Ian Tong, MD
Clinical Assistant Professor
Department of Medicine
School of Medicine
Stanford University
Stanford, California
Internal Medicine

Jennifer Tong, MD
Hospitalist, Galen Inpatient Physicians
Department of Internal Medicine
Santa Clara Valley Medical Center
San Jose, California
Internal Medicine

Lisa Vargish, MD, MS
Attending Physician
Jewish Home of Rochester
Rochester, New York
Family Medicine

Stephanie E. Weiss, MD
Chief, Adult Brain Tumors and Radiosurgery
Brigham Women's/Dana Farber Cancer Institute
Harvard Medical School
Boston, Massachusetts
Radiation Oncology

Lisa Yerian, MD
Assistant Professor of Pathology
Medical Director, Continuous Improvement
Cleveland Clinic
Cleveland, Ohio
Pathology

Tomasz Zabiega, MD
Neurologist
Joliet Headache and Neuro Center
Joliet, Illinois
Neurology

PREFACE

Twelve years ago I was a confused third-year medical student, not having any idea about the next step in my education and professional training. Deciding on a career in medicine was easy; choosing a specialty, on the other hand, was agonizing. Like my classmates, I felt overwhelmed by the number of choices. I imagined myself as a future surgeon or emergency medicine physician, but after extensive research and clinical experiences, I soon discovered that anesthesiology was the perfect fit. I realized at the time that medical students need a good written resource to guide them through this difficult career-defining decision. This is when the idea for *The Ultimate Guide to Choosing a Medical Specialty* was born. Today's doctor-in-training requires as much information as possible to make a confident decision, but has little time to gather it. A single comprehensive resource, this book provides detailed insight into each field and allows students to quickly and easily compare specialties under consideration.

SPECIAL FEATURES

- An "insider's look" into different areas of medicine—specialty chapters written by physicians just out of residency training
- Candid and revealing descriptions of each specialty, including the pros and the cons, plus salary information, employment data, match statistics, and much more
- Profiles of the major medical specialties, including those to which medical students may receive little exposure, such as radiation oncology
- A concise up-to-date guide to the residency application and matching process, including a separate chapter dedicated to the "Couples Match"
- A special chapter with explicit advice to help medical students maximize their success in obtaining a residency position in each field

ORGANIZATION

This book is organized into two major sections. Part 1, "Planning Your Medical Career," delves into the main issues surrounding the choice of one's medical specialty. These 12 chapters provide everything you need to begin making this major decision—how to research each specialty, what to do if you remain undecided, how to apply for a residency position, and much more. This section is especially valuable if read early during your medical education. In Part 2, "Specialty Profiles," a chapter is devoted to each of the 20 major medical disciplines, all following a similar format and exploring common themes. Interspersed throughout the text are special inserts—"Vital Signs" and "The Inside Scoop"—that provide easy-to-read factoids such as salary information and match statistics.

AUDIENCE

Most readers interested in this book are current medical students—allopathic and osteopathic, and those who attend medical school in the United States and abroad. But you do not have to be a medical student in order to get something out of this book. Many residents have second thoughts about their chosen specialty and wish to change fields. In addition, premedical college students, as well as anyone considering medicine as a possible career, will find this book helpful.

FEEDBACK

For comments and suggestions about the book, you are invited to contact the author by e-mail (nerveblock1@yahoo.com) or by regular mail:

Brian S. Freeman, MD
c/o McGraw-Hill Medical
1221 Avenue of the Americas, 45th Floor
New York, NY 10020

Your feedback is invaluable for continuing to make this book a must-have resource for future medical students. If you have questions regarding specific areas of medicine, you may e-mail the contributor of that specialty chapter. Their biographical and contact information can be found at the end of each chapter.

ACKNOWLEDGMENTS

Many people helped make this book a reality. I first would like to acknowledge my mother, Ellen, for all her guidance, love, and support throughout my life. I also owe a huge debt of gratitude to the following people who shared their encouragement and advice: Eric Freeman, Gertrude Eichschlag, the Spiro family, Dr Russell T. Wall, and Dr William McDade. A special "meow" goes out to our Cornish Rex cats who kept my lap warm on cold winter nights while writing and editing this book.

In the medical publishing division of McGraw-Hill, a fantastic team of editors helped bring this book into creation. For the first edition, Shelley Reinhardt, the editor-in-chief, went out of her way to nurture a new author. Susan Meigs offered unparalleled editing expertise and countless useful suggestions that were right on target. For the second and third editions, my new editors, Marsha Loeb and Kirsten Funk, were incredibly helpful in paving the way for an even stronger book. The entire copy-editing and production team turned words and thoughts into a reader-friendly and fun package.

I especially thank the extraordinary writers who contributed chapters on their specialties for the second and third editions of this book. Even while under the stress and hardship of being a resident then attending, their passion for their chosen careers shines through in their work. This special group of physicians includes Vicki Anderson, Kathleen Ang-Lee, Gregory Borschel, Kelly Elmore, Amy Farmer, Derek L. Fimmen, Jeremy Graff, Arjun Joshi, Jennifer Lamb, John Langland, Jane M. Lewis, Michael Mendoza, Aaron Miller, Ashish Raju, Andrew P. Schwartz, Kiarash Shahlaie, Neil Tanna, Ian Tong, Lisa Vargish, Stephanie Weiss, Lisa Yerian, and Tomasz Zabiega.

Brian S. Freeman, MD
Washington, DC

1
PLANNING YOUR MEDICAL CAREER

1

CHOOSING A SPECIALTY: THE MOST DIFFICULT DECISION OF YOUR CAREER

"Is it true that gynecologists have the worst sex lives of all doctors?"

"Are you going to be a neurosurgeon like your mother?"

"Why don't you look into dermatology? It's got easy hours and you'll make good money."

Throughout their education, medical students never stop hearing these kinds of comments. Starting from the moment of acceptance into medical school, these questions continue well into the final year of earning the MD. As they undertake the first major professional decision of their career, medical students often struggle to come up with a good answer. After all, it seems like just about everyone has a strong opinion on the "best" specialty for a future doctor. That person could be an advisor, parent, supervising physician, or even Aunt Betty at the annual family reunion. From anesthesiology to urology, there are more than 60 specialties and subspecialties (Table 1–1). How will a medical student make an educated decision?

"MD" REALLY STANDS FOR "MAJOR DECISIONS"

Medicine is a profession that requires overwhelming sacrifice and commitment. You have to spend more than $200,000 for 4 years of rigorous education, followed by many long, tough years of on-the-job training. Like life in general, many

3

TABLE 1–1

RECOGNIZED MEMBERS OF THE AMERICAN BOARD OF MEDICAL SPECIALTIES (ABMS)

Specialty Board	Year of Founding
Allergy and immunology	1971
Anesthesiology	1941
Colon and rectal surgery	1949
Dermatology	1932
Emergency medicine	1979
Family practice	1969
Internal medicine	1936
Medical genetics	1993
Neurological surgery	1940
Nuclear medicine	1971
Obstetrics and gynecology	1930
Ophthalmology	1917
Orthopedic surgery	1935
Otolaryngology	1924
Pathology	1936
Pediatrics	1933
Physical medicine and rehabilitation	1947
Plastic surgery	1941
Preventive medicine	1949
Psychiatry and neurology	1935
Radiology	1935
Surgery	1937
Thoracic surgery	1970
Urology	1935

Data from American Board of Medical Specialties.

important decisions line the road to becoming a doctor. Think back to the day when you decided on a career in medicine. Whether you were a college student, trying to pick between medicine, engineering, and public policy or perhaps an older, nontraditional applicant who chose to leave a well-paying—but unrewarding—job for a new calling in medicine, it was one of life's biggest decisions. After slogging through tedious premedical courses and the application process, you then made the choice of where to attend medical school.

Now, another career-defining challenge awaits. The medical school experience is more than just memorizing all the branches of the facial nerve, holding retractors during surgery, and learning how to use a stethoscope. Each and every medical student has to go through 4 years of grueling examinations, sleepless nights on call, and tough clinical rotations. Despite these hurdles, most medical students see eye to eye on what is really the greatest challenge of all—choosing one's medical specialty. Figuring out what type of doctor to be is, in many ways, more difficult than deciding to become a physician. Once medical students settle on a specific niche within medicine, they become more than just future doctors. They start to take on a new *identity*—that of a pediatrician, forensic psychiatrist, endocrinologist, orthopedic surgeon, or interventional neuroradiologist.

The specialties themselves are quite diverse. Graduating doctors have the freedom to choose from a wide variety of medical fields. Some are based strictly on an organ system, like the brain (neurosurgery and neurology), the heart (cardiology), and the male genitourinary system (urology). Others provide comprehensive medical care for specific population groups, such as women (obstetrics–gynecology) and children (pediatrics). Another set of specialties share in common the fact that they are hospital-based services. Its members include radiology, pathology, anesthesiology, and emergency medicine. Medical specialties can also generally be divided into two main groups: primary care (long-term comprehensive care) versus secondary/tertiary care (referral-based care). Generalist specialties such as family practice, internal medicine, and pediatrics are considered primary care fields. More specialized areas such as gastroenterology, dermatology, and cardiothoracic surgery fall into the latter category.

Everyone knows that medical school has many rigorous demands: patient care, lectures, rounds, examinations, and call schedules all compete for a medical student's time, often crowding out sleep and a personal life. As a result, most students have even less time for the proper self-assessment, research, and exploration required to choose the right specialty. Every medical student agrees that it is the most difficult professional decision that they will have to make. Yet most will probably spend more time researching what kind of car to buy! In the end, many hastily choose their lifetime careers without having all the information they need to make an educated decision.

This book is designed to help medical students make an informed choice by the time senior year rolls around. Deciding on a field of medicine is often described as matching oneself with the characteristics of a particular specialty, such as lifestyle, intellectual challenge, technological focus, and research potential. Because of these factors, there is much confusion, frustration, and uncertainty involved in this defining moment of a young physician's career. Poor decision making can have considerable implications for one's professional happiness later in life.

INTERNSHIP, RESIDENCY, AND FELLOWSHIP

Medical school is only the first step in learning how to become a competent, caring physician. There are three different types of on-the-job training that commence immediately following graduation from medical school. These avenues take young, inexperienced doctors and turn them into well-trained specialists, ready to cure disease and save lives. Choosing a specialty determines what form of further professional training is required after medical school. Today's medical student, therefore, needs a clear understanding of the structure of postgraduate medical education.

Medical students have to commit to their specialty to begin the next phase in training: residency. During the past 70 years, rapid advancements in medical science created a greater demand for specialists, which residency programs expanded to meet. Depending on the specialty, residency consists of 3 to 7 years of additional formal training and study (under physician supervision). Medical school provides only a broad clinical foundation. Residency takes it one step further and confers the skills, knowledge, and experience necessary to practice medicine unsupervised in a given specialty. Being a resident physician is like working as an indentured servant. You work long hours for little pay and spend many nights sleeping in the hospital. In fact, residency earned its name from the old days when house staff physicians actually lived on hospital grounds, as residents.

Through the National Resident Matching Program, graduating medical students may enter residency training in 20 different specialties. You actually have even more options. Here is why: The American Board of Medical Specialties (ABMS) recognizes 24 official specialty boards. But every year, statistical data from the residency match show that nearly all medical students enter 1 of only 20 areas. What about the remaining four? Three of the specialties—medical genetics, preventive medicine, and nuclear medicine—offer such a small handful of residency positions (13 total in 2011) that few students really consider them as options. The other disciplines—allergy medicine and thoracic and colorectal surgery—are really considered subspecialties of internal medicine and surgery, respectively. (Psychiatry and neurology both share the same specialty board, and radiation oncology falls under the jurisdiction of radiology.) In addition, students may also select more than one specialty through the combined residency programs described in Chapter 7. Doing the math, these 14 available options bring the grand total to 34 choices.

After deciding on a specialty for residency, many physicians later choose to subspecialize further by obtaining a fellowship, which can last any number of years. Subspecialties exist for nearly every specialty. Examples include rheumatology or infectious disease (internal medicine), vascular surgery (general surgery), pain management (anesthesiology), and retinal surgery (ophthalmology). Because of all the subspecialties, there are more than 60 different kinds of doctors out there! You can be an adolescent medicine specialist, critical care physician, or interventional radiologist. The choices seem endless. Because areas of subspecialization are primarily of interest to current residents in training, they will not be a major focus of this book. It is important to remember, however, that these fields are all potential career paths. Do not exclude them from your mind while you are contemplating and exploring the 20 basic specialties. Having so many additional options just means that the decision gets even tougher.

Where does internship fit into all this? In the old days (prior to 1970), all graduating medical students completed a 1-year rotating internship before entering residency. This busy year consisted of all the core specialties: internal medicine, surgery, pediatrics, obstetrics–gynecology, and psychiatry. The goal was to provide broad hands-on training that would enable a new physician to work in the community as a general practitioner. After the demise of the formal internship in 1970, only the lingo lives on today. Internship is now simply considered the first postgraduate year (PGY-1) of residency. In most hospitals, newly minted MDs, fresh out of medical school, are usually known as first-year residents rather than interns. The old internship does still exist in a disguised form: the transitional year residency. This track (along with other 1-year programs) is discussed further in Chapter 9.

WHY HAS CHOOSING A SPECIALTY BECOME SO DIFFICULT?

Medical Students Are Faced with More Choices than Ever

Back in the old days of medicine, the career options for a graduating medical student were pretty simple: become a general practitioner, or . . . become a general practitioner. Medicine has changed quite a bit since that era. New discoveries in science, advancements in medical care, and high-tech innovations paved the way for the growth of more specialties. Radiology, for instance, prospered greatly from the introduction of computed tomography (CT) scans and magnetic resonance imaging (MRI). The discovery of inhalation anesthetics gave birth to anesthesiology, progress in drug therapy revolutionized psychiatry, and the development of the colonoscope created gastroenterology. The list goes on and on. Today, with nearly 60 specialties and subspecialties of medicine, narrowing the choices down to one is more challenging than ever.

Clinical Clerkships Have Many Limitations

After making it through 2 hard years of basic sciences, medical students have to complete a series of clinical clerkships (rotations). The purpose of this hospital experience is twofold: (1) to acquire a basic fund of clinical knowledge in that specialty and (2) to explore whether or not that field of medicine may be one you want to pursue. For the latter goal, clerkships prove inadequate for many reasons. Most rotations only last from 2 to 8 weeks. During this short period of time, medical students get limited exposure to that specialty. It feels more like an overview or introduction.

Anxiety over clerkship examinations and grades takes both time and mental energy away from focusing on the merits of the specialty. During a rotation, many students spend more time studying for the test or worrying about their daily performance on rounds instead of discussing the pros and cons of that specialty with residents and attendings. When the clerkship ends, the evaluations and grades often subjectively influence a medical student's final impressions. More often than not, your enjoyment of a particular rotation does not correlate with what you really think and feel about that specialty. This usually happens because bad evaluations from bitter residents or tough attendings leave a negative lasting impression, making a student less inclined to choose that specialty. Having a rough experience in a single month-long rotation, however, should not influence your decision. It is possible to have a bad rotation but still end up choosing that specialty for a career.

Most clinical rotations are completed within the setting of an academic medical center or teaching hospital. Here you receive an unbalanced, biased view of that particular specialty. The academic environment is vastly different than the private practice setting of most doctors. Take the internal medicine clerkship, for example. Most medical students spend weeks gaining internal medicine experience by seeing sick patients admitted to the medicine wards. They primarily get a solid grasp of the inpatient side of this specialty. In reality, most private practice internists, whether generalists or specialists, spend the majority of their time in clinic. There, they practice ambulatory medicine, seeing a large number of patients a day. They complete tons of paperwork and haggle with insurance companies. Thus, the internal medicine clerkship does not give you a good sense of what a typical day is really like for an office-based internist.

Medical Students Have Little First-Hand Experience

It is hard to know whether a specialty is the right fit until you have a chance to immerse yourself completely in it. In a typical clerkship, medical students—who possess little practical knowledge—act more as observers than they do as physicians. They write notes in the chart that no one really reads and spend long hours in the operating room holding retractors during surgery. Many future surgeons, for example, commit to a career of slicing, cauterizing, and sewing without ever having the chance to truly operate. (Retracting tissue for the attending surgeon does not count as operating.) Of course, there are good reasons to prevent medical students from writing medication orders, performing anesthesia, operating on patients, and delivering babies alone. But these constraints make it harder to figure out if you would actually like doing those things for the rest of your working life.

In the old days, medical students did not have this problem. They were able to gain first-hand experience in different specialties through the rotating internship. During this time, they actually used their newly earned MD to work as a doctor and could perform more tasks and procedures unsupervised. The internship year also allowed more time to choose a specialty, building on the 2 years of clinical exposure in medical school. This was the year when interns had to apply to residency programs. The formal rotating internship was eliminated in 1970, when residency training swallowed up PGY-1.

There Is Not Enough Time to Explore Every Specialty

Because of the overwhelming number of specialties, it is impossible for medical students to gain exposure to all of them. This failing is a direct result of the structure of American medical education. After briefly rotating through different specialties (both required and elective), students have to decide early on a field of medicine—after just over a year! Hypothetically, being a diligent student and doing month-long rotations in every specialty would take almost 2 years. So new doctors necessarily commit to a specialty without having rotated through all of them. Many students graduate without having any idea of what physical medicine and rehabilitation is all about, for instance, or what radiation oncologists do on a daily basis. They may end up making hasty, ill-informed decisions.

To meet federal accreditation requirements and maintain high standards, medical schools have to ensure that their students obtain basic clinical knowledge in several core disciplines. Whether they like it or not, all third-year students spend their entire year rotating through seven fundamental specialties: internal medicine (12 weeks average length), surgery (12 weeks), pediatrics (8 weeks), obstetrics–gynecology (6 weeks), psychiatry (6 weeks), family practice (6 weeks), and neurology (4 weeks).[1] Some medical schools have additional requirements, such as emergency medicine and anesthesiology. All these requirements mean that there is little to no elective time during the crucial junior year. In the end, you will definitely not have clerkship experiences in every specialty that you might possibly consider for residency training.

Having so many required third-year rotations leaves just a few months in the senior year for electives in other specialties before applying for residency. Students have to commit to their desired specialty early (by late summer) in the senior year. Residency applications are typically submitted in September and October of the final year. This time frame gives medical students only a year or so to explore different specialties and make the big decision. Once fourth year begins in July, it is time to start thinking about subinternships, collecting letters of recommendation, writing the personal statement, and researching residency programs. Students who use the beginning of fourth year for additional career exploration may find themselves rushed during the application process. The stressful time crunch is even worse for medical students interested in checking out one of the "early match" specialties, such as ophthalmology or urology. For them, applications are due even earlier (around midsummer)!

With only 1 year to make up their minds, the pressure is intense for many medical students. The need to make such an early (and important) commitment creates high levels of stress, frustration, and anxiety. It has progressed to the point where first- and second-year students are now worrying about this decision, too. Instead of focusing their energy on mastering the basic sciences, they rack their brains over what specialty lies in the not-so-distant future.

Medical Schools Offer Little Career Planning

Some students enter medical school certain of the type of doctor they want to become. "I was born to be a neurosurgeon," they insist. Perhaps, they want to follow in the footsteps of a parent and feel ordained to live up to their expectations.

Other medical students have vague ideas about their careers, such as knowing they want to perform procedures or have an office-based group practice. A third group (probably the largest) declares itself undecided. Its members are the students who are always changing their minds during medical school about their future specialty. One day, they wake up thinking about psychiatry, and the next month, a career in dermatology begins to sound appealing.

No matter which group you feel you belong to, not many medical schools have adequate resources to help you make this decision. Many students go for 4 whole years without anyone ever sitting down with them to offer career advice and information on specialty selection. Some schools just leave a dusty box of outdated printed information in some unused closet. Students are left on their own to do independent research and to seek out medical professionals for advice.

A few medical schools, however, are better when it comes to career planning. These rare exceptions hold workshops, career fairs, presentations, private counseling sessions, and "Q&A sessions" sponsored by different departments. But too many students fail to take advantage of these resources because of the more immediate demands of medical school—taking overnight call, studying for examinations, and preparing presentations for teaching rounds. Without good career advice, today's medical students have even less information on which to base their specialty decision.

WHAT ABOUT CHOOSING THE "WRONG" SPECIALTY?

Is there really such a thing as the perfect specialty? Most doctors would probably argue against this idea. After rotating through various areas of medicine, most medical students find themselves drawn to a number of them. In their decision-making process, students typically first rule out the list of disciplines that they are sure they are not interested in, for whatever reason. The remaining options under consideration, though, would probably all lead to a rewarding, intellectually stimulating medical career. Because of the similarities among certain groups of specialties, there is almost always more than one potential choice that might meet your criteria. If you want to be a behind-the-scenes doctor's doctor, consider radiology or pathology. If you want to know a little bit about everything in medicine, consider family practice or emergency medicine. If lots of procedures are more your style, think about cardiology, interventional radiology, or surgery.

You cannot choose a medical specialty without taking a closer look at career satisfaction among today's doctors. In the United States, the majority of physicians are basically satisfied with their medical careers. However, a recent study of more than 12,000 doctors found that only 40% of physicians are very satisfied with medicine, with a significant proportion (20%) feeling completely dissatisfied.[2] Why such negative feelings toward medicine? Many cite the encroachment of managed care on their practices as a major influence. Others are less satisfied because of their long work hours, declining income, practice location, or for other personal reasons.

One of the most significant factors contributing to physicians' satisfaction is their choice of specialty. Ill-informed decision making can lead to a lifetime as an unhappy doctor. The same study, therefore, looked at differences in physicians' satisfaction across the medical specialties and came up with important conclusions. Surprisingly, the highest proportions of dissatisfied doctors are those practicing some of the procedure-oriented specialties, such as obstetrics–gynecology, otolaryngology, ophthalmology, and orthopedic surgery. These are areas of medicine with traditionally high income and prestige. They may have lost their luster due to years of managed care and Medicare reimbursement reform, which led to less autonomy, higher liability insurance premiums, and declining income. On the flip side, more cognitive-oriented specialties—pediatrics, geriatrics, infectious disease, and neonatology—are filled with very satisfied physicians. Perhaps, these fields gained the most benefits from all the recent changes in health care delivery in the United States.

In a 10-year follow-up to this data, the same authors surveyed more than 6000 physicians to verify whether the desire for more controllable lifestyles had changed specialty satisfaction.[3] Each specialty was compared with the satisfaction score for family medicine, the field with the greatest number of physicians. Compared with the previous cohort, there were several similar findings. The specialties with significantly lower satisfaction levels were neurosurgery, pulmonary and critical care medicine, nephrology, and obstetrics–gynecology. The specialties with significantly higher satisfaction levels were pediatric emergency medicine, geriatric medicine, other pediatric subspecialties, neonatology, combined internal medicine–pediatrics practice, pediatrics, dermatology, and child and adolescent psychiatry. Not surprisingly, the same variables explained some of these differences: higher income levels, work hours, and expectations versus practice realities. So how can we improve career satisfaction among specialties that consistently score low? Changes in reimbursement and delivery of care can only occur at the level of the policy makers in Washington, DC. All medical students should, therefore, learn how to contribute to their specialty's political action committee.

The results of these surveys reiterate an important concluding point: choose your medical specialty thoughtfully and carefully. Finding the right area of medicine for you will have a huge bearing on your future career satisfaction. Moreover, physicians' contentment correlates strongly with patients' satisfaction and their outcomes.[4] It goes without saying, then, that happy doctors end up being better doctors for their patients.

REFERENCES

1. Barzansky, B., Etzel, S.I. Educational programs in U.S. medical schools, 2001–2002. *JAMA.* 2002;288(9):1067–1072.

2. Leigh, J.P., Kravtitz, R.L., et al. Physician career satisfaction across specialties. *Arch Intern Med.* 2002;162(14):1577–1584.

3. Leigh, J.P., Tancredi, R.L., et al. Physician career satisfaction within specialties. *BMC Health Services Res.* 2009;9(166):1–12.

4. Haas, J.S., Cook, E.F., et al. Is the professional satisfaction of general internists associated with patient satisfaction? *J Gen Intern Med.* 2000;15:122–128.

2
THE SPECIALIZATION
OF MEDICINE

For all medical students, the area of specialization they choose will shape the nature of their careers. Some will become pediatricians or neurologists. Others may find themselves drawn to callings in orthopedic surgery, emergency medicine, or family practice. But over time, the popularity of any given specialty follows a cyclical pattern among medical students. One year, it seems like everyone is clamoring for internal medicine, while the next year, radiology becomes the hot field. Today, nearly all doctors identify themselves in terms of their specialties first and as physicians second.[1] When did medicine become specialty oriented? Is it possible anymore for a doctor to be, well, just a doctor? Why are there so many options for today's medical students?

The answers to these questions are complicated. Unlike other professions, medical education has shifted from general training to a fractionated system of specialties and subspecialties. Throughout the twenty-first century, the rapid growth of new scientific knowledge led to a steady rise in the number of medical specialties. Amazing new drugs or fancy magnetic resonance imaging (MRI) scanners, however, do not protect any specialty from the economic, political, and social forces that have changed the delivery of health care. The current managed care climate has particularly affected certain areas of medicine. So before choosing a specialty, every future physician needs a solid appreciation of how medicine became a fragmented profession. In consideration of the busy lives of premed and medical students, this history lesson will be kept short and concise.

IN THE BEGINNING THERE WAS GENERAL MEDICINE

During the first half of the twentieth century, almost every doctor practiced general medicine. At the time, aspiring young physicians entered medical school

intending to become general practitioners (GPs). Very few completed postgraduate training. After graduating from medical school, they spent 1 to 2 years in
an apprentice-like internship with a more experienced physician. Just like today's
family practitioner, the GP took care of patients of all ages, from infants to the
elderly. They treated medical problems, delivered babies, and performed surgery.
As respected members of the community, they even made house calls on their
patients. Because there was a limited amount of clinical knowledge to master,
GPs could capably manage most medical and surgical problems.

Although GPs dominated the medical scene, several specialties were in the
early stages of development. But additional formal training in these areas—such as
ophthalmology and otolaryngology—was practically nonexistent. The postgraduate internship prepared new physicians for general practice only. If an American
doctor wanted to gain more expertise in a narrow field of medicine, a few nonstan-
dardized options were possible. Some worked as apprentices to the small number
of established specialists. Others took formal coursework at freestanding graduate
medical schools or entered one of the few available residency programs. This path
represented the culmination of training through the pursuit of specialized knowledge. The majority, however, went to Europe, where they learned the latest skills
in established medical centers, particularly those in Germany. Because there was
no uniformity or consistency across the different forms of specialty training, some
specialists received better preparation than others.

Specialists were initially met with a great deal of skepticism by the well-
established GPs, who viewed them as "quacks." Although GPs outnumbered the
small but growing cadre of specialists, more doctors were returning from abroad
with new knowledge and technology. They also brought with them the research
skills for making life-changing medical discoveries, which further hastened the
trend toward specialization. Patients now had new drugs, chemotherapy, insulin,
and vitamins in their treatment regimens, which meant that GPs were competing with specialists for mastery of these agents. By the early 1930s, there were
roughly ten areas of specialization within medicine: general surgery, orthopedics,
otolaryngology, internal medicine, pediatrics, psychiatry, dermatology, urology,
ophthalmology, and obstetrics–gynecology.[2] The growing use of x-rays, electrocardiography, and blood transfusions added to the tension between specialists and
GPs. Making matters worse for the GP, new surgical specialties and procedures
developed with the introduction of anesthesia and sterile operating conditions.

As the United States prepared to enter World War II, the medical community
was still centered on the GP. In the 1940s, only 24% of physicians officially
considered themselves to be specialists.[3] In fact, the average American citizen

regarded his or her doctor as a "trusted bedside physician"—not a high-tech hospital-based specialist.[4] Despite the growing popularity of specialties, medical schools continued extolling the virtues of general practice. But with more scientific innovations on the horizon, there was no stopping the trend toward specialization. The start of World War II added even more fuel to this movement, leading to a dramatic change in the medical landscape.

WHO WANTS TO BE A SPECIALIST?

American physicians drafted into the military in 1942 were responsible for the first great surge of interest in specialty medicine. Soldiers with wounds inflicted during conflict required the latest medical care, and only specialists could best meet this crucial need. Accordingly, being a specialist became associated with higher prestige. Board certification in a medical specialty led to higher pay, higher ranks, and better war assignments than the GP. This disparity in the armed forces widened the already growing rift between the two types of physicians. Treating severely wounded soldiers gave the GPs exposure to new techniques and skills. For instance, those who worked alongside specialists in orthopedic surgery were inspired to pursue their own careers in orthopedics after the war. Back home, there was also a developing need for all types of specialists, such as rehabilitation doctors and plastic surgeons, to care for the returning wounded veterans.

The high volume of specialized medicine practiced in the military had a noteworthy influence on the postwar career decisions of many medical officers. After release from active duty, most of the doctors (even the older ones) wanted to go straight into residency for specialty training, rather than returning to general practice. The GI Bill, which considered residents as students, made it easy to go back for training by providing living expenses, tuition stipends, and hospital subsidies. The demand greatly exceeded everyone's estimates. Hundreds of recently discharged physicians applied for residency positions. In response, residency programs in the 15 specialties expanded greatly, eventually to the point where the number of positions outnumbered the number of applicants. After 1945, higher enrollments in existing specialties, rather than from the approval of new specialties, shifted the interest of physicians to specialization.

After the war veterans returned home, the acute demand for residency positions did not drop off. Instead, it seemed like every doctor wanted to specialize in something. The war effort had directed millions of dollars into biomedical and clinical research, which eventually yielded substantial improvements in medical technology and new discoveries in the basic sciences. Wanting to be a part of this high-tech side of medicine, graduating medical students stampeded from general practice to specialty medicine. They believed that GPs could no longer master the wealth of new information and therapies, and therefore they turned to specialization as a means of gaining expertise. To them, the future of medicine lies in the direction of their specialist role models. In their minds, specialists were the ones who cured rare diseases, treated complicated conditions, and became experts at performing difficult procedures.

THE NEED FOR BOARD CERTIFICATION

The explosive growth of medical specialties also presented the challenge of developing a system to confirm — and to assure patients — that a specialist was actually a qualified physician. After all, would you want abdominal surgery performed by untrained hands? Some areas — such as general surgery and obstetrics–gynecology — were not as well defined as others. To address this problem, each specialty formed its own examination and certification board. These organizations promoted cohesion among their physician members by raising standards and setting qualifications. Based on their success, leaders among the specialties got together to form a national system of standardization — the American Board of Medical Specialties (ABMS). This association has the final say in approving any new specialties (and subspecialties) to its 24-member group.

With a standardized system of board certification in place, more medical students began entering fields of specialization. For newly trained specialists, becoming certified means successfully joining the ranks of their peers. After finishing residency, candidates for certification submit their credentials to the respective specialty board, which then rules whether a physician is "board eligible." If he or she meets the requirements of the certifying board, the physician may sit for the certification examination. A passing score leads to full certification as a "diplomat" of that specialty board. Although certification is not required to practice medicine, this accomplishment adds prestige and confers the professional status of expert. Depending on the specialty, board certificates last from 6 to 10 years, after which recertification via examination is necessary.

SPECIALISTS VERSUS GENERALISTS

Over the next several decades, medicine continued to diversify. Bucking tradition, new physicians wanted their specialty training, and residency programs were more than happy to oblige. Soon, however, even 3 to 5 years in residency were not enough to prepare young doctors in an area of expertise. To make matters worse, the ABMS began strictly limiting the approval of new specialty boards. The end result? A proliferation of more narrowly defined subspecialties. These areas of medicine, such as rheumatology and pediatric cardiology, required additional training through fellowships. Although the focus of residency shifted to clinical learning and patient care, fellowships placed more of an emphasis on reading, research, and scholarly work (which was the purpose of residency back in the old days). Along with learning new diagnostic tests and procedures, taking care of patients was still an integral part of a fellowship.

Medicine continued to give birth to new specialties and even more subspecialties. Since the dawn of modern anesthesiology in the 1930s, anesthesiologists have advanced the limits of surgery by permitting operations that were scarcely conceivable before. As a result, surgery flourished. Much of the original domain of the general surgeon was subjugated to board-certified specialists in otolaryngology (ear–nose–throat–neck), neurosurgery (brain), orthopedic (bone and joint), and cardiothoracic (heart and lungs) surgery. Internal medicine, now considered a specialty, acquired a slew of subspecialties, as new technical procedures were devised in the 1950s. Medical centers began training gastroenterologists to perform endoscopy and colonoscopy, pulmonologists to master bronchoscopy, and cardiologists to implant pacemakers and perform catheterization. The hospital-based specialties also expanded. The explosion of imaging techniques overwhelmed the field of radiology, which then split into diagnostic radiology, nuclear medicine, and radiation oncology. Improvements in molecular techniques and histologic stains led to the division of pathology into over a dozen subspecialties. In more recent years, new specialties such as medical genetics and emergency medicine have also come into being.

Twenty years after veterans of World War II raced to residency training, the passage of Medicare in 1965 inspired another surge of interest in specialized medicine. This historic initiative enabled the nation's elderly to receive government-funded medical insurance and benefits for expensive health services, thus protecting their limited savings. By influencing decisions regarding health care for the first time, the American public helped to pave the way for more professional flexibility among physicians. With Medicare, doctors could now treat their elderly patients without worrying about either bankrupting them or not getting paid for their expensive specialist services. With their salaries assured from treating so many sick patients with multiple medical problems, graduating physicians continued to enter specialties and subspecialties. Fewer medical students were attracted to a noble career in general practice, and residency programs ballooned to meet the demand for specialty training. Specialists became influential within the American Medical Association, pushing out GPs from positions of power. Now that medical students no longer headed out into general practice after internship, most residency programs began incorporating internship into the first postgraduate year of training. By 1970, all rotating internships were finally eliminated.

Why were students no longer interested in becoming GPs? Most began to realize that the staggering amount of new medical knowledge made specialty training a necessity. Despite the increased length of training, they wanted to become experts in a particular organ system or disease area. Higher social prestige and increased compensation (from performing lots of procedures) attracted many graduates to careers of cardiology, surgery, and gastroenterology. New technology such as colonoscopes, respiratory ventilators, and MRI machines fell under the expertise of the specialty-trained physician. At the same time, the National Institutes of Health began granting tons of money to the university-based specialists, not GPs, for biomedical research projects. Despite the tension between the two physician groups, these advancements in medical science helped to improve the lives of every patient suffering from illness.

Although the number of GPs rapidly dwindled after World War II, as medical school graduates went into the specialty disciplines, a core group of dedicated physicians continued to believe in the merits of general medicine and its wider scope of practice. In 1969, they achieved partial victory through their newly defined specialty—family practice—and its corresponding specialty board. Additionally, internists and pediatricians (who were also considered generalists) came together in 1967 and agreed to sponsor certification of combined residency training in both internal medicine and pediatrics. Many years later, generalists finally got their much-deserved moment in the limelight. In the 1990s, health care reform was at the top of the political agenda, and generalists were an important part of this movement.

First, experts in the health care industry accepted the conclusion that there was an oversupply of specialists. Several powerful organizations, including the Graduate Medical Education National Advisory Committee and the Bureau of Health Professions, predicted that specialists would continue to outnumber generalists, leading to a massive specialist glut by the turn of the century. To improve the skewed distribution, they recommended increasing the ratio of generalists to specialists to an equal 50:50 proportion. This would also alleviate the tight job market that existed for specialists at the time. Believing that more patient care by generalists would improve access to health care, many politicians, bureaucrats, and lobbyists agreed with this assessment.

Specialists were also assigned the blame for rising health care costs. They prescribe fancier (and more expensive) drugs and perform costly procedures. Many felt that specialists drive up the cost of health care, rapidly increasing its percentage of the gross national product. But patients with insurance were also held responsible, because they took advantage of the lack of regulation over specialist services. Many went shopping for specialists based on self-diagnosis and referral, such as the middle-aged woman with chronic migraines who went straight to a neurologist instead of first seeing her generalist. Combined with high inflation, these factors contributed to escalating health care costs. What was the solution? Managed care. This movement sought to reduce medical expenditures by deferring the bulk of health care to generalists rather than specialists.

The encroachment of managed care led to renewed efforts to produce more generalist physicians—internists, pediatricians, and family practitioners. (Psychiatry and obstetrics–gynecology are also sometimes considered primary care specialties.) Health maintenance organizations (HMOs) are among the most common forms of managed care because employers like their lower rates and broader coverage. But these groups attempt to reduce medical costs by limiting patients' access to specialists. Patients have to see their primary care physician (PCP) first for diagnosis and treatment. If the generalist cannot handle the problem, he or she refers the patient to a specialist. Patients belonging to an HMO essentially have to get permission from their PCP to see a specialist. Generalists, therefore, were assigned the new role of gatekeeper.

With support thrown behind it, managed care did, at first, achieve its goals. Combined with the fear of there being an oversupply of specialists, the managed care health system was a boon for generalists. In the mid-1990s, medical schools nationwide began encouraging their graduates to choose careers in primary care. Seeking to fulfill the 50:50 ratio, their efforts kindled renewed interest in family practice, internal medicine, and pediatrics. Driven by the need for more primary care gatekeepers, medical students raced to these generalist specialties. At the same time, medical schools were discouraging students from entering fields such as anesthesiology, cardiology, and pathology. Many deans believed that the current glut of specialists, as well as all the talk about primary care, meant that future employment prospects were dismal. Specialists began to lose more than just autonomy and income; they also lost promising new medical school graduates.

THE CYCLE TURNS AGAIN: WHO WANTS TO BE A SPECIALIST?

The resurgence of the generalist physician that managed care sparked only lasted for a short time, however. In response to the hype about greater opportunities, medical students' interest in primary care peaked by the late 1990s but then declined. Managed care systems quickly fell out of favor among health care consumers as their restrictions began to affect patient care. The PCP gatekeeper was now seen as a barrier to the best medical care. To increase physician productivity in primary care, managed care groups hired hundreds of nurse practitioners and physician assistants. This led to subtle discussions among prospective candidates about the intellectual stature of primary care. Reading between the lines and keenly aware of the problems facing primary care, more medical students entered specialized areas again in the new millennium. In fact, in 2002, there was a 5.6% decline in primary care residency matches.[5]

Once again, newly minted MDs are choosing careers in highly specialized areas of medicine, and the trend to specialization will likely continue. In fact, many academicians believe that currently there is a significant shortage of specialists.[6] Despite new formulas that lowered the incomes of specialists and raised generalists' salaries, insurance reimbursements still favor the specialist, who make much more money. Specialists are also back in demand because of the problems of the aging baby boomers. Who is going to perform their screening colonoscopies, stent their hearts, look at their suspicious moles, and replace their hips and knees? This is why there is a pressing need for more gastroenterologists, cardiologists, dermatologists, and orthopedic surgeons. The general fields of medicine face many challenges in the face of scientific advances in the more technical specialties. Perhaps discouraged by the daunting amount of information that is there to master in general practice, most internal medicine residents (over two-thirds) pursue fellowship training, especially in procedure-oriented fields such as cardiology and gastroenterology.[7]

Although specialization (and subspecialization) is inevitable, not every physician supports it. Some doctors see this phenomenon as "both a prerequisite and a logical outcome of human ingenuity in understanding and combating disease; others attack it as unnecessarily fragmented, expensive, dehumanizing, and confusing for patients."[2] Whatever one's perspective, patients still receive the highest quality of medical treatment possible within this fragmented system. For example, a subspecialist (eg, endocrinologist) may now assume care of a patient with complicated clinical material (eg, hyperthyroidism) rather than the appropriate specialist (general internist). With better coordination between these types of doctors, medicine may finally become well integrated once again.

Many uncertainties surround the rate of specialization in the future. Fueled by the pace of scientific research in medical diagnosis and treatment, more sub-specialties will likely continue to form. There is, however, one certainty: with all the choices that lay before them, today's medical students have a much more difficult decision to make.

REFERENCES

1. Langsley, D.G., Darragh, J.H. *Trends in Specialization: Tomorrow's Medicine.* Evanston, IL: American Board of Medical Specialties; 1985.

2. Donini-Lenhoff, F.G., Hedrick, H.L. Growth of specialization in graduate medical education. *JAMA.* 2000;284(10):1284–1289.

3. Ludmerer, K.M. *Time to Heal: American Medical Education from the Turn of the Century to the Era of Managed Care.* New York: Oxford University Press; 1999.

4. Stevens, R. *American Medicine and the Public Interest: A History of Specialization.* Berkeley: University of California Press; 1971.

5. Schroeder, S.A. Primary care at a crossroads. *Acad Med.* 2002;77(8):767–773.

6. Cooper, R.A. There's a shortage of specialists. Is anyone listening? *Acad Med.* 2002;77(8):761–766.

7. Lyttle, C.S., Levey, G.S. The national study of internal medicine manpower, XX: The changing demographics of internal medicine residency. *Ann Intern Med.* 1994;121: 435–441.

3
TEN FACTORS TO CONSIDER IN SPECIALTY SELECTION

The proliferation of specialties (and subspecialties) means that every physician practices a different type of medicine. Even within the same specialty, no two doctors are
alike. Faced with all this diversity, how do medical students commit to a single specialty? Many go through a "process of 'trying on possible selves' (ie, projecting themselves into hypothetical career and personal roles)."[1] Others prefer to choose through
a process of elimination—tossing out specialties that do not meet their predetermined
criteria.

No matter how each medical student goes about picking a specialty, everyone
takes into account a long list of variables. An analysis of the 1993 graduating
medical school class found that the following factors were the most influential in
choosing a specialty:

- The type of patient problems encountered.
- The opportunity to make a difference in people's lives and to help others.
- The intellectual content of the specialty.[2]

Further down on the list, some students look closely at malpractice insurance
costs, or worry about overcrowding in a given field, and others seek specialties
that offer the opportunity to pursue research. One of the most unifying variables,
ranking at the top of the list, is a good personality match between student and
specialty (see Chapter 4). The relative weight of any of these factors, of course,
varies for each student.

When it comes down to the final decision, young physicians often choose
their specialty based on less noble factors than the ones the study cites. Today's

25

debt-ridden medical student—who experiences first hand the economic and legal domination of medicine—ascribes more value to practical variables. This chapter examines some of these less idealistic factors, such as quality of life, income potential, and job opportunities. Although they are less influential, each factor may still make a student think twice about committing to one specialty or another. When contemplating a possible specialty, keep the following ten variables in mind, determine their order of importance, and apply them to each field you are considering.

GENERALIST, SPECIALIST, OR NONE OF THE ABOVE

The 20 medical and surgical disciplines can be further subdivided into three major specialty groups: generalist, specialist, or supportive. Before committing to a specialty, future physicians first need to decide what type of doctor they would like to become.

The generalist specialties are those in which physicians practice primary care medicine. Classically, these have always included family practice, internal medicine, and pediatrics. For many, psychiatrists and obstetrician–gynecologists also fall within this category. All generalists have broad medical knowledge, encompassing a variety of common (and often chronic) problems in their community. An integral part of their patients' lives, they provide long-term continuous care in a single setting, referring their patients to specialists only when necessary. Preventive medicine—a major part of their job—can catch early signs of disease and keep patients from ending up in the emergency room with serious problems. As the first doctor to see a patient, a generalist must have greater tolerance for the unknown, especially when dealing with signs and symptoms that may not fall into a neat diagnosis. Generalists also have to cope with the pressure to know just about everything. Swamped with dozens of medical journals, they need to read daily to keep up with the latest advances in their fields.

Although pediatrics, for instance, is still considered a specialty, a true specialist, by definition, cares for a specific region of the body or a narrowly defined area of medicine. Ophthalmologists, cardiologists, urologists, and neurologists—just to name a few—all fit this description. As practitioners of secondary or tertiary care medicine, specialists prefer action-oriented patient interactions. Within their narrow scope of practice, they perform many technical procedures, like cataract surgery or cardiac catheterization. As consultants, nearly all practice on the basis of patient referrals from primary care physicians. After solving the clinical problem at hand (eg, left hip replacement), specialists usually schedule infrequent follow-ups, leading to less long-term involvement in their patients' lives. Most practice in the clinic and the hospital. Many are affiliated with large medical centers.

Several specialties are neither medical nor surgical—they function independently as the supportive disciplines of medicine. Radiology, physical medicine and rehabilitation, pathology, anesthesiology, radiation oncology, emergency medicine, and nuclear medicine fall within this category. They are all hospital-based specialties. Although not front-line doctors, these physicians still play a crucial role in patient care. Without them, patients would not make it through surgery alive, receive accurate diagnoses from imaging and biopsy studies, or receive the correct doses of radiation therapy to treat their cancer. Because of their anonymous roles and minimal patient contact, these behind-the-scenes doctors tend not to get the recognition they deserve from their patients. Without external rewards, they instead have to derive their professional satisfaction from within.

INTELLECTUAL CONTENT AND CLINICAL ISSUES

Radiologists cannot operate on a patient's heart, dermatologists cannot administer general anesthesia, and neurosurgeons should not be delivering babies. Because the subject matter and type of patient care differ quite a bit across the specialties, every doctor practices a distinctive brand of medicine. Take ophthalmology and rehabilitation medicine, for instance. Lying on the opposite ends of the specialty content/patient care spectrum, these two fields almost seem like completely different professions!

At the most fundamental level, with all other factors aside, medical students should love the intellectual content of their specialty. Students with a genuine interest in the underlying clinical material and basic science of a certain discipline will find themselves voraciously reading its textbooks and journals, wanting to know more about the specialty's diagnostic challenges. To gauge the appeal of the clinical problems found in a specialty, read the current literature for 1 week. If you love clinical pharmacology and physiology, then perhaps a career in anesthesiology is your destiny. If studying anatomy brings up bad memories from your first year of medical school, then stay away from surgical specialties, radiology, and pathology. Above all, you should never have to force yourself to love an area of medicine.

Making a good match depends on the "discovery and comparison of information about three distinct domains: one's self, the others practicing in a specialty, and the content of that specialty."[1] When it comes to the third domain, nearly all students rely heavily in the end on their gut feelings. After much deliberation, you will become aware of feeling at home in certain fields of medicine. Those who like immediate interventions, technical skills, and urgent problems find themselves drawn to surgical specialties or medical subspecialties. Students who prefer lots of interpersonal contact, a diverse patient population, and preventive medicine usually select a primary care specialty.

AMOUNT OF PATIENT CONTACT

All physicians-in-training choose careers in medicine, perhaps the noblest of all professions, because they want to help people—to take care of sick patients, cure disease, and make a difference in people's lives. Yet until medical students finally spend hours with patients in the hospital while on clinical rotations, they really have no idea what this experience is like. Most love talking with patients, forming relationships with them, and examining them for signs of disease. Others, however, find that interacting with sick people is less appealing than they had imagined. They do not like performing physical examinations, for example, or dealing with gushes of body fluids or the smell of infected wounds.

No matter what your colleagues might say, wanting a specialty with more (or less) patient contact has no bearing on how good a physician you will be. There is a place for everyone in medicine—even for those who decide to work behind the scenes. Radiologists and pathologists, who have basically no contact with patients, are equally as righteous doctors as internists, who interact with and examine patients in every single encounter. Every specialist or subspecialist has an important role in patient care; some just have more face time with patients than others.

You should decide how much patient contact you want in your career and rule out specialties that may not meet your needs. If long-term relationships and continuity of care are important, consider areas like internal medicine and family practice. If you like getting down and dirty, think about careers in emergency medicine, obstetrics–gynecology, and surgery. In some specialties, like urology and orthopedic surgery, doctors only have to perform focused physicals (instead of examining everything). Cleaner specialties—those with lots of patient interaction but not much physical contact—include psychiatry, ophthalmology, and radiation oncology. In fields like emergency medicine and anesthesiology, contact with the patient is typically short and to the point.

TYPE OF PATIENTS ENCOUNTERED

Every physician—including pathologists working in the laboratory—interacts with patients in some way. (One cannot practice any form of medicine without patients!) Many aspiring doctors forget to factor the different types of patients into their specialty decision. Take a closer look at the typical patient in the specialty you are considering. Ask yourself whether or not you could thrive both emotionally and professionally in that type of doctor–patient relationship. Emergency medicine physicians, for instance, are always dealing with many angry patients with nonemergent complaints who have been kept waiting for hours on end. Pediatricians have to interact with demanding, concerned parents in addition to sick infants and children. Oncologists (medical, surgical, and radiation) have patients with mortal diseases that typically lead to poor outcomes despite aggressive treatment. Although these examples seem like stereotypes, the maxim that all doctors are not equal also holds true for their patients.

Medical students often wonder about the risk of facing a malpractice suit within their chosen specialty. Some patients are more litigious than others. Obstetricians, for instance, manage a group of patients who could slap them with a malpractice suit for any minor defect in their baby. A recent study took a closer look at specialty-specific malpractice risk.[3] Specialties with the highest probability of facing a malpractice claim include neurological, cardiothoracic, general, and orthopedic surgery; those with the lowest include family medicine, pediatrics, and psychiatry. However, no correlation between lawsuit risk and indemnity payment size was found. The average plaintiff payout for low-risk specialties like pediatricians and pathologists were actually much greater than those of high-risk specialists like neurosurgeons and obstetricians. Regardless of specialty, medical students should be aware that nearly all physicians face at least one malpractice suit by the end of the careers. The cumulative career risk is quite high, unfortunately.

PRESTIGE, STATUS, AND SOCIAL EXPECTATIONS

The selection of a specialty should be your own choice. Think about the areas of medicine in which you are the happiest and forget about how others (family, friends, and colleagues) might view your chosen specialty. Always remember that every type of doctor has an important role in the big picture of medicine, and the idea that one specialty garners more respect and prestige than another is really just a matter of personal opinion. Because all medical students have excelled academically their entire lives, those who subscribe to these beliefs find it hard at this point to stop being the best. For them, a career in family practice or psychiatry may not carry as much social status as being a world-renowned neurosurgeon or earning a position in ophthalmology, an ultracompetitive specialty. Yet, as a soon-to-be physician, it is no longer necessary to prove yourself. By putting aside external influences such as social prestige and others' expectations, you will likely choose the right specialty and end up a much happier doctor.

LIFESTYLE CONSIDERATIONS

Medicine has always been a demanding profession. After working long hours in the hospital or clinic, physicians end up taking calls in the middle of the night to deliver a baby, remove an appendix, or admit a patient. Tired of delayed gratification and ungodly schedules, many of today's doctors-in-training want careers that leave room for other interests or allow more time for their families. Compared to previous generations of physicians, the millennium medical student seeks a much better balance between life and work. They desire less night call, fewer hours spent in the hospital, and more control over their work schedules. Many are even willing to give up income and professional aspirations to have better personal lives and more free time. The current focus is now shifting to specialties with more controllable lifestyles and higher incomes relative to the length of training.

What accounts for the higher priority of quality-of-life issues in a medical career? The dean at one prestigious medical school believes that the change mirrors a general shift in societal values and professional goals. "Residency program directors were brought up to honor the Christian work ethic. Delayed gratification and unremitting toil were the rules of the day, and residency programs were built on that model. But young people coming through now want to spend more time with their families," she commented.[4]

Perhaps this change reflects the composition of the current generation of medical students. Today nearly half of all graduating doctors are women, most of whom want flexible careers with time to raise children and maintain a normal family life. In addition, the average age of entering medical students has increased. Many older students left behind careers in business and technology, where they could have earned more money with much less stress. For them, "medicine, once aspired to as both a noble profession and a guarantee of financial security, strikes many current students as simply a stressful and poorly paid job."[4] Instead of focusing solely on good patient care, today's physician has to cope with more insurance paperwork, lower reimbursements, overnight phone calls from patients, loss of autonomy due to managed care, and the ever-growing threat of malpractice litigation. Certain areas of medicine, particularly the primary care specialties, have more of these problems than others. Medical students, therefore, are turning to specialties that afford better lifestyles and minimal hassles.

As medical students began to reject fields with more grueling lifestyles (like internal medicine and obstetrics–gynecology), one workaholic specialty particularly suffered: general surgery. In the past, only the most elite students—those within the upper tier of their class—went into surgery. A highly competitive specialty for decades, general surgery is the gateway to high-status careers in vascular, cardiothoracic, oncologic, and plastic surgery, among others. But the current generation of students seems less concerned with prestige. The poor quality of life and years of personal sacrifice are discouraging many top medical students from surgical careers. These shrewd students "do their cost-benefit analysis and surgery is the loser."[5] General surgery began to hurt for qualified students. In 1981, 12.1% of all US seniors went into general surgery; by 2005, the numbers were predicted to decline to just 4.8%, with only 76.6% of available positions filled by American medical graduates.[6] Fortunately, surgery programs have accommodated these lifestyle concerns. No longer are the best and brightest US seniors committing to other specialties. In the 2011 Match, 99.8% of all available positions in general surgery (categorical) were filled—and with the majority by US senior medical students. General surgery is back to being quite competitive once again.

So which are the so-called lifestyle specialties that the most academically successful students are selecting? They include radiology, dermatology, emergency medicine, anesthesiology, pathology, ophthalmology, physical medicine and rehabilitation, and neurology (among others), all of which allow you to control the number of hours you devote to your practice. You could potentially have a career with adequate family and leisure time, less stress, a more regular schedule, and an income commensurate to the workload. Although any specialty can offer job satisfaction, today's medical student believes that only certain specialties allow enough time for family and recreational activities (instead of an overly taxing workload). The evidence is in the numbers: by 2002, the fill rate of programs in anesthesiology and physical medicine and rehabilitation increased by 7% and 13%, respectively.[7] Diagnostic radiology added 44 new positions (a 6.3% increase) and filled all of them. The 2011 NRMP Match shows that high fill rates in these "lifestyle specialties" continue today.

LENGTH OF RESIDENCY TRAINING

Keep in mind that certain specialties require more years of residency training than others. In general, the shortest programs (3 years) are fields of primary care—internal medicine, pediatrics, family practice, and certain emergency medicine programs. Surgical specialties require much longer training, anywhere from 5 to 8 years. Within this spectrum, 4 to 5 years of residency training are necessary for careers in anesthesiology, pathology, dermatology, and radiology, for example. If you want to become a subspecialist, plan on adding even more years of training in a fellowship (Table 3–1). Cardiologists, for instance, spend a total of 6 years learning the discipline before entering practice (a 3-year internal medicine residency plus a

TABLE 3–1

LENGTH OF RESIDENCY TRAINING IN YEARS

Anesthesiology	4
Dermatology	4
Emergency medicine	3–4
Family medicine	3
General surgery	5
Internal medicine	3
Neurology	4
Neurosurgery	6
Obstetrics and gynecology	4
Ophthalmology	4
Orthopedic surgery	5
Otolaryngology	5
Pathology	4
Pediatrics	3
Physical medicine and rehabilitation	4
Plastic surgery	6
Psychiatry	4
Radiation oncology	5
Radiology	5
Urology	5

Data from American Medical Association.

3-year fellowship). Some doctors even "super-subspecialize," such as the cardiologist who undertakes an additional fellowship year to master echocardiography. You could potentially be a physician-in-training forever!

This variable should only have limited influence on your choice of specialty. Yet some medical students are more concerned than others about the number of years residency training requires. Tired of delayed gratification, these students are quite anxious to finish training, practice medicine unsupervised, and start earning a real salary. Older, nontraditional students—especially those with children—often fall into this group. Others simply want to finish training so that they can devote time to outside interests. In any case, never forget that the arduous, low-paying years of residency and/or fellowship are only temporary. Medical students should not select a less-preferred specialty just because the residency training is shorter. Otherwise you may spend a lifetime as a rather dissatisfied physician. Is it really worth it?

DIFFICULTY OF OBTAINING A RESIDENCY POSITION IN THAT SPECIALTY

Over the past 10 years, several new medical schools opened, current class sizes increased, and larger cohort of graduates sought nearly the same number of residency positions. Correspondingly, the increasing competitiveness of many fields of medicine has become a daunting obstacle. Because entrance into certain specialty programs is much more difficult than others (see Chapter 11), medical students must be well aware of their chances. Unfortunately, just because your heart is set on becoming a plastic surgeon or an ophthalmologist does not necessarily mean it will be possible for everyone. For many specialties, there are far more applicants than available positions. Medical students should be careful about basing their decisions on predictions such as, "I can only match into pediatrics," or "I'm not going to bother with radiation oncology because I know I won't get into it."

Before contemplating any specialty of choice, take an honest assessment of your academic competitiveness. Compare the difficulty of obtaining a training position in that specialty with your chances of matching into it. Medical students interested in highly competitive specialties need a great deal of flexibility when making these choices. You might need a backup specialty (second or third choice option) if the field you want is slightly beyond your academic reach. By factoring in this variable, future physicians will match with the most appropriate specialty.

Unfortunately, scores on Step I of the United States Medical Licensing Exam (USMLE) play a very important role in the direction of medical careers. This difficult examination of the basic sciences is typically taken after the second year of medical school. In 2011, the minimum passing score for Step I was 188.[8] All students who pass the exam begin a multistep pathway to becoming licensed physicians; however, those with the highest scores have more specialty options from which to choose. This discrepancy has defeated the primary purpose of the exams—to provide a shared pass–fail evaluation system for individual medical licensing authorities.

But faced with large numbers of highly competitive applicants, certain specialty programs have little choice but to screen candidates for interviews based upon their USMLE Step I scores. Many medical schools have "honors–pass–fail" grading systems, which means that the USMLE provides the only standardized objective measure by which to compare students. In a survey of national program directors on their selection criteria, across all specialties, directors ranked the USMLE Step I score as second in importance (after grades in required clinical clerkships).[9] Step I scores carried more weight than Step II scores (ranked fifth). Similar to the emphasis on MCAT scores for medical school admissions, it is not surprising that so much weight is given to a single examination performance. The Electronic Residency Application Service (ERAS) will automatically submit USMLE score transcripts to applicants' chosen residency programs.

Published results from the National Resident Matching Program in 2011 confirm the very important role of the USMLE Step I score.[10] These results are summarized in Table 3–2. In general, the average Step I score correlates with specialty competitiveness. You can see how lower board scores will make it much more difficult for medical students to obtain entrance into the more competitive specialties. In a recent letter to the most preeminent journal within academic medicine, one senior dean believes that "it is a travesty that student affairs deans are annually forced to explain to perfectly capable, sometimes truly outstanding, medical students that their career dreams of being in "X" specialty are categorically eliminated simply because their USMLE Step I scores were insufficiently high."[11] As an assistant program director, I agree with this assertion. I would argue that the results from the USMLE correlate weakly with clinical success in residency and performance on that specialty's board certification exam. Unfortunately, without other evaluation tools, this practice is likely to continue for the near future. Students who are displeased with their Step I scores should focus on achieving outstanding clerkship grades, collecting superb letters of recommendation, and studying for a high Step II score (see Chapter 11).

TABLE 3–2

AVERAGE USMLE SCORES OF MATCHED APPLICANTS BY SPECIALTY

Plastic surgery	249
Dermatology	244
Otolaryngology	243
Orthopedic surgery	240
Radiation oncology	240
Radiology	240
Neurosurgery	239
Ophthalmology	237
General surgery	227
Anesthesiology	226
Internal medicine	226
Pathology	226
Neurology	225
Emergency medicine	223
Pediatrics	221
Obstetrics and gynecology	220
Physical medicine and rehabilitation	214
Psychiatry	214
Family medicine	213

Data from National Resident Matching Program.

FUTURE INCOME AND EARNING POTENTIAL

According to the Association of American Medical Colleges, the average educational debt of a recent medical school graduate was roughly $100,000. In fact, 21% carried loans of over $150,000. The issue of financial rewards, therefore, becomes very important during the senior year when it comes to select a specialty. At this point, the amount of debt has reached its peak. After 4 years of paying exorbitant tuition, coupled with the prospect of many low-paying years of residency training, graduating physicians are very concerned about their future income potential. With massive amounts of debt, they often put their altruistic motives aside and focus instead on economic realities.

As a result, future reimbursement is an influential factor in some students' decisions to enter a given specialty. New physicians with huge amounts of indebtedness are shunning the primary care fields because of their low earning potential. Others want to pay off their loans right away, and therefore they lean toward specialties that shell out high starting salaries, like radiology, anesthesiology, and orthopedic surgery. But once loans are out of the picture, remember that you will practice in that specialty for the rest of your professional life. For that reason, financial remuneration should be only a less influential variable. No amount of income can make up for a lifetime of miserable days in the wrong specialty.

No matter the specialty of choice, all physicians will earn a comfortable salary. Table 3–3 ranks the average compensation per specialty according to a single

TABLE 3–3

MEDIAN COMPENSATION BY SPECIALTY

Neurosurgery	$548,186
Orthopedic surgery	$476,083
Radiology	$438,115
Radiation oncology	$413,518
Urology	$389,198
Plastic surgery	$388,929
Anesthesiology	$366,640
Otolaryngology	$365,171
Dermatology	$350,627
General surgery	$340,000
Ophthalmology	$325,384
Obstetrics and gynecology	$294,190
Pathology	$285,173
Emergency medicine	$267,293
Physical medicine and rehabilitation	$236,800
Neurology	$236,500
Psychiatry	$208,462
Internal medicine	$205,441
Pediatrics	$202,832
Family medicine	$197,655

Data from American Medical Group Association.

survey. Keep in mind that compensation also varies depending about geographic location (metropolitan vs. rural) and practice model (solo, group, managed care, hospital). As you can tell, the "doing" specialties generally receive a higher level of compensation than the "thinking" specialties. This discrepancy is partly due to the current Medicare physician payment schedule known as the resource-based relative value scale (RBRVS). In this system, reimbursement is calculated by the resource costs necessary to provide those services. With the shifting emphasis on outcomes in upcoming health care reform measures, it remains unclear how physician reimbursement may actually change.

JOB OPPORTUNITIES AND PREDICTIONS ABOUT THE SPECIALIST WORKFORCE

There is plenty of erroneous information out there about physician workforce projections and employment patterns. One day, students hear rumors about pathologists having trouble finding jobs; the next week they read an article in the newspaper about significant shortages of cardiothoracic surgeons. Many of the published expert workforce studies have significant flaws in their methodology. Who, then, should everyone believe? Because it is impossible to predict the nature of the specialist job market, medical students should not base their specialty choice on any workforce projections. This ill-advised approach is full of inherent problems.

The challenges anesthesiologists faced in the 1990s, when this specialty lost some of its allure, serve as a word of warning. In this case, medical students heeded the wrong advice of supposed experts, leading to drastic changes within the specialty. In response to national discussions about an oversupply of specialists, the American Society of Anesthesiologists commissioned an outside consulting group to evaluate the relative glut of new anesthesiologists and their future manpower needs. Patterned after other flawed studies, their report recommended decreasing the number of anesthesiologists entering the workforce. Private practices immediately reacted by dropping their starting salaries and hiring fewer partners. Discouraged by their advisors and by reports about the specialty's economic future in newspapers like the *Wall Street Journal*,[12] medical students responded by shunning anesthesiology.

With fewer applicants, and underestimating the future need for anesthesiologists, residency programs drastically slashed the number of training positions. Today there is nearly an 11% shortage of anesthesiologists, a substantial deficit that will continue for years to come.[13] Private practice groups are fighting over residents by offering incredibly lucrative salaries. Because of the aging population, greater involvement in the intensive care unit and pain clinic, and advancements in surgical technology, anesthesiology is rapidly returning to its competitive status.

The recent changes within anesthesiology illustrate an important take-home point. In this case, the miscalculation of demand in an influential study, combined with declining incomes, left students fearful of selecting this field. It is hard to make career plans in an uncertain economic world. Even the supposed experts — who have been wrong many times before — cannot predict these kinds of changes, whether in the scope of practice of competing mid-level health providers or in the turf wars between specialists over shared procedures and tests. When choosing their dream specialty, students should pay little heed to its current or projected state of job opportunities. Shortages and surpluses can change rapidly by the end of residency training; therefore place this variable low on your list of influential factors. After all, have you ever heard of any unemployed, starving physicians?

REFERENCES

1. Burack, J.H., Irby, D.M., et al. A study of medical students' specialty-choice pathways: Trying on possible selves. *Acad Med.* 1997;72(6):534–541.

2. Kassebaum, D.G., Szenas, P.L. Factors influencing the specialty choices of 1993 medical school graduates. *Acad Med.* 1994;69(2):164–170.

3. Jena, A.B., Seabury, S., et al. Malpractice risk according to physician specialty. *NEJM.* 2011;365(7):629–635.

4. Weiss, B. Primary care? Not me. *Med Econ.* 2002;79(14):42, 48–49.

5. Gelfand, D.V., Podnos, Y.D., et al. Choosing general surgery: Insights into career choices of current medical students. *Arch Surg.* 2002;137:941–947.

6. Bland, K.I., Isaacs, G. Contemporary trends in student selection of medical specialties: The potential impact on general surgery. *Arch Surg.* 2002;137:259–267.

7. Data and Results — 2002 Match. National Resident Matching Program. Washington, DC: American Association of Medical Colleges.

8. The United States Medical Licensing Examination. Accessed December 13, 2011; http://www.usmle.org/transcripts

9. Green, M., Jones, P., et al. Selection criteria for residency: Results of a national program directors survey. *Acad Med.* 2009;84(3):362–367.

10. National Resident Matching Program; Association of American Medical Colleges. Charting outcomes in the match. Accessed December 13, 2011; http://www.nrmp.org/data/chartingoutcomes2011.pdf

11. Wong, J.G. The role of USMLE scores in selecting residents. *Acad Med.* 2011; 86(7):793–794.

12. Anders, G. Numb and number: Once a hot specialty, anesthesiology cools as insurers scale back. *Wall Street J.* 17 March 1995.

13. Schubert, A., Eckhourt, G., et al. Evidence of a current and lasting national anesthesia personnel shortfall: Scope and implications. *Mayo Clin Proc.* 2001;76(10): 995–1010.

4

PERSONALITY ASSESSMENT: ARE YOU MY TYPE?

"Orthopedic surgeons are all jocks."

"Only nerds become internists."

"Psychiatrists are as crazy as their patients."

"Pathologists are so socially inept that they only like working with dead people."

These are just a few of the stereotypes that abound in the world of medicine. During your hospital clerkships, you will overhear these and many more statements from residents and attending physicians. Underlying each caricature is a common theme: personality type.

As you learned from Chapter 3, there are many important factors to take into account when choosing a medical specialty. Yet one very decisive variable— personality types within each discipline—was left out because it deserves a separate in-depth discussion. In fact, most medical students say they chose a particular specialty based on their gut feeling—meaning, often, how comfortable they feel with the doctors in that field. Each specialty requires a set of skills, a circle of qualities, and a certain type of disposition. Some of these intangibles are unique to that area of medicine, while others overlap across many disciplines. But these traits and affinities define a physician's personality—the factor that is perhaps the single most important consideration in choosing a medical specialty.

Unfortunately, most students do not spend much time thinking about their own personality type or considering how it might match with the specialties that interest them. Lectures, studying, and patient care all place huge demands on a medical student's time. But at some point during medical school, take some time out for an honest assessment of your values, character, and temperament. By taking a closer look at the specialties that best match your personality type, you will gain valuable information to help you make your decision.

PERSONALITY TYPE AND MEDICAL SPECIALTY

What makes you tick? How do you handle stress? What gives you satisfaction and fulfillment? How do you interact with your peers? These are all dimensions of a doctor's personality. Discerning your personality type is not simply finding a stereotype that fits. Instead, it means identifying your distinctive attributes, values, and affinities and finding the natural comfort zone where your true preferences lie as a physician.

Although it is especially important for doctors-in-training to select a specialty that is the best match with their personality, best match does not mean it has to be perfect. Take a hard look at the physicians you have met and make sure that your personality type is well represented (rather than underrepresented) in the specialty that interests you. The notion that opposites attract will probably not lead to a long, satisfying medical career. For instance, most physicians would not dispute the idea that empathic, laid-back medical students make better psychiatrists, and strong-minded, authoritarian, no-nonsense ones should become surgeons. In these examples, students find themselves most comfortable working side by side with other physicians who share their personality traits. When you get along well with your colleagues, patients end up receiving the best medical care possible.

Many physicians have studied the relationship between a doctor's personality and chosen specialty. A group of surgeons sought to determine whether there were differences in the characteristics and temperament of physicians in three types of medical careers: surgical, primary care (family practice, internal medicine, and pediatrics), and controllable lifestyle specialties (anesthesiology, dermatology, emergency medicine, neurology, ophthalmology, pathology, psychiatry, and radiology).[1] Most students think of surgeons as dominant, uninhibited, and aggressive. They tend to overlook the fact that surgery requires a certain type of person who can handle its tasks and challenges. Are you one of them? Their study found that surgeons tend to score higher than other specialists on being extroverted, practical, social, competitive, and structured. At the same time, however, surgeons were less creative than their colleagues in controllable lifestyle specialties (who were found to be the most withdrawn and rebellious). Neither group differed significantly from the primary care physicians. This particular study, therefore, helps to support the idea that a physician's satisfaction in a given specialty has a lot to do with personality factors, such as temperament and sociability.

Another landmark study surveyed a group of medical students to determine any relationships between personality type and specialty choice.[2] Students entering the hospital-based specialties (anesthesiology, radiology, or emergency medicine) had less tolerance for ambiguity and preferred highly structured environments with fixed guidelines and immediate closure to every patient encounter. Future obstetrician–gynecologists saw themselves as warm and helpful, but they were also emotionally vulnerable, uncomfortable around others, and very concerned about appearances and making a good impression. Future pediatricians, who sought warm and close interactions with their patients, were the most extroverted and sociable people. In contrast, the introverted students with fewer social connections—particularly the ones who had been in psychotherapy themselves—became psychiatrists. The study also found that students interested in surgery were more likely to be competitive, aggressive, and highly confident. They were the doctors-to-be who carried a strong conviction that their actions could rapidly influence the course of events.

When checking out all the different choices, medical students should keep in mind that more than one specialty could meet their preferences. For every personality type, it is possible to find a satisfying match with more than one area of medicine. If you are a visually oriented person, consider specialties such as pathology, dermatology, and radiology. For students who want to speak only the language of medicine every day as a doctor's doctor, radiology and pathology are ideal choices. Primary care specialties, such as internal medicine and family practice, are great opportunities to have long-term, intimate patient relationships. If you prefer an action-oriented specialty that gives immediate gratification, then consider anesthesiology, any surgical subspecialty, and emergency medicine. Some areas overlap considerably—such as the great variety of medical problems encountered in both family practice and emergency medicine. But at the same time, they can have significant differences—such as the long-term follow-up nature of family practice versus the acute, "stabilize the patient and move on" style of emergency medicine. Thus, to make the best decision, you have to know yourself and your desires well.

THE MYERS–BRIGGS TYPE INDICATOR

First developed in the 1950s by Isabel Briggs Myers and Katherine Briggs, the Myers–Briggs Type Indicator (MBTI) has become the most popular and widely used psychological test in the world. In fact, Isabel Myers was particularly interested in career development within the medical profession. Medical students were the subjects of her first longitudinal study. Based on Carl Jung theory of personality types, the MBTI was designed to analyze personality in a systematic, scientific manner. Where other questionnaires (type tests) only illustrate type, the MBTI precisely identifies a person's personality-type preferences.

The MBTI can help medical students to choose the right specialty for their personality and temperament. The test enables you to learn more about how you perceive and judge others, whether in an occupational or social situation. It identifies your strengths and weaknesses and shows whether you value autonomy or prefer interdependence.

Medical students usually take the MBTI at some point during the first 2 years of medical school. It is a very understandable and useful test for health professionals. Your Dean of Students Office will use the valuable information for career planning and development purposes—especially when it comes to figuring out which specialty might be the best one for you. For those who have not yet taken the MBTI, now is the perfect time to do so in conjunction with reading this book. Many Web sites offer different versions of the MBTI. You can do an Internet search for these, or simply log on to the official site of the Center for Applications of Psychological Type at *www.capt.org*. For a fee, they will send you the official test and provide personalized expert feedback over the telephone about your results and how to use their interpretation. When taking the test, be sure to answer every question truthfully; honesty is the only way to yield the most accurate results and help you pick the most appropriate specialty.

BREAKING DOWN THE MBTI: SIXTEEN PERSONALITY TYPES

According to the theory behind the MBTI, every individual falls into 1 of 16 types of personality. These personality types are derived from the four main indices of the MBTI. Each index represents one of the four basic preferences (described by Jung) about how every individual perceives and processes external stimuli and then uses that information to make some kind of cognitive judgment. As part of one's overall personality, this judgment guides behavioral preferences in any situation involving other people—such as colleagues or patients. The four dimensions measured by the MBTI are as follows:

1. *Extroversion (E) versus Introversion (I):* How do you relate to others? Where do you best derive your energy—from yourself or from others? Introverts prefer to focus their interest and energy on an inner world of ideas, impressions, and reactions. Being introverted does not mean being asocial. Instead, introverts prefer interactions with greater focus and depth, with others who are also good listeners and who think before they act or speak. Extroverts, on the other hand, derive their energy from external stimuli and tend to focus their interest on the outside world. They prefer dealing with facts, objects, and actions. Not all extroverts are the life of the party, however. They simply prefer being engaged in many things at once, with lots of expression, impulsivity, and thinking out loud.

2. *Sensing (S) versus Intuition (N):* What kinds of stimuli do you prefer when collecting, processing, and remembering information? Sensors are the ones who are drawn to the hard, immediate facts of life—practical details and evidence that can be taken in through one of the five senses. They are sensible, matter-of-fact people who look at the reality of the world around them, rely on prior experiences, and take things literally. Intuitives, on the other hand, look beyond the facts and evidence for meanings, possibilities, connections, and relationships. They are more imaginative and creative people who like to see the big picture and abstract concepts. Using intuition often means relying on a hunch or gut feeling rather than past experience. They eschew facts for theories and look beyond simply the obvious.

3. *Thinking (T) versus Feeling (F):* How do you make decisions and come to conclusions? This index concerns the kind of judgment you trust when you need to make a decision. Thinkers make their decisions impersonally, based mainly on objective data that makes sense to them. As analytical people motivated by achievement, they always consider the logical consequences of their decisions. Unlike thinkers, feelers rely on personal, subjective feelings in their decisions. As empathetic, compassionate, and sensitive people, they take the time to consider how their decision might affect others. Feelers like pleasing others and tend to get their feelings hurt rather easily.

4. *Judgment (J) versus Perception (P):* How do you order your life? What kind of environment makes you the most comfortable? This index describes how a

person deals with the outside world. Those who prefer judgment are serious, time-conscious individuals who live by schedules. They like things orderly, planned, and controlled. Judgers need a world of structure and predictability to have a sense of control over their environment and to be their most organized and productive. Judgers work hard, make decisions quickly and decisively, and sometimes can be closed minded. On the other hand, perceivers are much more open minded, relaxed, and nonconforming. They are much more aware of ideas, events, and things. Their flexibility and spontaneity, however, can sometimes lead to irresponsibility. Although judgers need to finish projects and settle all issues, perceivers tend to gather information in a leisurely way before making a final decision. Perceivers prefer to experience as much of the world as possible, and so they like to keep their options open and are most comfortable in adapting.

According to the theory behind the MBTI, personality type indicates an innate preference (similar to hand dominance) toward one of the two poles in each index, meaning that a person is probably never a 100% introvert but may lie closer to the introversion pole (the dominant or leading process) on a continuum scale, while still having some qualities of extroversion (which in this case would be considered the nondominant or auxiliary trait). When you take the MBTI, you receive a score that shows the strength and consistency of your natural tendency in each of these four dimensions. It is the interplay between the four poles that ultimately gives us our individual personality and temperament. Thus, the test classifies you as 1 of 16 different personality types combinations: INTP, ESTJ, ENFJ, ISTP, and so on. A complete description of the 16 personality types can be found on the Web site of the Center for Applications of Personality Type.

HOW THE MBTI CAN WORK FOR YOU

At this point, you are probably thinking "Enough with all this psychology stuff! How does this help me choose a specialty?" The best approach is to take the MBTI and identify your specific personality type. Use the expert feedback and interpretation of your results to learn more about the types of people with whom you work best. Then, as you rotate through the different fields of medicine during the junior year, look closely at each specialists and try to discern their personality type. Do pediatricians seem more like introverts? Are surgeons judgers or perceivers? What do specialties chosen by your personality type have in common? The overall goal is to make sure you know yourself well before determining which specialty is right for you.

Ideally, medical students should think about taking the MBTI more than once, because personality type may change over time (especially in young people). Personal growth and new experiences can often change the way a person interacts. Introverts may become more extroverted, or thinkers might become feelers from 1 year to the next. In fact, one study compared MBTI results in a group of medical students who took the test during their first and fourth years of school.[3] The authors found that nearly 57% of students had changed their personality-type preferences on one or more of the MBTI indices.

The MBTI has been studied quite extensively within the medical profession to draw conclusions about the relationship between personality type and career choice. One study examined whether the results of the MBTI taken in the first year of medical school accurately predicted the choice of medical specialty in the postgraduate year.[4] The authors found that three out of the four type indices (S–N, T–F, J–P) were predictive of future specialty choice: Students who were sensing, feeling, and judging types selected family practice. Students who were sensing, thinking, and judging types chose obstetrics–gynecology. Students who were intuitive, feeling, and perceiving types undertook careers in psychiatry.

Another study looked closely at the association between these two variables for medical students deciding between primary care and nonprimary care specialties.[5] The authors found that the E–I and T–F axes were the most statistically significant MBTI predictors with regard to specialty selection. Introverts and feelers were more likely to choose primary care, a highly service-oriented area of medicine with the rewards of long-term patient relationships. For graduates who chose nonprimary care fields, extroverted thinkers preferred surgical specialties, which is to be expected given the nature of surgical practice—high patient volume, less long-term continuity of care, and clinical situations that require rapid decisions based on facts.

Recently, researchers at Louisiana State University updated the original longitudinal study done by Myers in the 1950s (see Table 4–1) with new data on doctors graduating between 1988 and 1998.[6] They, too, found that I–N types are more drawn to fields such as internal medicine and neurology, whereas surgical specialties attract E–S types. Introverts and feeling types are more likely to choose primary care because of its nurturing, compassionate aspects. Within primary care,

TABLE 4–1

MEDICAL SPECIALTIES BY TEMPERAMENT

Introverted–Sensing–Thinking–Judging (ISTJ)

Dermatology

Obstetrics–gynecology

Family practice

Urology

Orthopedic surgery

Introverted–Sensing–Feeling–Judging (ISFJ)

Anesthesiology

Ophthalmology

General practice

Family practice

Pediatrics

Introverted–Sensing–Thinking–Perceptive (ISTP)

Otolaryngology

Anesthesiology

Radiology

Ophthalmology

General practice

Introverted–Sensing–Feeling–Perceptive (ISFP)

Anesthesiology

Urology

Family practice

Thoracic surgery

General practice

Introverted–Intuitive–Feeling–Judging (INFJ)

Psychiatry

Internal medicine

Thoracic surgery

General surgery

Pathology

Extroverted–Sensing–Thinking–Judging (ESTJ)

Obstetrics–gynecology

General practice

General surgery

Orthopedic surgery

Pediatrics

Extroverted–Sensing–Feeling–Judging (ESFJ)

Pediatrics

Orthopedic surgery

Otolaryngology

General practice

Internal medicine

Extroverted–Intuitive–Feeling–Perceptive (ENFP)

Psychiatry

Dermatology

Otolaryngology

Psychiatry

Pediatrics

Introverted–Intuitive–Thinking–Judging (INTJ)

Psychiatry

Pathology

Neurology

Internal medicine

Anesthesiology

Introverted–Intuitive–Feeling–Perceptive (INFP)

Psychiatry

Cardiology

Neurology

Dermatology

Pathology

Introverted–Intuitive–Thinking–Perceptive (INTP)

Neurology

Pathology

Psychiatry

Cardiology

Thoracic surgery

Extroverted–Sensing–Thinking–Perceptive (ESTP)

Orthopedic surgery

Dermatology

Family practice

Radiology

General surgery

Extroverted–Sensing–Feeling–Perceptive (ESFP)

Ophthalmology

Thoracic surgery

Obstetrics–gynecology

Orthopedic surgery

General surgery

Extroverted–Intuitive–Thinking–Perceptive (ENTP)

Otolaryngology

Psychiatry

Radiology

Pediatrics

Pathology

Extroverted–Intuitive–Feeling–Judging (ENFJ)

Thoracic surgery

Dermatology

Psychiatry

Ophthalmology

Radiology

Extroverted–Intuitive–Thinking–Judging (ENTJ)

Neurology

Cardiology

Urology

Thoracic surgery

Internal medicine

Data from McCaulley, M.H. *The Myers Longitudinal Medical Study (Monograph II)*. Gainesville, FL: Center for Applications of Psychological Type; 1977.

feeling types are more likely to choose family practice over internal medicine (which has a more technological focus). Anesthesiology seems to attract more ISTPs and ISFPs, and pediatrics appeals more to ESFJs and ESTJs. Sensors—who love more technological, direct approaches with well-learned skills—are more common in surgery (general and orthopedic) as well as obstetrics–gynecology. Intuitives prefer complex diagnostic challenges and problems with subtle nuances, and therefore they are more likely to become psychiatrists. INT types, who enjoy the challenge of medicine without ever seeing a patient, are attracted to pathology and research due to their ability to detach personally. Thinking types prefer caring for patients where impartiality and stamina are required. They also flock to the surgical specialties, where rapid decisions are needed based on hard evidence and facts.

LOOKING AT THE BIG PICTURE

The MBTI is a useful tool for identifying aspects of your personality, which can help you to find a compatible medical specialty. Remember the more you understand your temperament and motivations, the less likely you will allow other variables (such as those discussed in Chapter 3) to overshadow them. At the same time, medical students should not rely too heavily on personality type. Simply be aware that working with people with the same personality preferences is an important variable to consider. Typically, a physician who switches to a new specialty chooses one in which his or her own personality type is much more common. After all, medicine is a wonderfully broad profession in which there is an appealing specialty for every personality type!

REFERENCES

1. Schwartz, R.W., Barclay, J.R., et al. Defining the surgical personality: A preliminary study. *Surgery*. 1994;115(1):62–68.

2. Zeldow, P.B., Daugherty, S.R. Personality profiles and specialty choices of students from two medical school classes. *Acad Med*. 1991;66(5):283–287.

3. Brown, F., Peppler R.D. Changes in medical students' Myers-Briggs "preferences" between their first and fourth years of school. *Acad Med*. 1994;69:244.

4. Friedman, C.P., Slatt, L.M. New results relating the Myers-Briggs type indicator and medical specialty choice. *J Med Educ*. 1988;63(4):325–327.

5. Stilwell, N.A., Wallick, M.M. Myers-Briggs type and medical specialty choice: A new look at an old question. *Teach Learn Med*. 2000;12(1):14–20.

6. Wallick, M.M., Cambre, K.M. Personality types in academic medicine. *J La State Med Soc*. 1999;151:378–382.

5
FINDING THE PERFECT SPECIALTY

Medical students often make the mistake of believing that they will find the perfect specialty out of sheer luck or good fortune. Unfortunately, it is not always so easy. Choosing the ideal field of medicine requires time, research, and a great deal of thought and investigation. It should be an active process—almost like shopping, in a way. Whether you are a first- or fourth-year medical student, you need to put in the time to research every specialty under consideration. Hard work and effort forms the path to success and happiness. Procrastination will only lead to a more stressful (and ill-informed) decision—one that may end up being the wrong specialty!

This chapter addresses the potential opportunities for students to go about researching medical specialties. Use the different resources and options available to immerse yourself fully in a specific area of medicine. By interacting with other clinicians, you will find out whether that specialty makes good use of your interests, preferences, talents, and values. The list may seem daunting, but every student has four years in which to take advantage of the many sources of information. These are the only means by which doctors-to-be can figure out answers to many questions: What types of patients do you prefer? Can you handle diagnostic ambiguity or do you require absolute certainty? What kind of lifestyle do you want? Do you need to be an expert in your field? By pursuing as many of these options as possible, medical students will better determine their needs and preferences regarding each important variable in specialty selection.

This discussion is particularly beneficial for first- and second-year (preclinical) medical students. Compared with their upperclass peers, these medical students' exposure to patients, doctors, and the hospital is extremely limited. Instead, they are immersed in the rigorous demands of studying anatomy, pathology, microbiology, and other basic sciences. Although preclinical students gain little practical

51

knowledge or clinical exposure, they have ample opportunity outside the classroom and laboratory to explore different specialties.

Yet, first- and second-year medical students, just like juniors and seniors, also agonize greatly about what type of doctor to become. Most of them mistakenly believe that there really is no way to start learning about the different specialties until they start clinical rotations in the hospital. This is a misconception. By actively engaging in each of the following opportunities, all medical students — whether first year or fourth year — will help alleviate some of their apprehension about specialty choice as the time to make the decision approaches.

BASIC SCIENCE (PRECLINICAL) COURSES

The first 2 years of medical school consist of courses designed to provide a solid foundation in the scientific basis of medicine. You spend long days in the classroom and laboratory, memorizing anatomic terms, studying biochemical pathways, and reading about bugs, drugs, and diseases. During these years, students rarely step foot inside the hospital (except to learn how to take patient histories and conduct physical examinations under resident supervision).

Without direct clinical experience and exposure, is it possible to figure out which specialty may be right for you? Yes. Believe it or not, the basic science courses also give you insight into areas of medicine that may be a possible match for you. Every specialty represents a clinical discipline that draws upon a particular group of basic sciences as its scientific foundation. Some of the broader fields of medicine — such as emergency medicine, family practice, and internal medicine — make use of nearly all of the basic sciences in the diagnosis and treatment of disease. Other specialties focus on one or two fundamental sciences within their clinical spectrum. For instance, if you thoroughly enjoyed the course in neuroscience and neuroanatomy in the first year of medical school, there are many ways to study the diseases of the brain as a clinician. You could become a neurologist, neurosurgeon, psychiatrist, or physical medicine/rehabilitation specialist. If you absolutely thrived on the study of gross anatomy, then specialties such as diagnostic radiology and surgery are perfect for you. Take a closer look at Table 5–1.

By the end of the second year of medical school, you will have a much better idea of which basic sciences thrill you — and which ones bore you to death. During the clinical years, pay close attention to how each specialty makes use of the basic sciences. This will reinforce whether or not that field of medicine is right for you.

TABLE 5–1

SUBJECTS AND SPECIALTIES

If You Loved...	...Then Consider
Anatomy	Surgery, radiology
Histology	Pathology, dermatology
Biochemistry	Internal medicine
Neuroscience	Neurology, neurosurgery, psychiatry, physical medicine and rehabilitation
Immunology	Pathology, infectious disease
Physiology	Surgery, internal medicine, anesthesiology
Behavioral science	Psychiatry
Genetics	Pediatrics
Molecular biology	Pathology
Microbiology	Infectious disease
Pathology	Pathology
Pharmacology	Anesthesiology, internal medicine

"CAREERS IN MEDICINE"

To help medical students choose their specialty, the Association of American Medical Colleges (AAMC) offers a Web-based self-evaluation program titled "Careers in Medicine" (formerly known as "MedCareers"). This excellent career planning tool allows medical students to assess their skills, interests, talents, and personality characteristics. Starting right from the beginning of medical school, you can access it at *www.aamc.org/careersinmedicine*. Students will get the most out of this program if they use it repeatedly (ideally once or twice per year) as they refine their decision. After all, each educational experience during medical school can shape your ideas about which specialty is the perfect one. For this reason, Careers in Medicine is a superb way to create an honest and interactive self-assessment.

The actual program consists of four components: (1) personal career assessment—figuring out your values, interests, and long-term career aspirations; (2) career exploration—collecting information and learning about the different medical specialties and career options; (3) decision making—applying the results of your personal assessment with the information gathered about career options to select a single specialty; and (4) implementation—explaining how to go through the residency application, interview, and matching process. In essence, the entire system is an interactive questionnaire full of easy-to-use tools.

As you complete the different structured steps in the Careers in Medicine workshop, the AAMC recommends reassessing and reviewing previously answered questions. In fact, the system allows the user to store and update his or her personal profile and answers to different aspects of the program at any time. Using its decision-making tools, students can approach their choice in a systematic manner. To log in to the system and begin the program, medical students must obtain an access code from the appropriate AAMC liaison at their medical school.

CLINICAL ROTATIONS

Nearly all medical students base their choice of specialty on their third- and fourth-year clinical experiences. These are the years during which students complete their required clerkships, elective rotations, and subinternships in different medical and surgical specialties. Most schools require a set of core rotations in the basic areas of medicine in which all students must gain solid knowledge: internal medicine, pediatrics, surgery, obstetrics–gynecology, psychiatry, family practice, and neurology. The rotations last anywhere from 2 weeks to 3 months. During the surgery and internal medicine clerkships, you will have an opportunity to spend time in some of the relevant subspecialties, such as cardiology, orthopedic surgery, and neurosurgery.

Unlike the basic science courses, clinical rotations allow students to gain first-hand experiences and inside looks into a medical specialty. As full members of teams in each department, medical students have the important responsibility of knowing in detail every single aspect of their assigned patients' medical care, such as their test results and medications. As a subintern, a fourth-year medical student receives even more responsibility by functioning at the level of a first-year resident (or intern) in that specialty. These are the only times in medical school when you will immerse yourself in what specialists do on a daily basis—the kinds of problems they face, the tests they order, the procedures they perform, and the kinds of patients they treat.

During each clinical rotation, take the time to talk in depth with your attending physicians and residents. Find out what made them choose their specialty. As you meet new physicians, ask them a lot of tough, probing questions, such as

"Would you pick your field again if you had the option?" "What do you dislike about your specialty?" Write everything—especially your own impressions and thoughts about these experiences—down in a journal that you can refer to once the third year is over and it is time to choose a specialty. Hospital rotations are your only opportunity to gain a real-world perspective about the many different areas of medicine. Medical students, therefore, should use their limited elective time wisely to explore a specialty if they feel their previous exposure to it was inadequate.

Although clinical rotations are the best way to learn about the options available for every medical student, they are certainly not perfect. Take this time to review the section in Chapter 1 that discusses the limited value of the clinical clerkship in specialty selection.

GLAXO PATHWAY EVALUATION PROGRAM

Similar to Careers in Medicine, the Glaxo Pathway Evaluation Program (cosponsored by Duke University and GlaxoSmithKline, a major pharmaceutical company) is designed to help medical students undergo the specialty selection process. This innovative career planning program—endorsed by both the American Medical Student Association (AMSA) and the US Department of Health and Human Services—is an important part of medical education. The program consists of an interactive workshop, self-assessment exercises, and CD-ROM resources (such as specialty surveys and profiles). Diligently taking part in each component allows students to carefully evaluate their many options and to make a better-informed decision about their future career direction. Medical students who are completely clueless about what specialty to choose (or who are deciding between multiple specialties) find this program particularly helpful. It can give them an excellent start on the whole decision-making process.

The main component of the Glaxo Pathway Evaluation Program is a $3\frac{1}{2}$-hour workshop for third-year medical students. The program facilitator is a faculty member from your medical school. The program consists of a series of discussions, lectures, and interactive exercises, with an emphasis on informed, educated decision making. You will also interact with your peers while participating in both small and large discussion groups. Topics include factors in your decision such as the skills and talents that a specialty requires, the type of patient population, lifestyle issues, and so on. You will learn much about yourself and the specialty in which you are best suited.

Not everyone can participate in the Glaxo Pathway Evaluation Program. Your medical school has to set it up for you; therefore, get a group of students together and petition your Dean of Students Office to bring the program to campus. To obtain more information about the program, call 1-800-444-PATH or talk with any faculty advisor at your medical school.

GRAND ROUNDS

Throughout all 4 years of medical school, attending grand rounds is yet another way to check out what different specialties are like. Every department holds these hour-long meetings, typically once per week. They bring in a very prominent physician who gives a lecture about the latest advances in medical science related to his or her subject. Food is often served. Do not be bashful about showing up to listen to the talk. Everyone in the medical center is invited, and almost every member of that department—faculty, residents, and staff—makes a concerted effort to attend.

By going to grand rounds, medical students (particularly first and second years) will begin to expose themselves to new fields of medicine. It is a chance to hear about interesting cases, follow the thought processes of different specialists, and observe the interactions among faculty members and resident physicians. These talks are a great way to learn about a specialty by hearing about the newest research and other updates in the field. Although some topics may be technically overwhelming, grand rounds can give you an excellent sense of a discipline's clinical subject matter. If you find yourself nodding off, maybe that specialty is not the right one. If you find yourself excited and keenly interested in the discussion, perhaps that field should move to the top of your list.

INTERNET RESOURCES

Through the World Wide Web, medical students can obtain a wealth of information on any topic in medicine—especially the important issues related to any medical specialty under consideration. Want to know what the job market is like for anesthesiologists? Check out *www.gaswork.com*. What are today's practicing radiologists talking about? Check their discussion forums and chat groups on *www.auntminnie.com*. Wondering about the state of burnout among emergency medicine physicians? Then take a look at studies published in the online version of *Academic Emergency Medicine*. To find the specific piece of information you are looking for, simply run a keyword search on one of the many Internet search engines, such as the popular *www.google.com.*

One of the best starting points for gathering information about a particular medical specialty is its national professional association. For example, the American College of Surgery is the main entity for surgeons; their colleagues in anesthesiology belong to the American Society of Anesthesiologists. The Web sites of these organizations contain a wide variety of medical, professional, educational, and patient-related information. You could spend hours reading the articles and newsletters posted on these pages. It is an excellent way to learn about the latest issues and debates within that specialty. In addition, becoming a student member of these societies entitles you to a subscription to their monthly journals as well as invitations to national meetings. A complete list of the national specialty associations and their respective Web sites (as well as other highly recommended Internet resources) can be found at the end of this book.

MEDICAL JOURNALS

Each medical school has its own library that is stocked with nearly every single medical journal that exists. In your spare time, take a look at some of them. You are probably thinking, "What spare time?" From cramming for biochemistry examinations to preparing presentations for morning pediatrics rounds, the intense workload of medical school leaves little time for outside reading. However, reading the journals of different medical specialties can provide a nice flavor of the subject matter in that field—but on the same level that a practicing specialist would read. Instead of reading that surgery review/outline book, flip open *The American Journal of Surgery.* Do not be concerned about understanding every single word or unfamiliar topic. The point of this endeavor is to get an overall sense of the current research in each of the many specialties. These issues, in general, will have a different focus than the topics that students read about in their texts or outline books.

To help you choose a specialty, there are several noteworthy publications within every library's collection. Several times per year, the Journal of the American Medical Association (JAMA) publishes a series of articles of particular relevance to medical students and residents in its "msJAMA" section. Previous topics have included specialty selection, the match process, and women in medicine. The AMSA publishes a monthly magazine called *The New Physician*, which typically has features on choosing a specialty. Many faculty members read *Academic Medicine*, a well-respected publication that has featured many articles and studies about residency, medical school, specialty selection, and the match. These journals and others can provide illuminating information that most medical students might not otherwise come across.

MEETINGS: NATIONAL AND LOCAL

Attending national and local meetings is another excellent opportunity for medical students (especially first and second years) to meet physicians in various specialties. These conferences generally consist of lectures, discussions, poster presentations, and social events. Every national specialty association holds an annual, multiday meeting in a major US city—possibly one in which you currently attend medical school. For instance, every December, the meeting of the Radiological Society of North America draws radiologists and radiation oncologists from all over the country to Chicago. Interested in a career in internal medicine? Try to make it to the annual meeting of the American College of Physicians. Some meetings occur locally, such as the annual get together of the Massachusetts Society of Anesthesiologists. Others are even more specific, such as the National Conference of Family Practice Residents and Medical Students, sponsored by the American Academy of Family Physicians. Although some events may require an entrance fee, medical students are generally welcomed at each of them. By going to these meetings, you will see the specialty from a different perspective— similar to that of a private practitioner attending their annual continuing medical education conferences. Specialties hold their national meetings in different locations each year and so you will have to look them up on their respective Web sites.

MENTORS AND COLLEAGUES

It goes without saying that the physicians and future doctors-to-be with whom you interact on a daily basis are some of the best sources of information and advice. All medical students should make good use of any formal (and informal) career advising at their institution. Cultivate relationships with faculty members in various specialties and ask them questions about their areas of interest. Explore various specialty areas by establishing relationships with at least two mentors who will take a professional interest in you. Sharing in their professional, community, and family lives will provide great insight into what being a physician is like in their particular specialty of medicine. Of course, do not forget about your fellow upperclass students. They are also invaluable sources of inside information and personal experiences. Seek out these informal advisors and ask them a lot of questions about their specialty interests.

RESEARCH PROJECTS

Clinical and basic science researches are fundamental components of the medical profession. Many aspiring physicians enter medical school with varying degrees of research experience from college or other positions prior to beginning their medical education. Once in medical school, a fair number of students engage in research projects outside of their classroom and clinical work requirements. There are two types of research you can pursue — in the basic sciences (eg, microbiology, biochemistry) and clinical disciplines (eg, radiology, surgery).

Engaging in clinical research is a wonderful way to learn about a specialty. You will immerse yourself in the department, interact with faculty members, and have a chance to see their clinical and nonclinical activities every day. Moreover, you can become familiar with the subject matter of that discipline. If you are un-decided about a specialty, then seek out research projects that deal with topics that cross multiple specialties, such as diabetes, asthma, or hypertension. For instance, many students conduct clinical research projects in the emergency department, where they get to talk to patients, take surveys, and see what emergency medicine specialists do down in the trenches. The early exposure to specialties through research projects may help you rule in or out particular ones. In the end, even if taking part in research does not help you select a specialty, it is still a valuable experience. You will learn how to critically interpret the scientific literature and ask probing questions — skills essential for all types of specialists.

On a specialty-related side note, getting involved with medical research has the potential to strengthen your application. A few residency programs will invite only those applicants who completed extensive research for an interview; there-fore, consider your options carefully (see Chapter 11 for specifics). Residency selection committees like to see students with excellent achievement — and noth-ing looks better than a publication in a major medical journal. This is partic-ularly true for the most competitive specialties, where anything that makes you stand apart from the crowd is helpful. In fact, some specialties — such as radiation oncology — almost require students to have completed research projects. (Keep in mind, however, that it looks best to continue any research started during the summer following first year. One-time projects have less influence.)

Most medical students initiate the pursuit of research during the summer between the first and second years of medical school. By this point, they have become familiar with their university, its departments, and its faculty members. Many medical schools offer funding or generous stipends for their students to stay at their institution and conduct research within one of the departments. Some students leave for other medical centers. There are several sources of outside funding for medical students through a competitive application process. These include the National Institutes of Health, the Howard Hughes Medical Institute, and AMSA. See your Dean of Student Affairs Office for more information.

At the most prominent research universities, a small cadre of students participates in the "Medical Scientist Training Program" (MSTP), an ultracompetitive program in which students simultaneously pursue both MD and PhD degrees. Sponsored by grants from the National Institutes of Health, the MSTP aims to train the next generation of physician-scientists for careers in both biomedical research and clinical practice. What kind of specialties does these physician-scientists select? A survey of all MSTP graduates from 2004 through 2008 found that the top five specialties chosen were internal medicine (24.6%), pathology (10.3%), pediatrics (10%), diagnostic radiology (6.9%), and dermatology (5.9%).[1] Clearly, MD/PhD graduates were much less likely to pursue training in the surgical specialties and subspecialties. Perhaps, the five most commonly chosen areas have many strong physician-scientist role models who encourage careers in academic medicine.

SHADOWING RESIDENTS AND ATTENDING PHYSICIANS

First- and second-year medical students spend very little time in the hospital and clinics. Aside from learning how to take patient histories and perform physical examinations, you rarely interact with many specialists during these 2 years. For this reason, get a head start in checking out different areas of medicine by spending your free time shadowing physicians—either residents or attendings. Many hold weekend clinic hours in which you can tag along with them as they see patients. Most residents will not mind if you want to attend daily rounds in the hospital, too. Get some practical volunteer or work experience in the hospital or neighborhood clinic. Hang out in the emergency department, where the doctors will teach you how to suture wounds and perform other minor procedures. The time you spend with specialists in different areas of medicine may ultimately give you the necessary exposure to help make a final decision in the next year. Moreover, you will begin to get to know physicians who may write letters of recommendation in support of your residency applications.

SPECIALTY INTEREST GROUPS

During medical school (especially in the preclinical years), almost every student gets involved in many kinds of medically related extracurricular activities. There are lots of options from which to choose—giving tours to prospective applicants, teaching elementary school students about how the heart works, or coordinating the delivery of medical supplies to third-world countries. To help you to figure out what specialty might be the best match (before you head out on the wards in third year), consider taking part in a specialty interest group as one of your extracurricular activities.

Medical students often get together and form an interest group based on a particular specialty, such as the Emergency Medicine Interest Group or Pediatrics Interest Group. The purpose of these unique and valuable groups is to bring together medical students, residents, and faculty physicians who share the same interest in that specialty. As a member, you can set up time to shadow physicians, attend special lectures, get ideas and make contacts for research projects, meet with clinicians outside of the hospital in social situations, perform services for the local community, and much more. This educational resource provides time to ask questions to more experienced physicians. Because there is no pressure to perform well and obtain a good evaluation, specialty interest groups are excellent ways to learn informally about a specialty before hitting the wards as an upperclass medical student.

Some specialty interest groups have even established a national presence on the Internet. Future family practitioners, for example, can take advantage of one of the best ones—the Virtual Family Medicine Interest Group. Modeled after successful campus specialty groups, this Web site provides information and resources to help students explore the specialty of family practice and all of its related topics (such as residency training and the match process). You can take a look for yourself at http://fmignet.aafap.org.

SUMMER BETWEEN MS-I AND MS-II

Unlike the best years of your life in college, medical school provides only a single summer vacation—between the first and second years. Most medical students agonize over what to do during this last free summer. They are not sure whether to work to make money, pursue research, read up before second year (!), hang out and relax, or do something that looks good on their resume—such as vaccinating all the children of Africa. After all, students are generally worried about what those residency program selection committees might think about how exactly they spent their summer vacation.

Your goal during this summer should be to attach yourself to clinicians (while at the same time taking a rejuvenating break from all the lecture and laboratory work from the first year). In these formative years of training in medical school, future doctors should seek out any and all experiences and chances to build a solid foundation of the best physician that they can be. So take this summer break seriously and do something productive at least the majority of the time. Early clinical exposure during this summer will give you a jump-start to specialty decision making before the crucial third year. By pursuing a structured activity, you can start thinking and learning about different areas of medicine, particularly the ones you might not have time to rotate through during third year, such as dermatology or ophthalmology.

There are a number of summer opportunities for career exploration, such as clinical externships, research programs, and community preceptorships. All of these paths can help you check out different medical specialties and start figuring out your preferences, likes, dislikes, and values when it comes to career options. Some medical students make informal arrangements to volunteer in community health clinics or shadow physicians (while also earning money through part-time jobs such as waiting tables). For motivated students who do not mind another round of applications, there are formal programs that provide more structured clinical experience. Following are some examples:

- The National Health Service Corps, a federal agency, offers a month-long rotation (funded with a stipend) to expose students to the practice of rural medicine and primary care in underserved areas. You might be placed in Alaska, Nevada, North Dakota, West Virginia, or other exotic locales. This program (called Student/Resident Experiences and Rotations in Community Health [SEARCH]) allows preclinical students to get a taste of clinical medicine, practice taking patient histories, and get a head start on their physical examination skills.
- On a more local level, many states offer summer externship programs. For instance, the Illinois Academy of Family Practitioners has a program for rising second-year students in which they are paired with a family practitioner for a month-long one-on-one preceptorship.
- You can obtain funded externships directly from medical centers. For instance, Thomas Jefferson University Hospital in Philadelphia sponsors

a 6-week experience in radiation oncology (The Simon Kramer Society Externship) for interested medical students.

• Want to get some clinical experience and learn how to speak Spanish? AMSA offers a summer program in many Latin American countries called SALUD — a Medical Spanish program abroad. Through classroom and practical clinical work, you learn about another country's health care needs and become proficient in another language.

Although not every specialty has its own organized clinical summer program, many do exist and more are established every year. Either conduct searches in the Internet or contact your Dean of Student Affairs Office to find out more information on these externship programs. Above all, make every effort to use this summer to gain early exposure to different specialties without having to commit yourself to any of them. It will help you to begin prioritizing some of the many factors that go into deciding on a specialty (and on what you want out of your medical career in general). Even if your heart has always been set on orthopedic surgery, use this last summer to check out primary care or family practice. You never know what kind of meaningful clinical experience may end up changing your mind.

REFERENCE

1. Paik, J.C., Howard, G., et al. Postgraduate choices of graduates from medical scientist training programs, 2004–2008. JAMA. 2009;302(12):1271–1272.

6

SPECIAL CONSIDERATIONS FOR WOMEN

Not too long ago, women only made up a tiny minority of physicians and medical students. Today that has changed dramatically. Medicine is no longer a profession heavily dominated by men. Instead, women now make up about half of the average medical school class. During the past two decades, the number of female doctors has nearly quadrupled.[1] In the 1990s, academicians predicted that more than one-third of all practicing physicians will be women by 2010.[2] A closer look at the number of female residents making up each specialty supports this prediction (Table 6–1).

The influx of so many women into medicine slowly changed the traditional take on doctors. The public no longer thought of physicians as wise, gentle men who made house calls. Instead, they began to have female doctors of their own — women who treated hypertension, performed cardiac bypass surgery, interpreted chest radiographs, and delivered babies. For many of these women physicians, their gender had an important role in their final choice of medical specialty.

CHALLENGES FOR TODAY'S FEMALE PHYSICIAN

Despite the encouraging numbers, gender inequality remains a fact of life in medicine. Across the medical specialties, the distribution of women is somewhat unbalanced. In 2011, for example, women made up only 13% of orthopedic surgery residents, compared with about 81% in obstetrics–gynecology and 73% in pediatrics.[3] In general, a much smaller proportion of women enter the highly technical specialties (such as surgery and radiology); the majority gravitate toward

TABLE 6-1

PERCENTAGE OF FEMALE RESIDENTS BY SPECIALTY

Obstetrics–gynecology	81.4
Pediatrics	72.7
Dermatology	63.7
Family medicine	55.4
Psychiatry	54.7
Pathology	53.8
Neurology	45.7
Internal medicine	44.7
Ophthalmology	41.6
Physical medicine and rehabilitation	40.6
Emergency medicine	40.2
Anesthesiology	37.2
General surgery	36.2
Radiation oncology	33.3
Otolaryngology	32.7
Radiology	27.8
Plastic surgery	23.2
Urology	23.2
Neurosurgery	13.9
Orthopedic surgery	13.2

Data from Brotherton, S.E., Etzel, S.I. Graduate medical education. *JAMA*. 2011;306(9):1015–1030; Appendix II, Table 2.

primary care fields such as pediatrics, family practice, internal medicine, and psychiatry.[4]

Why are women more likely than men to select a career in primary care? After all, many medical students think of these specialties as having lower status, perhaps because of the lower income and lack of emphasis on procedures. Typically, more women seem to be drawn to the primary care specialties because they are compatible with their practice styles. In general, women physicians perform more preventive medicine services, show more compassion and empathy, and spend more time with their patients, especially when it comes to just simply listening. One prominent female physician believes that "pediatrics and obstetrics–gynecology are related to mothering and child-bearing, which are very important for women in our society, and may be why these specialties seem consistent with the personality of women."[5] Another study agreed with the assessment that women are overrepresented in primary care specialties because of their maternal and nurturing qualities. The authors looked at variables influencing the decision to enter primary care and concluded that "it is possible that the emphasis on family values and needs that in our culture affect women as a group more than men would have a larger influence on a woman's decision to become a primary care doctor than would other factors."[6]

Even so, more women today are forging into areas of medicine that have been exclusively occupied by men in the past. By demanding equality, these pioneers make it easier for female medical students to follow in their paths. Although women and men now work side by side within every specialty, this does not necessarily mean that their lives and career paths are alike. Women may weigh different considerations when approaching their specialty choice. This may be in part because of a sociologic difference of perspective in what makes for a satisfying career between men and women. There are also practical concerns to consider, such as comfortably integrating the issue of pregnancy (and all of the decisions that come with it) and how its timing will affect their medical careers. Many women in medicine want a specialty that is family friendly — one that lends itself to having greater control over work hours and the possibility of working part-time when they have children. When deciding on her specialty of choice, every female medical student should spend some time honestly weighing these concerns and competing responsibilities. In doing so, you will likely choose the best specialty and have a rewarding professional career in medicine.

CAREER SATISFACTION AMONG FEMALE PHYSICIANS

There are a lot more women in medicine today, but are they all happy with their chosen profession? The majority of women (84%) are generally satisfied with their medical careers. But surprisingly, a solid number (38%) would choose a new specialty if they could do it all over again. Why such remorse? Many variables — work stress, degree of autonomy, work hours, income, and so on — affect how content a doctor is with his or her career. Choosing a medical specialty with the right balance, then, makes a big difference between a happy physician and a dissatisfied one. In fact, the same survey of female physicians revealed that work environment and stress (two factors directly related to their specialty) are the strongest predictors of career satisfaction.[7]

Certain types of female doctors have higher degrees of career satisfaction, according to this study. Dermatologists, psychiatrists, ophthalmologists, anesthesiologists, and surgeons were among the happiest of all female physicians. They were the least interested in changing their specialty. With the exception of surgery, these specific careers have the most controllable lifestyles in terms of work hours and on-call demands. Internists and general practitioners, on the other hand, had the strongest desires to change their specialty. But a cushier way of life does not necessarily mean career satisfaction. Take radiology, for instance. With its 8 to 5 workdays and limited call responsibilities, this field should be full of happy doctors. Instead, the same survey found that female radiologists had among the lowest levels of career satisfaction. This was especially surprising in comparison with their colleagues in surgery, who cope with a rigorous lifestyle, long hours, heavy on-call demands, and a male-dominated work environment. Yet despite these perceived lifestyle drawbacks, female surgeons had some of the highest levels of career satisfaction, and 76% even reported that they would definitely not want to enter a different specialty! Perhaps, this extraordinary contentment reflects a sense of pride in being a pioneer in surgery, coupled with higher income and more control in their everyday patient care.

To ensure the best chance for happiness, female medical students should ask themselves the following questions when thinking about their future career.

1. How Do You Envision Your Practice Style?

Some medical students prefer short patient interactions with no continuity, whereas others want to have life-long relationships with all those under their care. In general, women like spending more clinical time than men do with their patients, particularly regarding issues of counseling, preventive medicine, and psychosocial development.[8] If you share this preference, then consider careers in primary care fields. If you are more action oriented and like working at a fast pace, then think about emergency medicine, anesthesiology, or surgery. If you seek the latest technical gadgets, then cardiology, radiology, and radiation oncology may be the best specialties for you.

2. Could You Handle Working in a Predominantly Male Environment?

Certain specialties, particularly the more technical ones, are known to be boys' clubs. The most conspicuous are surgery (and surgical subspecialties), emergency medicine, radiology, and ophthalmology. Keep in mind that high levels of testosterone in the workplace can often lead to inappropriate comments, gender bias, and even sexual harassment. In the operating room, for instance, the perpetual locker room mentality often means that female surgeons tend to feel pressure to behave as one of the boys to fit in well with their male colleagues. Are you prepared for this type of working environment? No matter the specialty, it is essential to feel comfortable around the physicians with whom you will be working. Without a supportive atmosphere at work, patient care may suffer.

3. Will You Be Able to Take Maternity Leave, Have Children, and Raise a Family?

It is challenging, but certainly not impossible, for women to maintain a thriving professional career and have children. According to the aforementioned study, the happiest female physicians—no matter the specialty—were the ones who had children. Certain specialties more easily allow for maternity leave and time to raise children, particularly during the peak reproductive years surrounding residency training and initial employment. In a survey of women who entered pediatrics, for example, nearly half based the timing of pregnancy on their career stage, leading to a mean age of conception at 29 years (when most were just out of residency).[9]

So if you are planning to have kids (or already have a family), keep in mind whether or not your dream specialty will permit time for them. Take a closer look at whether physicians in your chosen specialty might penalize female physicians for maternity leaves or even actively discourage their pregnancies. For instance, hospital-based specialties such as radiology, anesthesiology, and emergency medicine offer more predictable schedules, ones in which you will rarely take work home with you. Unlike the trauma surgeon, gastroenterologist, or obstetrician, physicians in areas such as psychiatry and dermatology seldom get paged for emergencies in the middle of the night. These are all areas of medicine that might be more amenable to flexibility when it comes to timing a pregnancy.

For most women, stability within their specialty is just one of many factors that play a part in their happiness in medicine. In the workplace, female physicians often have to cope with sexual harassment, higher expectations, and salary inequity. In general, women in medicine earn less money than men because more are either clustered within the lower-paying primary care specialties or work part-time. Moreover, women have to tackle an inverted career pyramid, one in which they will devote more time to their careers only after bearing and raising children at a younger age. Outside the workplace, busy physicians have additional stressors. They have to juggle multiple responsibilities—practicing medicine, managing their office, and running their household. Most women still do proportionally more cleaning, cooking, and so on than their husbands, in some cases even after a long day of practicing medicine. Whether a radiologist, surgeon, or pediatrician, every female physician faces similar at-home challenges, which cannot be excluded from one's overall professional satisfaction.

SEX AND SURGERY: BEING A FEMALE PHYSICIAN IN THE OPERATING ROOM

To become a surgeon, you must love spending hours in the operating room more than anything else in the world. Most specialties are flexible enough to allow women physicians to have an outside family life and to raise children. The rigorous, sleep-deprived lifestyle of surgery, however, requires the greatest time commitment, particularly when it comes to the intensity and length of residency training. Partly because of this, surgery has traditionally been a rather male-dominated field. Excluding obstetrics–gynecology, only 18% of surgical residents are women.[10] Within this small group, each female surgeon undergoes considerable self-examination to prepare herself for the demands of a surgical career.

Initially, just like their male colleagues, many female medical students do find themselves attracted to a career in surgery. They are partial to the emphasis on technical procedures, the ability to save a patients' life, and the immediate gratification of performing a surgical operation. They love the thrill of delving into the internal anatomy of a fellow human being. They could actually see themselves becoming orthopedic surgeons, cardiothoracic surgeons, or surgical oncologists. Yet there is still a striking underrepresentation of women in the surgical specialties. Why do 76% of women who plan to pursue surgery lose their interest and commit to something else?[11] And why do only 6% of female students actually gain interest in surgery during medical school?

It is clear that certain barriers within the surgical profession end up discouraging women from entering. Many women are discouraged by the long hours, family sacrifices, and male-dominated operating room. Also, performing routine and emergency surgery on patients at all hours of the day and night does not lend itself well to being an available parent. Compared with other specialists, female surgeons are more likely to be single (but their divorce rate is equal to that of their male colleagues). And, because of strong professional aspirations and interests, they are also less likely than others to have children, or, if they do, more likely to have full-time childcare.[12] Moreover, the military nature of a surgical residency—degradation, humiliation, and rigid chain of command—is especially unappealing. On a lesser note, many medical students and residents have observed that female scrub nurses may have problems taking orders in the operating room because of their deferential role to another woman. Clearly, there are many variables that every potential female surgeon should think about carefully when considering a surgical career.

Surgery is the one specialty where female doctors have the most difficulty integrating themselves with their male colleagues. "Surgery is kind of a high testosterone battlefield, so when it comes time to give orders, women surgeons are sometimes taken less seriously," says a university-based female neurosurgeon. "When male surgeons 'take charge,' their behavior is usually interpreted as assertive and appropriate, but we women are often labeled 'aggressive and inappropriate.'"[13]

And yet, despite the decline in the number of medical students entering careers in general surgery today, a surprisingly higher percentage of women are deciding to become surgeons. General surgery, orthopedics, and neurosurgery are competing for these female applicants, all of whom are no longer discouraged by the rigorous training of the competitive tiers of medicine. As a way of helping their fellow women, many female medical students now aspire to become breast surgeons. Even the gentler surgical subspecialties—such as urology—are experiencing an influx of women. Despite the drastically skewed distribution of men to women, nearly all (94%) of female urologists would highly encourage other women to enter this boys' club specialty.[14] As pioneers in their specialty, today's female surgeons build on their self-confidence and end up with extremely high levels of career satisfaction.

CONSIDERING YOUR PRACTICE OPTIONS

In every specialty—whether it is psychiatry or surgery—all female physicians can arrange time to raise children, pursue outside interests, and have a productive medical career. These aspirations are not mutually exclusive. But to do so, you must carefully plan the type of practice you want. In the primary care specialties, such as pediatrics and family practice, female doctors have successfully led the way for innovative practice options, like working part-time or job sharing. Other specialties, however, have been slow to accept the following more accommodating career strategies.

1. Practicing Medicine Part-Time

By definition, working fewer than 40 hours per week is considered part-time. The primary care fields are among the most favorable to part-time work, especially because they are appointment based. Specialties with highly controllable hours are also as conducive, such as the shift work of emergency medicine, the case-by-case nature of anesthesiology, the scheduled hours of pathology and radiology, and the lack of off-hour emergencies in dermatology and ophthalmology. Even surgeons can work part-time. Breast surgeons, for instance, perform mainly elective surgery and can therefore schedule fewer cases and less clinic time each week. Another way to work part-time is to arrange for a shared-schedule position with another physician. In this format, each doctor works half time with alternating appointment schedules; together, they equal one practitioner. Some even arrange this system with their spouse if both are in the same specialty. In either situation, remember that working part-time means sacrificing higher salaries for flexibility. Another disadvantage is that part-time academic physicians are ineligible for tenure, and those in private practice often are unable to become partners or stockholders in the practice. Women should also keep in mind that many unsympathetic colleagues may be hostile to physicians seeking to change their schedules to fulfill parental roles.

2. Join Group Practices or Managed Care Companies

Through this practice option, a physician generally works 40 hours a week with little overnight call responsibility (shared among either the group partners or health maintenance organization [HMO] members). However, you will give up quite a bit of autonomy. Especially in an HMO, physicians have to submit to its rules, regulations, paperwork, and bureaucracy, which often dictate or constrain how you conduct patient care.

3. Work Out of Your Home

Many female solo practitioners, particularly those in psychiatry, opt to set up their office in their home. This allows for greater interaction with their family. The major disadvantage, of course, is the intrusion of patients, secretaries, nurses, and other staff members on your home property.

4. Enter Academics Rather Than Becoming a Private Practitioner

In the university teaching hospital, academic physicians devote less clinical time. They primarily supervise residents, who provide the majority of patient management. You will have greater job flexibility in this salaried position because of the additional time for teaching and research. Unlike private practice, there is much less emphasis in academic medicine on productivity and seeing as many patients as possible. In fact, female physicians practicing in medical schools and teaching hospitals reported the most happiness with their specialty choice.[7]

FIND A MENTOR—BE A MENTOR

To make the most informed decision, all medical students (both male and female) should try to find an advisor, role model, or mentor. Seeking advice from a respected faculty member is an essential part of choosing a specialty — form these relationships early in your medical training. Because women often have additional concerns when deciding on their specialty, a good female mentor can provide invaluable guidance. Remember, you do not have to establish an advisor–advisee relationship with lots of physicians, or even with ones who practice in the specialty under consideration. More importantly, female medical students should seek out other women who have already gone through the same decisions. These doctors usually have a wealth of information and personal experience about being female in a male-dominated profession. They should be more than happy to share their thoughts and answer questions from a younger version of themselves.

The best female mentor makes you feel comfortable enough to exchange ideas, personal thoughts, and concerns. She should always make herself available for discussing somewhat intimate issues, such as marriage, gender discrimination, career aspirations, and the best time to have children. In a study of role models within the specialty of internal medicine,[15] the most sought-after faculty mentors

- spend more than 25% of their time teaching students and residents,
- spend more than 25 hours per week teaching and conducting rounds when serving as an attending physician,
- always call attention to the psychosocial aspects of medicine,
- emphasize the value of the doctor–patient relationship, and
- served as chief resident.

Finding the perfect mentor may seem like the ultimate challenge. Regardless, female students should make it one of their top priorities during medical school. In the clinical years, seek out women faculty members in all departments, especially male-dominated specialties such as surgery, radiology, and emergency medicine.

Identify good role models and encourage them to take you under their wings (or rather, their white coats).

Why is having a first-rate mentor so important for female medical students? When choosing a specialty, inadequate (or nonexistent) exposure to role models can lead to high levels of career dissatisfaction in the future. After all, good clinical mentors exert considerable influence over medical students regarding the merits of a particular specialty. Take a female student rotating through the surgery department, for example. More women ended up committing to surgery as a career in cases where a higher proportion of women on the surgical faculty served as mentors during the rotation.[16] Similar conclusions can likely be drawn for other specialties, but first you have to seek out advisors within that department. These honest relationships can clear up misconceptions about career satisfaction and may even change students' specialty decisions. There are three ways to go about finding a female mentor in your specialty of choice.

1. Talk With Your Fellow Classmates or Dean

Your colleagues in medical school are usually the best source of advice. They can tell you which faculty members have traditionally served as excellent role models for women. Throughout the year, try to set up frequent meetings with them, keeping in mind that there are often a limited number of senior faculty physicians available. Not every female student finds a good mentor. In fact, at the typical academic medical center, 31% of men are full tenured professors of clinical medicine, whereas only 10.5% of women hold the same title.[17]

2. Become a Member of the American Medical Women's Association

Most medical schools have their own chapter of this excellent organization for female students. With members totaling more than 10,000 physicians, the American Women's Medical Association (AMWA) has been the voice of women in medicine since 1915. As the percentage of female physicians increased, AMWA expanded its scope accordingly. Having more women in medicine brought new issues to the forefront, such as gender equality among faculty appointments and the role of women in male-dominated fields. To help students cope with the specialty decision-making process, local AMWA branches often sponsor brown bag lunches. Chapter members invite respected female physicians to give a talk over the lunch hour about their careers and reasons for choosing their specialty. Speak to the president of your affiliated AMWA chapter for more information on how to get involved.

3. Contact Specialty Groups for Women Physicians

Nearly all specialties have affiliated women-only organizations, which are helpful sources of information. You can get in touch with them for names of doctors who may be willing to mentor female students and perhaps even allow for job shadowing. For a complete list of these organizations, visit the Web site of the American Medical Association (http://www.ama-assn.org/ama/pub/about-ama/our-people/member-groups-sections/women-physicians-congress/specialty-groups.page?).

REFERENCES

1. Barzansky, B., Etzel, S.I. Educational programs in U.S. medical schools, 2001–2002. *JAMA.* 2002;288(9):1067–1072.

2. Braus, P. How women will change medicine. *Am Demogr.* 1994;16:40–47.

3. Brotherton, S.E., Etzel, S.I. Graduate medical education. *JAMA.* 2011;306(9):1015–1030; Appendix II, Table 2.

4. American Medical Association. *Women Physicians by Specialty.* Accessed December 27, 2011, from http://www.ama-assn.org/ama/pub/about-ama/our-people/member-groups-sections/women-physicians-congress/statistics-history/table-5-women-physicians-specialties.page.

5. Bowman, M.A., Frank, E., et al. *Women in medicine: Career and life management.* New York: Springer-Verlag; 2002.

6. Xu, G., Rattner, S.L., et al. A national study of the factors influencing men and women physicians' choices of primary care specialties. *Acad Med.* 1995;70:398–404.

7. Frank, E., McMurray, J.E., et al. Career satisfaction of U.S. women physicians: Results from the women physicians' health study. *Arch Intern Med.* 1999;159:1417–1426.

8. McMurray, J.E., Linzer, M., et al. The work lives of women physicians. *J Gen Intern Med.* 2000;15:372–380.

9. Sells, J.M., Sells, C.J. Pediatrician and parent: A challenge for female physicians. *Pediatrics.* 1989;84(2):355–361.

10. Kwaka, K., Jonasson, O. The longitudinal study of surgical residents, 1994–1996. *J Am Coll Surg.* 1999;188:575–585.

11. Novielli, K., Hojat, M., et al. Change of interest in surgery during medical school: A comparison of men and women. *Acad Med.* 2001;76:S58–S61.

12. Frank, E., Brownstein, M., et al. Characteristics of women surgeons in the United States. *Am J Surgery*. 1998;176:244–250.

13. Jones, V.A. Why aren't there more women surgeons? *JAMA*. 2000;283:670.

14. Bradbury, C.L., King, D.K., et al. Female urologists: A growing population. *J Urol*. 1997;157(5):1854–1856.

15. Wright, S.M., Kern, D.E., et al. Attributes of excellent attending-physician role models. *N Engl J Med*. 1998;339:1986–1993.

16. Neumayer, L., Kaiser, S., et al. Perceptions of women medical students and their influence on career choice. *Am J Surg*. 2002;183(2):146–150.

17. Bickel, J., Clark, V. Encouraging the advancement of women. *JAMA*. 2000;283(5):671.

7

COMBINED RESIDENCY PROGRAMS

C hoosing your dream specialty from 20 possibilities is hard enough. The dilemma becomes even more complicated for medical students trying to decide between two equally appealing fields of medicine. For instance, many doctors-in-training love taking care of the medical problems of both children and adults. After months of soul searching, they still cannot decide between a career in pediatrics or internal medicine. Both highly intellectual disciplines draw upon the same fundamental clinical skills, such as performing physical examinations and interpreting laboratory tests. So, why not do both?

TWO SPECIALTIES FOR THE PRICE OF ONE

The average medical student does not know that a unique integrative career option exists: becoming a physician trained in two specialties (Table 7–1). Any doctor can complete two separate residency programs and earn board certification in both disciplines. For example, a small subset of anesthesiologists, who have already completed 1 internship year of general medicine, also finish the two final years of internal medicine residency and become board certified in anesthesiology and internal medicine. Likewise, in other areas of medicine, different specialists take their own approaches to treating the same disease, such as the management of dementia by psychiatrists versus neurologists.

To train physicians in overlapping skills and knowledge, selected hospitals offer combined residency programs. Currently, there are 15 accredited types of these distinctive pathways. Upon completion of the accelerated training, a physician becomes board certified in both specialties and practices as a dual-trained

TABLE 7–1

COMBINED RESIDENCY PROGRAMS

	Length (Years)	Number of Accredited Programs
Emergency medicine–family medicine	5	2
Internal medicine–dermatology	5	9
Internal medicine–emergency medicine	5	12
Internal medicine–emergency medicine–critical care	6	3
Internal medicine–family medicine	4	2
Internal medicine–neurology	5	4
Internal medicine–pediatrics	4	77
Internal medicine–physical medicine and rehabilitation	5	2
Internal medicine–preventive medicine	4	6
Internal medicine–psychiatry	5	14
Neurology–diagnostic radiology–neuroradiology	7	2
Pediatrics–anesthesiology	5	4
Pediatrics–emergency medicine	5	3
Pediatrics–medical genetics	5	16
Pediatrics–physical medicine and rehabilitation	5	4
Pediatrics–psychiatry–child and adolescent psychiatry	5	10
Psychiatry–family medicine	5	7
Psychiatry–neurology	5	7

Data from Accreditation Council on Graduate Medical Education.

specialist. These programs have transformed the physician workforce. Now, medical centers are producing internist–psychiatrists, pediatrician–emergency medicine doctors, and psychiatrist–neurologists, among others.

In the past, combined residency programs were few in number, so many medical students failed to consider them in their career planning; however, more and more hospitals are now offering these double residencies. Despite the rigor and length of training, their popularity among medical students has started to pick up remarkably. Because many students cannot make up their minds on a particular specialty, one program director recommends combined programs as "ideal for the chronically undecided."[1]

There is one caveat, however. While in training, attrition rates are generally the highest during the transitional period between departments. Rather than choosing this route out of sheer indecision, medical students should be equally committed to both specialties from the very beginning. Otherwise, the odds of dropping out to a single specialty become much higher.

With a rigorous compressed structure, combined residency programs shave a year or two off the time it would take to complete two separate residencies. Despite the shortened training time, all combined residency programs adequately train residents to be competent in both specialties. In the end, their skills are equivalent to those of their counterparts in categorical programs. Board passage rates provide the best evidence for clinical competence following residency. For example, graduates of combined internal medicine–pediatrics (IMP) programs achieved a slightly higher pass rate on the pediatric specialty boards (81.8%) compared with the scores of their colleagues who trained only in pediatrics (75.9%).[2] With this excellent dual training behind them, young physicians can now meet the challenge of being innovative, collaborative practitioners.

WHY TRAIN IN TWO SPECIALTIES?

You Will Become a Better Physician

The exponential growth of clinical information within medicine requires life-long learning. Doctors with training in two specialties can better meet this challenge. In every patient interaction, dual-trained physicians integrate their knowledge base from two different fields, leading to better patient care. For example, a physician certified in both neurology and psychiatry commented, "I can think 'neurologically' and 'psychiatrically' about each patient."[3] Most important, learning one discipline well enhances one's mastery of advanced knowledge in another area. Internist–pediatricians, for instance, can easily manage difficult fluid and electrolyte problems in adults because of their understanding of weight-based pharmacologic and nutritional issues in children. Thus, combined training leads to the natural development of synergistic skills.

You Will Have Greater Career Flexibility

After completing a combined residency program, graduates may further diversify their experiences through fellowship training. Double-boarded doctors can subspecialize in one (or both!) of their primary fields. For instance, a graduate of a combined IMP program could elect to subspecialize in adult nephrology or pediatric endocrinology while also practicing general medicine and pediatrics. Some physicians add even more variety to their careers by pursuing accelerated dual fellowship training, such as adult and pediatric cardiology, after completing a combined residency. As long as a program supports the idea of fellowship training in both disciplines, the possibilities are limitless.

Your Marketability Will Increase Job Opportunities

The comprehensive training of combined programs quickly propels new physicians' careers. Having two board certificates under your belt opens many more doors for young doctors than training in only one specialty. It is, after all, a good investment for employers to have doctors with so many great skills. For instance, graduates of internal medicine–psychiatry programs can choose from many options—general medicine–mental health clinics, academics, primary care medicine, or psychiatric consultations for private medical groups.

You Will Save Valuable Training Time

All combined programs eliminate 1 to 2 years of training compared with completing two separate residencies. You can use the additional time saved to enter practice right away, pursue fellowship or other advanced subspecialty training, or engage in research.

DISADVANTAGES OF A DUAL-SPECIALTY RESIDENCY

Physicians who have completed a combined residency program believe that there is little difficulty in integrating both specialties into a rewarding career. They insist that the only negative aspects of double-specialty training are found during the actual years spent in residency. After all, getting two independent academic departments to work together toward a common goal can be a challenge.

A combined residency has the following drawbacks:

- Because of the limited number of double-boarded doctors, there are few role models and mentors in combined residency programs.
- One department may be much stronger both clinically and academically than the other one.
- Residents have less flexible elective time to complete subspecialty rotations due to the shortened training.
- By belonging to two departments instead of one, residents often feel like they have no true home base.

- Being a member of two departments often leads to scheduling conflicts, particularly those unrelated to direct clinical work, such as journal clubs, informal gatherings, parties, and so on. Your faculty members could perceive absence at these events as a way of showing a lack of commitment.

THE BIG THREE: A CLOSER LOOK AT SELECTED COMBINED RESIDENCY PROGRAMS

Internal Medicine–Pediatrics

Blending together the principles of internal medicine and pediatrics, med–peds (or IMP) is the largest and most popular combined program. Since its creation in 1967, an estimated 1800 physicians now practice both internal medicine and pediatrics.[4] In response to the generalist health care initiative of the last decade, the number of IMP programs increased dramatically. IMP offers an alternative choice for physicians-in-training who wish to treat patients of all ages but do not want to become family practitioners. Recent data attest to the popularity of IMP among today's medical students. Between 1990 and 1997, the number of US seniors choosing IMP increased by 165% (as compared with 65% for family practice).[5] In fact, among the primary care specialties, IMP currently ties with general pediatrics for the highest percentage of US graduates.[6]

IMPs provide intellectual stimulation, rewarding patient relationships, and a broad range of career possibilities. Across the entire spectrum of age and development, these doctors are superb diagnosticians and patient advocates. Becoming an internist–pediatrician makes you just like an old-fashioned general practitioner who takes care of everyone. IMP physicians fit in well with today's changing managed care system, in which there is a perceived need for well-trained primary care doctors. After completing the 4-year program, they are eligible to sit for board certification examinations in both internal medicine and pediatrics. Even better, they can further subspecialize if desired. Across both specialties, there are more than 20 possible fellowship options, from infectious disease to rheumatology. IMP not only provides exceptional primary care training, but it also leaves open the option of completing a fellowship in pediatrics, internal medicine, or both.

So what are the differences between IMP and family practice? Family practice has a wider scope, while IMP has greater depth. Through comprehensive primary care, an internist or pediatrician cares for the entire person. A family doctor, in addition, must also be competent in obstetrics, gynecology, and minor office-based surgery. However, according to the American Association of Family Practice, only 24% of family practitioners still offer obstetric or surgical services. Discouraged by high malpractice liability and rising insurance premiums, disenchanted medical students can now turn toward IMP programs. Here, they believe that they will obtain more practical and rigorous education in medicine and pediatrics. Instead of rotations in obstetrics, gynecology, and surgical subspecialties, IMP residency provides additional training in inpatient and critical care experiences involving both adults and children. Today, the majority of US seniors desiring a career in primary care for all age groups still choose family practice. However, IMP remains an increasingly popular option.

Internist–pediatricians provide the highest quality primary care to patients of all ages. It is possible for patients and families to meet all their health care needs in the same setting with the same doctor. You could potentially take care of the same patient from birth to middle age! Adolescent medicine illustrates this strength of specializing in both medicine and pediatrics. Normally, patients switch from a pediatrician to an internist around the age of 18. Knowledgeable in development concerns and health issues of young adults, the familiar IMP is rather inviting to a teenager as their adult physician. This continuity of care is particularly beneficial for children with chronic illnesses, such as cystic fibrosis, Down syndrome, or congenital heart defects, as they transit into adulthood.

With a broad understanding of medical issues in many age groups, internist–pediatricians can adapt well to the needs of their community, whether there is more of a need for a pediatrician, or patients require the skills of a good internist. This adaptability makes IMP physicians very appealing in a lot of primary care settings for many communities.

Many career opportunities exist for graduates of combined IMP programs. They can become urban or rural primary care doctors, hospitalists for adults and children, academic physicians, or subspecialists bridging both fields. In the largest survey of IMP graduates to date, nearly all practice both specialties and care for patients of all ages, from infants to the elderly.[7] Most were involved in direct patient care in small community practices, devoting only a small amount of time to research, teaching, or administration. A large majority (81.6%) are board certified in both internal medicine and pediatrics. Of the few dual-trained doctors who pursue fellowship, only about one-third spend more than 20% of their practice on subspecialty care. In fact, a higher percentage of IMP residents go on to practice primary care than internal medicine or pediatrics residents. They truly live up to the generalist ideal of this combined residency program.

In the 2011 National Resident Matching Program, 99.2% of the 365 IMP positions were filled.

Internal Medicine–Psychiatry

In every primary care clinic in the country, a large number of patients seeking medical care also walk around with a significant amount of undiagnosed psychopathology. Many conditions, such as chronic fatigue syndrome and fibromyalgia, require treatment based on an understanding of psychology, social issues, and general medicine. There is a great need, therefore, for physicians who can manage people with both psychiatric illnesses and coexisting medical conditions. To meet this challenge, medical students can pursue a combined program in both internal medicine and psychiatry. Many of these doctors wanted to specialize in psychiatry but were reluctant to give up the opportunity to practice clinical medicine. It is a career path growing in both popularity and professional recognition.

A rather academic field, internal medicine–psychiatry focuses on the mind–body interface. In the last decade, psychiatry has shifted to a more biological focus, with pharmacologic therapy as effective as traditional medical treatment for organic diseases. Moreover, underlying medical illness can precipitate or worsen psychiatric disorders. At some point, the two forms of disease become inseparable. There is no one better to understand and sort out these diagnoses than a double-boarded internist–psychiatrist. In theory, each discipline complements the other. These doctors manage both primary medical conditions and psychiatric problems all in one setting. They even help teach nonpsychiatrist colleagues about the management of mental illness without having to refer their patients to a psychiatrist. Whether the problem involves an understanding of internal medicine or psychiatry, doctors double boarded in these specialties provide superior consultative services. They understand and articulate well the interaction between psychiatric and medical complaints.

The internal medicine–psychiatry combined program is rigorous, fun, and challenging. After training, graduates earn full board certification requirements in both disciplines. Because this residency is relatively new, little is currently known about the practice patterns of the graduates. Do they practice both internal medicine and psychiatry, only general psychiatry, or serve as consultants? Most patients with psychiatric illnesses present to their primary care physician rather than directly to a psychiatrist. Providing specialized care of psychiatric disorders in this primary care setting reduces health care costs by removing the need for outside consultation. As a result, job opportunities abound. Many rural areas of the country have a great need for both primary care doctors and mental health professionals.

Based on a recent survey of program directors, most internist–psychiatrists practice both specialties in an academic setting.[8] A smaller group works in the private sector, particularly outpatient clinics and integrated treatment programs. Those who work in state psychiatric facilities focus heavily on psychiatric diagnosis while also managing chronic medical diseases such as diabetes and hypertension. Regardless of practice setting, combined training in internal medicine and psychiatry provides focused, in-depth, biopsychosocial training while expanding and sharpening primary care skills.

In the 2011 National Resident Matching Program, 89.5% of the 19 internal medicine–psychiatry positions were filled.

Internal Medicine–Emergency Medicine

Since 1991, these 5-year combined programs have prepared medical students for a career in both acute and chronic medicine. Training lasts for 30 months in each area and includes the minimum requirements for that specialty. Internal medicine–emergency medicine (IM–EM) specialists can treat a broad spectrum of disease and injury that range widely in presentation — acute, nonurgent, emergent, and chronic. They are experts in the diagnosis, treatment, and rehabilitation of all kinds of patients.

Is it possible for internist–emergency medicine physicians to practice both fields? After all, their work schedules are rather different. Internists typically spend their days in a clinic and on-call overnight, whereas emergency doctors work varying shifts — whether days, afternoons, or nights. A recent survey of graduates found that most (65%) are active in emergency medicine only, and 30% still practice both fields.[9] Those who do integrate both specialties well often balance a part-time emergency department schedule with shifts on the wards as hospitalists. Instead of spending time in clinic, hospitalists are internists who work 12- to 24-hour shifts as inpatient physicians. Ten years later, a follow-up survey of another graduate cohort also confirmed these results.[10] Roughly 55% of the respondents practiced emergency medicine only, 7% internal medicine only, and 37% both emergency medicine and internal medicine. The majority (88%) was highly satisfied with their careers and would complete the 5-year residency program again. In the same survey, most IM–EM specialists identified the academic teaching hospital as their primary clinical setting. Here, several could be directors of observation units for patients under consideration for admission to the wards from the emergency room.

Although most graduates believe that their combined training provided excellent preparation for the clinical practice of emergency medicine, most (93%) felt it was only marginal training for the practice of internal medicine.[11] These results perhaps indicate that most students entering this combined program are more motivated to become emergency medicine physicians than internists.

In the 2011 National Resident Matching Program, 100% of the 26 IM–EM positions were filled.

THE TRIPLE BOARD PROGRAMS: MASTERING THREE SPECIALTIES

Pediatrics–Psychiatry–Child and Adolescent Psychiatry

Would you like to devote your medical career to the physical and mental health of children and adolescents? This combined residency program may be for you! The goal of this pathway is not necessarily to train someone to become all three types of doctors. Instead, the program strives to create a unique type of child and adolescent psychiatrist. Many pediatricians and psychiatrists have difficulty collaborating when it comes to certain patients with multiple medical and mental problems. Since 1986, the triple specialty residency has helped to bridge the gap between two worlds by creating a group of child psychiatrists with solid medical training in clinical pediatrics.

Currently, there is a national shortage of physicians with specialized training in child and adolescent psychiatry. The curriculum of this program consists of 2 years of pediatrics, 18 months of general psychiatry, and 18 months of child and adolescent psychiatry fellowship. Upon completion, physicians are eligible to take board certification examinations in pediatrics, general psychiatry, and child and adolescent psychiatry. Graduates of this program tend to remain in academics and practice all three specialties. As pediatric psychiatrists, they believe that it is impossible to separate the medical and biological aspects of children from their behavioral and developmental issues. Triple-boarded pediatricians provide this needed, well-balanced medical and mental care.

Neurology–Diagnostic Radiology–Neuroradiology

Interested in diagnosing and treating diseases of the brain and nervous system? This new combined residency program leads to triple board certification in neurology, radiology, and the subspecialty of neuroradiology. Graduates of these programs have the clinical and therapeutic skills of a neurologist, the diagnostic abilities of a general radiologist, and the specialized interventional techniques of a neuroradiologist. They are experts in cerebral angiography, myelography, positron emission tomography (PET) scans, head computed tomography (CT), and brain magnetic resonance imaging (MRI). Unlike other radiologists, these physicians maintain a high level of patient contact through their neurology practice. The residency program consists of 6 months of general medicine, 2 years of neurology, 2½ years of radiology, and 2 years of neuroradiology (typically a fellowship). These triple-boarded specialists are academic leaders in treating diseases of the nervous system.

REFERENCES

1. Lee, M.C. Weighing the benefits of combined residency programs. *JAMA*. 1991; 266(13):1867.

2. Onady, G.M. Med-peds—Three decades of the generic primary care physician. *Acad Med*. 1996;71(11):1144–1145.

3. George, M.S. Doing a combined residency. *JAMA*. 1990;263(12):1628.

4. Ciccarelli, M. The clinical philosophy of medicine-pediatrics. *Am J Med*. 1998; 104(4):330–331.

5. Campos-Outcalt, D., Lundy, M., et al. Outcomes of combined internal medicine-pediatrics residency programs: A review of the literature. *Acad Med*. 2002;77(3): 247–256.

6. Data and Results—2011 Match, National Resident Matching Program, Washington, DC.

7. Lannon, C.M., Oliver, T.K., et al. Internal medicine-pediatrics combined residency graduates: What are they doing now? Results of a survey. *Arch Pediatr Adolesc Med*. 1999;153:823–828.

8. Doebbeling, C.C., Pitkin, A.K., et al. Combined internal medicine-psychiatry and family medicine-psychiatry training programs, 1999–2000: Program directors' perspectives. *Acad Med*. 2006;76(12):1247–1252.

9. Munger, B.S., Ham, H., et al. Careers of graduates of combined emergency medicine/internal medicine programs. *Acad Emerg Med*. 2000;7(5):450.

10. Kessler, C.S., Stallings, L.A., et al. Combined residency training in emergency medicine and internal medicine: An update on career outcomes and job satisfaction. *Acad Emerg Med*. 2009;16(9):894–899.

11. Flaherty, J.J., Kharasch, M.S., et al. Evaluation of dual residency training in internal medicine/emergency medicine. *Acad Emerg Med*. 2001;8(5):472–473.

8
OPTIONS FOR THE UNDECIDED MEDICAL STUDENT

Within the first few months of your senior year, a final decision about specialty selection must be made. What happens if an overwhelmed medical student simply cannot decide? Because of the myriad of options, the pressure can lead to hasty and uncertain decisions. And residents unhappy in their chosen specialty may have to switch fields, hunt for a new residency, or even repeat years of grueling postgraduate training!

Choosing a specialty is tougher than ever. Although most make the big decision near the end of the third year of medical school, in recent years more and more students are finding themselves undecided at residency application time. After 4 rigorous years and a formidable financial investment, these students generally refuse to commit to a particular specialty unless they are absolutely 100% certain. Compromise is certainly not part of their lexicon.

The undecided student believes that it is better to hold off on making a final decision than to select the wrong one and become an unhappy, dissatisfied doctor. They would rather do it right the first time or not do it at all (by delaying the decision). Putting off a final commitment is one of several options for an undecided medical student. You should keep in mind, however, that simple procrastination is not necessarily going to make the big decision any easier when the time comes around again to make a commitment.

If you are a fourth-year medical student and still undecided about what specialty to choose, you have several options. You can delay making your choice and seek refuge in a year of research or internship only. Or, you can tackle your indecision head on and apply to more than one specialty or apply to a combined residency program. Either way, the undecided student should not be overwhelmed by the idea that choosing the wrong specialty is the end of the world. Most students would be happily satisfied in more than one specialty. And after all, no matter what field of medicine you end up in, you will still be a practicing physician.

This chapter addresses the needs of undecided students who, because of these fears, want additional time to reflect on the specialties before making the important choice. By pursuing these options, newly minted MDs will feel much more confident about their specialty decision.

ENTER A 1-YEAR INTERNSHIP PROGRAM ONLY

Let us say you are torn between several specialties that are quite distinct from each other, such as radiology, pediatrics, and surgery. If you find it impossible to make up your mind, then consider only applying for general internship positions (with no further postgraduate commitment), rather than a complete residency. After all, this is what nearly every physicians did back in the old days (before 1972) to decide upon their eventual specialty. By entering a 1-year internship, the undecided graduating medical student still earns credit for postgraduate training while at the same time continuing to explore other specialties. The intention, of course, is to reapply to residency programs to start hopefully as a postgraduate year 2 (PGY-2) resident in that specialty. Sounds like a perfect idea, right? Well, read on.

There are three types of internships, all of which are described in further detail in Chapter 9. In a transitional year internship, you receive broad exposure to many fields of medicine, such as internal medicine, surgery, pediatrics, and obstetrics–gynecology, plus electives. It is similar to the third year of medical school, but you are now a full-fledged first-year resident, with all the responsibilities that go along with that status. If undecided students can at least make up their minds about where they stand on the medicine–surgery dichotomy, then the other internships will suit them well. A preliminary medicine internship is equivalent to the first year of a complete internal medicine residency, whereas a preliminary surgery internship is identical to the first year of a categorical general surgery residency.

There are many advantages to this option for the undecided student. During the internship year, you will have many new clinical experiences and the right specialty may present itself. At the same time, while earning PGY-1 credit, you stay immersed in clinical medicine, keep your knowledge and decision-making skills up to date, and gain more patient care responsibility.

Undecided students should be forewarned that seeking refuge from the big decision through a 1-year internship position has its many drawbacks as well. In reality, you are really only delaying your decision for 1 more year (from the beginning of senior year to the early months of internship) compared with the rest of your classmates. Remember, in early fall, the residency application process starts up again. In the end, you will have only about 3 months of internship experiences on which to make that important career decision (this excludes, of course, any clinical rotations from the fourth year of medical school). Not to mention the fact that internship is much more difficult and time-consuming than the senior year of medical school. How will you have the time and energy to spend on making the decision and the application process? Will a program director really give you time off from internship to fly around the country for interviews?

One of the main caveats about applying only for internship positions is the possibility of having to repeat this first postgraduate year. This really depends on the type of internship taken and the specific field of medicine sought. For instance, internal medicine, pediatrics, and surgery programs will not accept transitional year internships for PGY-1 credit. Categorical programs such as psychiatry and obstetrics–gynecology may require you to repeat their own internship years, particularly if they were taken in internal medicine and surgery. Keep this important point in mind if you are considering this alternative path.

PURSUE A COMBINED TRAINING PROGRAM

Many confused and undecided senior medical students often waver between two different specialties, such as internal medicine and pediatrics, or neurology and psychiatry. A good choice for them might be the combined residency programs, in which you receive extended training (leading to dual board certification) in both specialties. Instead of having to decide on just one area of medicine, an undecided student can end up with the best of both worlds and be able to pursue a medical career in both specialties. Chapter 7 gives a detailed explanation of the advantages and disadvantages of entering a combined training program, as well as a thorough description of the possible choices. Although a combined residency program is an excellent option for an undecided medical student, positions are limited. Moreover, most programs combine similar fields, such as internal medicine and emergency medicine. If you are trying to decide between neurology and orthopedic surgery, no such combined program exists.

APPLY TO MORE THAN ONE SPECIALTY

Medical students who simply cannot decide between two fields (and for whom no combined residency program exists) also have the option of applying to both fields at once. This, in effect, delays the ultimate decision until late winter of senior year, when rank lists are due and the match process actually takes place. Aspiring physicians who are interested in both orthopedic surgery and radiology, for example, or doctors-to-be who could see themselves as either neurologists or neurosurgeons can use this option to delay making the final selection for another 6 months or so.

Be prepared, however, for twice the paperwork and effort (and financial expense!) in the application process. Both specialties will require their own set of recommendation letters, personal statements, and interviews. At rank list time, you will have to decide on the specific order of the programs. Thus, whatever specialty program is placed in the number 1 position, in a way, clearly indicates the undecided student's final preference. Why take your chances with the match computer to make your final choice? Many undecided students apply and rank multiple specialties every year and let the computer break the tie for them. If you simply cannot decide on a specialty, and do not mind surprises on Match Day, then consider this alternative.

ENTER A SPECIALTY TRAINING PROGRAM WITH THE INTENTION OF SWITCHING FIELDS LATER

Some undecided medical students end up applying to a desired (although not perfect) specialty, with the intention of switching fields later. Although these students may not feel committed to that specialty, they are willing to give it a try while at the same time keeping open the option of changing.

Several studies have found that specialty switching is not such an uncommon phenomenon. In fact, 20% of medical school graduates switch fields before completing their first residency, 15% change after completing residency, and nearly 20% of practicing physicians report a high level of unhappiness and career dissatisfaction with their chosen specialty. Every day, month, and year of clinical experiences can bring about a whole new phase of self-discovery (and its accompanying self-doubt)—a period of contemplation that may even lead to the conclusion that your chosen specialty just is not the right one or the best fit. To change fields of medicine, the simpler application process occurs out of the match. After deciding on a new specialty, physicians have to pick up the phone and start calling around to find out which residency programs have vacant positions.

Every physician should practice in a specialty for which they have passion and enthusiasm. However, there are several disadvantages to starting a residency program in one specialty with the intention of soon changing to another. Besides the recurring feelings of having wasted time, you (and possibly your family) will have to adjust again to a new hospital and a new life. The faculty at the first program may not appreciate your anticipated departure and may make the remainder of the year much more difficult. On a more practical note, you may also have difficulty securing funding for the entire length of the new residency. The federal government only reimburses teaching hospitals enough money for each resident to cover the number of years necessary to meet initial specialty board requirements (eg, 3 years for internal medicine) plus 1 year. If the total training time is beyond these limits, funding may not be available and you will have to petition the hospital of your second residency to provide the money for your paycheck. In these tough financial times, this is not always that easy to accomplish.

TAKE TIME OFF TO ENGAGE IN RESEARCH OR GAIN EXPERIENCE

If you are struggling to figure out your true direction within the medical profession, then taking time off is certainly a helpful option. Junior medical students can postpone graduation for 1 year and spend that time conducting clinical research, doing hospital rotations, and continuing personal self-assessment before applying to residency next year. This kind of decision needs to be made late in the third year of medical school.

Because any nonmedical time off from education on a resume can be a warning sign to selection committees, most students choose to do a year of clinical research before applying to residency. Many apply for special 1-year medical student research grants to work at the prestigious National Institutes of Health. Other worthy options include experiences in public health, such as a fellowship with the US Department of Health and Human Services. You could also potentially use this time to pursue another degree, such as a Masters in Public Health. Any of these types of experiences can provide time to help the undecided medical student figure out the perfect specialty and how to best plan a strategy for senior year electives and the residency application process.

AIMING FOR CONFIDENCE AND COMMITMENT

It should be obvious that these five options for an undecided student are all far from ideal. None of them allows for sufficient time to explore specialties further before having to make a final decision. This all stems from the compressed nature of American medical education and the very early start to the residency application process in the senior year.

Pursuing one of these options only defers the same crucial choice—commitment to a single specialty—which will still be there, no matter how hard you try to put it off. For this reason, all medical students should work hard during their 4 years to overcome any feelings of indecision or indifference. The best way to do so is by gathering as much information and experience as possible to make a definitive, informed, and confident decision. This commitment is an essential part of being a happy, satisfied physician for many long years to come.

9

APPLYING FOR RESIDENCY: AN OVERVIEW OF THE MATCH PROCESS

O nce you have reached this point in the long journey through medical school, the deliberation is over. You have confidently chosen the field of medicine that will become the focus of each waking day for the next 10, 20, or 30 years. Now it is time to enjoy the learning opportunities of senior year, fulfill graduation requirements, and continue exploring other disciplines of medicine before dedicating yourself to the specialty you have chosen.

INTRODUCTION TO THE MATCH

But the rite of passage is far from over. Every fourth-year medical student must enter the dreaded *Match* to be paired with a residency program. The United States is fortunate to have many excellent hospitals and academic medical centers. Yet, the quality, desirability, and reputation of training programs vary greatly. Every year, competition for the top programs—those with greater resources and a higher emphasis on teaching—is quite keen. As a result, the fourth year of medical school has evolved into a long year of playing the high-stakes residency-matching game.

Even for medical students, who are seasoned applicants, the residency application process seems unnecessarily complicated. There are lots of confusing acronyms to remember—National Resident Matching Program (NRMP), Electronic Residency Application Service (ERAS), letters of recommendation (LORs), and rank-order lists (ROLs). There are many detailed tasks to accomplish— collecting recommendations, writing personal statements, preparing applications, and scheduling interviews. Most medical students agree that the entire time-consuming process interferes with the remaining education of senior year.

Four years of hard work pay off in a single defining moment: Match Day. Ever since choosing medicine as a career, medical students eagerly await that emotion-filled third Thursday in March. With friends, family, and the local news teams watching, 17,000 medical students rip open the envelopes at exactly 12:00 PM EST to find out where they will complete their residency. The excitement and anticipation from waiting an entire year is intense. This is a moment of high drama—people cheering, laughing, and crying. Whether a student receives his first choice or last choice, Match Day is a singular milestone in the professional education of a new physician.

TYPES OF RESIDENCY PROGRAMS

The National Resident Matching Program (NRMP) offers three types of postgraduate training positions in the Main Match. Medical students should become familiar with the proper terminology. Every residency program has an assigned Accreditation Council for Graduate Medical Education (ACGME) identification number containing a single letter—C, P, or A.

1. *Categorical (C)*: These programs begin training at the first postgraduate year (PGY-1), which starts in July immediately following medical school graduation. Depending on specialty, they consist of 3 or more years of graduate medical education. Residents are expected to complete the entire length of training required for board certification. Specialties such as internal medicine, pediatrics, obstetrics–gynecology, and general surgery are primarily categorical tracks.

2. *Preliminary (P)*: These programs last 1 year, count for PGY-1 credit only, and are formally available through internal medicine, surgery, or transitional year. These positions exist to satisfy the 1-year prerequisite clinical training required by advanced specialty programs (see below).

3. *Advanced (A)*: These positions begin only at the level of PGY-2, after a year spent in a preliminary program. Specialized fields such as dermatology, ophthalmology, anesthesiology, and radiology are typically advanced tracks. Students apply to both advanced and preliminary programs at the same time, even though the advanced position does not commence for an entire year after the actual Match. (Your spot will be reserved.)

Match Day, and the application process that precedes it, is a relatively recent phenomenon in American medical education. After World War II, when the rapid pace of scientific advances in medicine influenced many students to specialize, competition for internships and residency programs became intense. To secure the best medical students, less-competitive programs offered binding contracts earlier and earlier in the application season—sometimes even in the second or third year of medical school—which soon resulted in a cutthroat free-for-all of offers and counteroffers. Some students felt pressured to commit to less-favored programs before they could consider more preferred options. Others reneged on their appointments once they received better offers from a more desirable choice. Students had to respond quickly to offers. In 1945, the typical offer expired within 10 days. Just 4 years later, students received a telegram and follow-up telephone call; a reply was then expected immediately.[1] Clearly, the system needed to reform.

THE NRMP: LET THE COMPUTER DECIDE YOUR FATE

To bring an end to the chaotic "free-for-all," a group of five organizations (including the American Medical Association and the Association of American Medical Colleges) joined forces in 1952 to cosponsor the formation of a centralized clearinghouse system known as the NRMP. It is a private, nonprofit corporation. Through the shared use of an ROL, medical students and residency programs submit a list of preferences from among those interviewed. A master computer in Washington, DC, running a 6-minute algorithm, generates a single Match between applicants and hospitals. Both parties learn of a mutually acceptable appointment on a common date and time. The match algorithm underwent a design change in 1997 to favor applicant ROLs over those of the residency programs. In the past 60 years, the Match has grown more complex. It now handles the joint ROLs of couples as well as supplemental ROLs for PGY-1 internships. Based on its success, many subspecialty fellowships have also started their own matches as well. The Medical Specialties Matching Program (MSMP) includes areas such as cardiology, colorectal surgery, hematology/oncology, thoracic surgery, and pulmonary medicine/critical care.

With this new system, the NRMP seemed to have achieved its purpose: uniformity and impartiality. For the first time, both applicants and residency programs could explore their options without intense pressure for early decision making. Medical students now were given a great deal of choice in deciding which residency program they would prefer. However, because both parties were still anxious over the relative uncertainty of the final Match outcome, students and program directors began to exploit other avenues that compromised the integrity of the Match, such as outside-the-Match contracts, pre-Match promises, audition electives, and second visits.

Despite these ethical violations, the NRMP does not stringently enforce its own rules. The result is that today the participants in the residency appointment system no longer believe each other. Nearly one-third of students felt that the residency program administrators had lied to them during the process, and 21% believed that program directors encouraged their unethical behavior in order to match.[2] Even the NRMP states that "the success of the match depends on a high level of trust among all participants." Apparently, a lot of people—medical students and program directors alike—seem to have missed reading the NRMP's Statement on Professionalism.

Take the out-of-Match contract, for example. During the application season, residency programs are not supposed to offer these binding commitments to US seniors. They are intended only for any highly desirable independent applicants, a large group that consists of anyone who is not currently a US senior, such as foreign-trained graduates, US graduates, osteopathic students, and Canadian students. Specialties such as internal medicine, pediatrics, psychiatry, family medicine, and pathology tend to select some residents outside the Match. If a medical student accepts a position outside the Match, the applicant commits himself to that program and is officially required to withdraw from the Match. Yet, some US seniors are even offered these under-the-table contracts. Certain specialties, particularly extremely competitive ones such as radiation oncology and dermatology, are more likely to engage in this behavior. In either case, these agreements have a detrimental effect on the application process for the average medical student. Any residency program that signs applicants outside the Match is supposed to contact the NRMP and reduce the number of positions (its quota) published in its online directory. Most programs, however, do not. For the average candidate, it becomes much more difficult to plan an application strategy for positions that may not even exist!

Pre-Match promises and informal commitments, which will be discussed again later in this chapter, also add to the unethical gamesmanship of the residency appointment process. Program directors and applicants frequently send letters that imply, but do not guarantee, a commitment to each other. In addition, many institutions promise scarce residency spots to their own medical students, who then rank the program no. 1 and receive that desired Match. As positions become more competitive, this type of behavior undermines the integrity of the whole system. The two dermatology positions at a particular hospital, for example, may have already been promised to its own medical students and therefore be unavailable for the common applicant. The misleading numbers create uncertainty and insecurity and make it very difficult for advisors to counsel their students on how to obtain positions.

With this greater emphasis on networking and contacts, the residency Match game has become more and more unfair. Some students end up left on the sidelines. The NRMP has finally responded to the rampant unprofessional behavior and widespread policy violations with new stricter rules. Pre-Matches with independent applicants will soon become a remnant of the past. Starting in 2013, all programs participating in the Main Residency Match will have to register and attempt to fill *all* of their positions in the Match. They cannot have some positions in the NRMP and at the same time fill other slots with independent applicants (outside the Match). Programs will have to update their advertised quota of available positions. While there may be some possible exceptions, the NRMP Board "believes this policy will address remnants of the problems that led to creation of the NRMP by eliminating inequalities in how residency programs recruit U.S. allopathic senior students and other applicants while simultaneously reducing the risk of undue persuasion when residency programs offer positions outside the Match."[3]

ERAS: LET THE COMPUTER SIMPLIFY YOUR LIFE

The NRMP is the corporation that supervises the Match process, ensures its integrity, and runs the computer algorithm that pairs applicants with residency programs. To do so, the NRMP receives rank-order preference lists from both parties. However, the NRMP is *not* a centralized application processing service. This is where the *Electronic Residency Application Service* (ERAS) comes in.

Remember how you applied to college? For a long time, the residency application process worked the same way. Medical students had to contact each individual program for a paper application, address envelopes for their letter writers, and drag out the old typewriter from the closet. The process was time consuming and tedious, especially for medical students applying to 20 or more programs in very competitive specialties. In 1995, ERAS changed the way medical students submitted applications. At first, only obstetrics–gynecology participated in the service, using a system based on diskettes sent in the mail. Over the next few years, more specialties caught on, particularly as ERAS became an Internet-based application. Today, nearly all specialties participate in ERAS (exceptions include ophthalmology).

ERAS has streamlined the entire application process. Every year, ERAS electronically transmits tens of thousands of digitized documents: transcripts, recommendation letters, personal statements, application forms, and Dean's Letters. The Web-based format is extremely user friendly, making it very easy to apply to multiple specialties, add or delete programs, or customize which supporting documents to send to each program. By reducing the amount of paperwork for both applicants and hospitals, ERAS has lowered application fees ($85 for the first ten programs). Another feature is that medical students can track the transmission status of every single document online, 24 hours a day, through the Applicant Document Tracking System (ADTS). Most medical students rate the ERAS system very highly.

What about the disadvantages of ERAS? There is a significant one. This service is so easy to use that candidates can easily flood the application pool with far too many unnecessary applications. Students should think carefully about limiting the number of programs to which they eventually apply. With the click of a mouse, you can check a box and, on a whim, add more programs, particularly those you are not seriously considering. The excess applications cause the same students to receive most of the limited interview offers available for a given specialty, leaving others out in the cold. ERAS attempts to prevent this shot-gunning approach by increasing the fees for applying to more than 20 programs ($15 per program for 21 to 30 programs, $25 each for 31 or more programs). Realistically, very competitive specialties such as orthopedic surgery and dermatology encourage students to apply to more than 40 programs.

To set up a personalized MyERAS account, all medical students must obtain their preassigned ERAS token (a string of numbers and letters) from their Dean's Office. Enter this token to begin registration on the ERAS Web site. Although the process is relatively straightforward, always refer to the detailed instruction booklet provided with your token. Apply as early as possible, so you will never have to worry about individual program deadlines (which can vary). A completed ERAS application consists of the following parts:

1. *Profile*: This one-page form contains your name, identification numbers (social security, ERAS, NRMP, and United States Medical Licensing Examination [USMLE]), citizenship, medical school, and contact information. The entries can be changed at any time; an updated version is electronically sent to all programs.

2. *Common Application Form (CAF)*: This 12-page form consists of all the basic background information typically found in a resume—degrees earned,

research and work experience, extracurricular activities, hobbies, and publications. After completing the form and proofreading for typos, click on certify. The electronic certification process officially submits the CAF and locks out any further changes from being made. Until you cough up the money for your programs, ERAS will not allow supporting documents to be scanned and uploaded by your medical school.

3. *Personal Statement*: You should type, edit, and spell check the personal statement on a word processing program and then copy and paste it into ERAS. Simply create a blank new personal statement in the *MyDocuments* section. If you are applying to multiple specialties or preliminary programs, give it an easily recognizable title (eg, *Derm*). Program directors will not see your titles. To create multiple personal statements, just click on the *New Personal Statement* button. Because the formatting of your document in ERAS will not look exactly like your original, print out a copy to view its appearance.

4. *United States Medical Licensing Examination (USMLE) Transcript*: The National Board of Medical Examiners (NBME) will send an unlimited number of USMLE transcripts to residency programs via ERAS (for a flat fee, of course). You must send all current USMLE scores and then choose whether or not to retransmit *automatically* updated transcripts when they become available. However, your decision is irrevocable and binding. If in doubt, do not choose the automatic retransmission option. Most medical students prefer reviewing their USMLE Step II scores prior to submission (in case they are poor). Manual retransmission of these transcripts incurs no additional cost.

5. *Medical School Performance Evaluation (MSPE)*: This document (previously known as the "Dean's Letter") is scanned and uploaded by your medical school. It does not count as one of the four possible letters of recommendation. ERAS transmits the MSPE to all selected programs on October 1.

6. *Medical School Transcript*: The applicant's medical school also uploads this document.

7. *Photograph*: Students must provide their Dean's Office with a wallet-sized photograph for scanning and submission. However, residency programs are prohibited from accessing the photo until an interview has been granted.

8. *Letters of Recommendation (LORs)*: ERAS allows applicants to assign up to four LORs to each individual residency program. However, an unlimited number of LORs can be solicited, scanned, and uploaded into the ERAS system. In the *MyDocuments* section, simply create a new LOR for each

expected writer, clearly indicating the faculty person's name on the file. Print out the LOR cover sheet, check the appropriate box whether or not you waive your right to review the letter, and give the form to the writer. The faculty member returns the recommendation to your Dean's Office for scanning and submission. If you complete a stellar rotation in late summer or early fall, an LOR can easily be submitted after the others have been transmitted.

Selecting residency programs and assigning the appropriate documents is the final step in the application process. Your program selection list remains strictly confidential. For every program on the applicant's list, ERAS will automatically transmit the profile, CAF, medical school transcript, photograph, and Dean's Letter. At this point, some personalization comes into play. For every program, ERAS will prompt the applicant to assign one personal statement and up to four LORs from the total submitted files. This feature allows medical students to customize the supporting documents each program receives.

THE "EARLY" MATCH: NON-NRMP SPECIALTIES

Of the 20 fields of medicine chosen by graduating medical students, all, but two, participate in the NRMP. These two specialties independently coordinate their own match system on an earlier time frame. Applications are due in early August, interviews are conducted in the fall, and ROLs are due in early January. Match results are announced 1 to 2 weeks later. These lucky medical students will know their final destination about 2 months before the rest of their classmates.

Urology

In 1985, the American Urological Association (AUA) established its own matching program for all applicants seeking training for their first year of urology, regardless of their prior graduate medical education. The interview, ranking, and match process for urology applicants is similar to that of the NRMP. For a long time, all aspiring urologists had to contact each individual residency program to acquire an old-fashioned paper application. As of 2003, nearly all urology programs participate in ERAS. However, program directors and applicants still have to submit their rank lists directly to the AUA, instead of the NRMP. After announcing urology appointments in January, some programs require matched students to enter the NRMP. This step is simply a formality for matched students to acquire (via a single entry on the rank list) their guaranteed PGY-1 position in general surgery at the same institution at which they just matched for urology.

Ophthalmology

The specialty of ophthalmology participates in an organization known as the *San Francisco (SF) Match*. Just like the advanced (A) specialties of the NRMP, training in this specialty begins at the PGY-2—following an internship. Back in 1952, when the founders of the NRMP designed the new system for 1-year internships and for specialties that started at the PGY-1 level, budding ophthalmologists still coped with the old system of early, pressured offers. At the time, the NRMP could not process both types of program appointments in its algorithm. In the 1970s, a separate match, supervised in San Francisco, was formed, which later evolved to incorporate four specialties (neurosurgery, ophthalmology, otolaryngology, and neurology), as well as their respective fellowships.

The SF Match is similar to the NRMP except for the time frame. Be prepared for early applications, interviews, and matches. Fortunately, the SF Match has its own easy-to-use Internet application just like ERAS—the Central Application Service (CAS). Interested students have to provide only one standardized application form and one set of supporting documents.

For these two specialties, training begins at PGY-2. What about the PGY-1 position? If you are applying to nonintegrated residency programs (which do not include a guaranteed internship year), you must apply and interview separately for PGY-1 positions through the NRMP. The early timing of the SF Match allows applicants to learn their PGY-2 appointment in January, before the mid-February deadline for submitting NRMP rank lists. This enables better coordination (particularly geographical) between the two matches. If a student matches with an integrated program, the PGY-1 slot is guaranteed. However, some programs still require these students to submit a single PGY-1 rank list to the NRMP as a formality. The majority of ophthalmology programs require an outside search for PGY-1 positions (internal medicine, transitional, or surgery), while most neurosurgery programs have an integrating, or categorical, surgical internship.

INTERNSHIPS FOR SALE: HOW TO SECURE A PGY-1 POSITION

Many of the specialized fields of medicine, such as ophthalmology and anesthesiology, begin residency training at PGY-2. According to NRMP classification, these are the "advanced" specialties. They require entering residents first to complete 1 year of broad clinical training, which is similar in scope to the old freestanding rotating internship required of all fresh graduates before its demise in 1970. Medical students who select a specialty with advanced positions have some extra work on their hands. Fortunately, the same application and matching system can be used to secure an internship position.

To meet PGY-1 requirements, there are three possible types of preliminary programs from which to choose. You have to decide for yourself what you want to get out of your PGY-1 year.

1. *Preliminary Medicine*: This track offers a 1-year rigorous experience in internal medicine. In most hospitals, the differences between preliminary and categorical (3-year track) interns on the medicine wards are minimal. They have similar clinical responsibilities, share the same call schedule, and admit the same number of patients. The only distinction is that preliminary interns sometimes are able to secure a few more elective months. Both community hospitals and academic medical centers offer preliminary medicine positions. You will learn a great deal of general medicine and how to take care of sick patients, both on the floors and in the intensive care unit. Students entering advanced specialties that heavily emphasize internal medicine—such as anesthesiology, dermatology, and neurology—often find it extremely helpful to complete their base year in preliminary medicine.

TEN SURE-FIRE WAYS TO GUARANTEE THAT YOU WOULD NOT MATCH!

- Earn a USMLE Step I score of 180 (barely scoring above the 179 pass level).
- Choose a competitive specialty having earned mediocre grades in the corresponding rotation.
- Avoid doing an audition rotation or away elective because you are scared that they will think less highly of you.
- Apply only to the "top ten" programs in your specialty.
- Do not consult with a faculty member, advisor, or dean to help plan a realistic match between you and your possible list of programs.
- Failing to send a letter of intent to your top program stating that you plan on ranking them as your no. 1 choice.
- Not having an advisor or chairperson make any calls on your behalf because you are afraid of inconveniencing the program director.
- Rank fewer than five programs on your ROL.
- Shorten your rank list because you received a flattering recruitment letter making you believe that the residency program was going to rank you at the top of their list.
- Not selecting a preliminary year or other backup option to place at the bottom of your primary ROL (for very competitive specialties).

2. *Preliminary Surgery*: Similar to its medicine counterpart, a position in preliminary surgery offers the exact same experience as that of an intern in general surgery. You will have the honor of rounding very early in the morning, managing postoperative patients on the surgical floors, taking call every third or fourth night, and occasionally scrubbing in for cases in the operating room. Which new medical school graduate would subject himself or herself to such rigor? The answer is that most preliminary surgery positions are informally assigned outside the Match to applicants who have already matched into an early surgical specialty (urology, neurosurgery, and otolaryngology). This position serves as their general surgery internship. The remaining positions are sometimes chosen by students who believe that a surgical internship would best prepare them for residency, such as those in ophthalmology, emergency medicine, and anesthesiology. Realistically, many preliminary surgery positions are last-minute choices picked by scrambling students who failed to match into preliminary medicine or transitional year internships.

3. *Transitional Year*: Many medical students are confused by the role of transitional year programs. These highly competitive internships provide a diverse clinical experience that is fully accredited by the ACGME. Usually offered by community hospitals, transitional programs are cosponsored by two departments. The curriculum of a typical transitional year requires 4 months (minimum) of internal medicine, 1 month of emergency medicine, and 1 month of ambulatory medicine. Some programs also mandate months of surgery or obstetrics, while others require critical care rotations. Regardless, all transitional year internships allow for 2 to 6 flexible months of electives. Because of these many months of flexibility, competition for transitional year spots is quite intense. In the 2011 Match, only 3.5% of the 952 available positions were unfilled. One word of caution: Unlike preliminary medicine or surgery, transitional years only count for PGY-1 credit in advanced specialties. If you switch later to a categorical specialty (such as internal medicine or pediatrics) during the transitional internship, you will have to repeat another PGY-1 year.

After deciding on one (or more) of the PGY-1 alternatives, it is time to apply. There is one more important item to clarify. Many specialty programs also offer, in addition to their advanced PGY-2 track, several categorical positions that *include* the PGY-1 internship year, typically at the same institution or affiliated hospital. For example, in 2011, the anesthesiology residency at the University of

Chicago Hospitals, where I trained, offered nine advanced positions and eight categorical positions. All 17 residents started anesthesiology training as PGY-2s, but the advanced residents had to secure their own internships independently, whereas the categorical residents completed their PGY-1 year at the University of Chicago Hospitals. The bottom line: When making your final list of residency programs in these specialties, make sure to check carefully which ones offer both advanced and categorical slots.

The ERAS system makes applying for a PGY-1 internship quite simple. You simply transmit your application file to selected programs as if applying to multiple specialties (eg, dermatology and internal medicine; ophthalmology and transitional). Here are some final tips for this important part of the application process:

1. When applying to preliminary medicine or surgery positions, look up the program under the categorical listings, but make sure to check the box labeled preliminary track.

2. Most medical students apply for PGY-1 positions either in the location of their medical school or in the anticipated city of their desired PGY-2 residency. Do you really want to move twice? This approach also keeps the interview process simple, sane, and easier on the checkbook.

3. You do not have to write a new personal statement for these positions. Most students either submit the same statement written for their primary specialty or they modify it slightly to tailor it to preliminary programs.

4. The same LORs can also be assigned to PGY-1 programs. The directors all know that their interns will be leaving after 1 year. The more competitive preliminary medicine programs, especially those at academic medical centers, often prefer a Chairman's Letter from the Department of Medicine. Consult your advisor on how to obtain one.

5. Apply to a sufficient number of programs to ensure that you will match! Every year, qualified students who do not take this part of their application seriously find themselves unmatched for a PGY-1 position. If you do not want to scramble for a surgery spot, never gloss over the preliminary year as an afterthought. Hospitals are cutting back on the number of preliminary positions. The high numbers of competitive applicants in radiology, dermatology, and other highly desirable departments are all vying for the same cushy transitional internships. Do not find yourself left out. If you put an equal

amount of effort into both the primary specialty and the PGY-1 programs, there should be no surprises on Match Day.

APPLYING TO MORE THAN ONE SPECIALTY

Most advisors tell medical students who are interested in a very competitive specialty (such as orthopedic surgery or dermatology) to apply to a backup specialty as a safeguard. The following advice also applies to medical students who remain undecided between two specialties and want to postpone the decision until they create the final rank list.

Thanks to ERAS, applying to more than one specialty is actually quite simple. You simply have twice the amount of work to accomplish: two personal statements, additional subinternships and audition rotations, more LORs, and more interviews. Once these are completed, the electronic paperwork is easy. ERAS sends the same CAF to both specialties and allows the applicant to customize personal statements and recommendation letters for each specialty program. The NRMP is equally flexible. The computer ranking system is designed to accept multiple specialties, program types, and locations—all on a single primary ROL. For instance, an applicant applying to both dermatology and internal medicine could rank dermatology programs in the first five spots of the rank list and place the internal medicine programs in the next three positions.

AFTER THE INTERVIEW: COMMUNICATING WITH RESIDENCY PROGRAMS

The gamesmanship of the residency application process rears its ugly head particularly once the interview season ends. Just like for any job interview, most candidates send an appropriate thank you note to each of their interviewers. However, the NRMP explicitly prohibits applicants and program directors from asking the other party about their ranking commitment or implying that the final ranking depends on it. Instead, they can only voluntarily reveal their ranking interest. Both parties then start flooding each other with letters, e-mails, and phone calls in an attempt to convey interest and obtain assurance. They often push the boundaries of persuasion as stated within the "Match Participation Agreement" through improper interview questions ("How serious are you about our program?") or post-interview communications ("I intend to rank you at the top of my list"). With the pressure to play up their enthusiasm through second visits and written expressions of commitment, medical students often finish the application process with a great deal of bitterness.[4]

Opinions on whether these attempts actually influence final ranking decisions in their favor vary greatly within the academic medical community. The NRMP stipulates that both parties "can express a high degree of interest in each other but must not make statements implying a commitment." Unfortunately, nonbinding statements such as "We intend to rank you highly" or "We hope to work with you next year" are frequently misinterpreted as false promises. Both students and programs have experienced their share of disappointment. Now, neither group trusts the other.

After deciding on the dream program, many medical students send an official letter to that program informing the director of their intention to rank it as their first choice. They also compose letters to their next ranked programs to let them know they are "among their top choices." Do these letters actually make a difference when program directors sit down and rank students? Based on surveys evaluating the ethical behavior of both parties in this process, a recent study found surprising results.[5] Nearly 84% of program directors were skeptical of these informal commitments, because the majority had previously failed to match a top choice who sent in such a statement. In addition, most (91%) believed that applicants in some instances lied to them outright about their supposed interest.

A different study found, however, that residency programs are equally culpable. Nearly all (94%) program directors felt that the Match process encouraged dishonesty with applicants in order to match their preferred choices.[6] Because directors like to brag about filling their program without going far down the list of their top choices, many coerce students into revealing where they intend to rank that program. Even though programs have the right to convey that they are strongly interested in a particular student's candidacy, many send letters implying a high or guaranteed match. In spite of these words of encouragement, program directors, like students, often change their minds right before the Match and switch rankings. In the end, the medical students who ranked highly in those programs that assured them of a high ranking (or match) are disappointed. Applicants should never trust statements that they will be "ranked to match." The most highly ethical programs, which are probably few in number, have policies that state that all post-interview contacts would not affect an applicant's position within their ROL.

A STEP-BY-STEP GAME PLAN FOR THE MAIN MATCH

May–June (End of Third Year)

- Narrow specialty of choice.

- Plan senior year schedule.

- Arrange for audition rotations.

- Meet with dean to review academic record and discuss competitiveness.

- Talk with graduating seniors about specific residency programs.

- Select an advisor in the department of your chosen specialty.

July–August (Fourth Year)

- Begin drafting the personal statement.

- Take application photos.

- Contact faculty members who will be writing your letters of recommendation.

- Register online for the NRMP Main Match—$50 fee.

- Gather information in residency programs through the Internet. Use general search engines or FREIDA.

- Pick up your ERAS token from the Dean's Office to begin working on your online application (ERAS opens July 1)

September

- Complete final draft of personal statement.

- Finalize list of possible residency programs.

- Complete and submit the ERAS application online. The ERAS system does not allow electronic submission until September 1; however, it is in your best interest to apply as early as possible.

- Your Dean's Office will upload your transcript, recommendation letters, Dean's Letter, and application photo.

- Use ADTS, a feature of the ERAS Web site, to verify document transmission to each of your programs.

- Follow up on any missing documents.

October–January

- ERAS releases the MSPE to all applied programs on November 1.
- Respond to all interview offers promptly and arrange a schedule of dates.
- Complete all interviews.

February

- Discuss your highest program choices with your advisor or department chairperson and determine whether or not a phone call can be made on your behalf.
- Send letters to your highest-ranked programs.
- Complete ROL online through the NRMP Main Match Web site. Rank lists are due by midnight on the third Thursday in February.

March (Third Week)

- Monday: Un-Match Day—all applicants are notified of their match status (matched or unmatched).
- Wednesday: Supplemental Offer and Acceptance Program (SOAP) begins—unmatched applicants and programs offer rounds for unfilled positions.
- Thursday, 1:00 PM, EST: Match Day—all applicants find out where they have matched.

If you decide to submit a first-choice letter of intent, never send the same letter to your second, third, or lower choices in an attempt to improve your chances. Be sincere about your intentions. Many program directors, especially those in smaller specialties, talk among themselves about candidates for whom they are all competing. Residency programs often give a higher ranking to applicants who state that the program is their first choice. Directors are furious when they rank that candidate within their quota but fail to acquire him or her because he or she has either lied or changed his or her mind. They must then resort to matching with a less-desirable candidate or filling the vacant spot with a student from the bottom of the unmatched applicant pool.

There are potentially serious consequences for dishonest students. The residency program can report the infraction to your medical school dean and blacklist future applicants from your school (by not offering interviews). The director can also give details about your dishonesty to the program at which you matched. The ensuing stigma could affect future fellowships and jobs, and follow you around for the rest of your professional career. The bottom line: If you choose to play the love letter game, always be honest!

CREATING YOUR RANK-ORDER LIST

Once the final interview is over in late January or early February, the next step is to assemble the official ROL. Of course, you can only rank those programs at which you interviewed. At the same time, program directors are ranking some (or all) of the candidates they have seen throughout the application season. The final preferences of both parties determine the Match outcome between applicants and programs.

In mid-January, the Main Match section of the official NRMP Web site will open rank lists for creation. This is the same Web site at which you registered sometime during the previous summer. The system closes exactly at 11:59 PM EST on the third Thursday of February. The NRMP recommends that all applicants enter their ROLs early to avoid online inaccessibility due to server overload. By inputting programs well before the deadline, students will have enough time to reflect on their choices in case any last minute changes need to be made. The system allows applicants to modify the rank lists as many times as necessary before the deadline. The ROL is not officially submitted to the NRMP until the student electronically certifies the list and receives immediate confirmation via e-mail.

Types of Rank-Order Lists

PRIMARY ROL This is the main list on which students place their desired specialty programs in order of preference. The programs can range from a simple list of psychiatry programs in New York to a complicated mix of different specialties and program types (categorical, advanced, or preliminary). It all depends on the applicant's preferences and needs. Students applying in very competitive specialties, such as dermatology, often rank preliminary medicine programs at the bottom of the primary rank list (after the dermatology programs) as a backup in case they find themselves unmatched in their desired specialty.

SUPPLEMENTAL ROL This list is used only by students who rank programs with advanced (A) positions on their primary rank lists. These applicants need to supplement the advanced programs with a PGY-1 position in preliminary medicine, surgery, or transitional. The NRMP allows for flexibility when creating supplemental lists. Students can use one supplemental rank list for all of their advanced programs or, at the other extreme, even create multiple supplemental lists—one customized for each advanced position. This convenience enables applicants to match the geographic location of their preferred PGY-2 positions with their corresponding PGY-1 rankings. Remember, it is still possible to secure an advanced program and fail to match to a PGY-1 position from the corresponding supplemental list. If that happens, you are committed to attending the PGY-2 program and must scramble for unfilled PGY-1 slots on Scramble Day.

List Guidelines

1. RANK THE PROGRAMS IN ORDER OF YOUR TRUE PREFERENCES Always place your number one dream program, even if it is a long shot, in the no. 1 rank position. The student-favored computer algorithm (a product of the 1997 revision) will first scan the applicant's rank list in an attempt to match the highest choice. It is impossible to predict your position on a program director's rank list. And where you rank a program on your list will in no way affect where you stand on that program's own list. Never place any program above the one that you really want simply because you think your chances for matching at your second choice are better. Because it is impossible to game the system with such a strategy, always follow your heart and make a ROL based on the order that will make you happy. Medical students who speculate too much about program directors' rankings, or who place too much trust in their promises, often find themselves burned on Match Day.

2. DO NOT RANK A PROGRAM ON YOUR LIST THAT YOU WOULD NOT ATTEND UNDER ANY CIRCUMSTANCES All medical students are committed to entering the residency program at which they matched. Choose wisely. Do not place an undesirable program on your list simply for the sake of extending the length of the ROL. A long rank list does not affect the likelihood of matching to programs high on the list.

3. DO NOT SHORTEN YOUR RANK LIST BECAUSE OF PROMISES MADE FOR POSITIONS Every year, there are disappointed medical students who failed to match into programs despite having been verbally assured of their very high ranking. Be appreciative of positive feedback, but never take verbal commitments seriously. Students should always create a rank list without these promises in mind. After all, program directors, who have to interview about ten applicants for each position, are anxious to make every applicant feel special.

4. No Matter What Specialty, Rank Enough Programs to Ensure That You Will Match All medical students should rank at least five programs (of any type) on the primary ROL. The NRMP allows applicants to rank up to 15 programs before incurring additional fees of $30 per program. In 2011, matched US seniors ranked an average of 10.55 programs; unmatched applicants had ranked 6.36 programs.[7] (Interestingly, the average ROL length has increased by about two programs over the last 10 years.) The actual number of ranks on your list really depends on the competitiveness of the intended specialty, the competitiveness of the desired programs, and the qualifications of the applicant. Even for noncompetitive specialties, such as pathology or physical medicine and rehabilitation, there is fierce competition for the highly sought after top programs.

THE MATCH ALGORITHM: THE LONGEST 6 MINUTES OF YOUR LIFE

The NRMP uses a supercomputer to process tens of thousands of ROLs, submitted by medical students and residency programs, in just 6 minutes. A newly revised algorithm creates the final matches. By starting at the top of the applicant's ROL, this student-optimal algorithm is on your side — not the programs'.[8] The following example illustrates how the applicant's primary ROL powers the action.

Medical Student XX is applying for internal medicine, and her top three choices are (1) University Hospital, (2) County Hospital, and (3) Suburban Hospital. The computer processes all the rank lists in a completely random order. When this student's ROL comes up for scanning, the computer looks first at her number one choice. The algorithm then scans the rank list from the internal medicine program at University Hospital. At this point, there are two possible pathways:

- If there are open spots in the program, a tentative match is made.
- If there are no available spots (meaning all positions have been tentatively matched already), then rankings are compared.
  1. If the student's rank on University Hospital's list is higher than that of the lowest-ranked applicant already in a tentative match with University

Hospital, student XX will replace that less-preferred applicant and obtain the tentative match.

2. If the student's rank on University Hospital's list is lower than that of the lowest-ranked applicant already in a tentative match with University Hospital, the computer moves on to the student's second choice (County Hospital) and repeats the process until the applicant finally obtains a temporary match or until there are no more programs on her ROL.

The cycles continue over and over, running every applicant through the algorithm, making and breaking provisional matches. If a more highly ranked applicant replaces another student in a tentative match, the computer immediately attempts to create another temporary match for that bumped student, beginning at the first choice. The same process occurs with programs on supplemental rank lists (the algorithm only scans supplemental ROLs if an applicant is tentatively matched with an advanced program). Once the computer runs through all applicants, the temporary matches are finalized. Your destiny is printed out on a piece of paper, stuffed into an envelope, and then given to you exactly 1 month later.

BREAKING THE RULES: HOW TO PREVENT MATCH VIOLATIONS

When medical students or program directors officially register with the NRMP, both participants electronically sign an agreement to abide by the rules of the Match. In a recent interview, the director of the NRMP admits, "it is impossible to police something as big as this."[9] Match violations are common, but few are reported. This is why the NRMP believes that, despite making more than 21,000 matches in 2002, "the vast majority of people are behaving with integrity."[9] Yet most would agree that this is not the case. Program directors desperately want to fill their programs with the best students, and medical students anxiously pine for their number one choice. Because medicine has traditionally been a competitive profession, we can assume that both groups have the potential to behave unprofessionally in an attempt to achieve their goals. A single breach of agreement negatively affects all applicants and programs.

Participants in the NRMP most commonly violate the following rules:

•   Neither party may solicit or pressurize the other to reveal their rank status or other form of commitment. But the NRMP allows both groups to express interest in the other or to willingly share ranking information.

- Program directors cannot sign contracts with US seniors prior to Match Day.
- Program directors cannot pressurize applicants to rank them no. 1 by guaranteeing these candidates a ranking within the program's quota.
- Unmatched applicants cannot begin contacting unfilled programs outside of the Supplemental Offer and Acceptance Program (SOAP).
- Both program directors and applicants must honor the binding commitment of the final Match result. The listing of a program or applicant on an ROL indicates a commitment to accept the appointment (provided that a match is made). Residency programs will release students from their Match agreements only in individual cases of serious hardship.

Because Match violations are rarely reported, most students are unaware of the consequences. For residents who are no-shows at their matched programs, the NRMP stipulates that "failure to honor this commitment will be a material breach of this agreement, and the NRMP is authorized to inform all interested parties, including the Dean of Student Affairs of the applicant's medical school, of such breach." To remedy the widespread problem of unreported violations, the NRMP is now considering stiff penalties. Match violators—both programs and applicants alike—are identified in the NRMP's database and even prohibited from participating in future NRMP matches for a given number of years. Residency programs could lose their accreditation for repeated offenses, and medical students may acquire a mark on their permanent licensure record. The Match system can only be fair and ethical when everyone—students and directors alike—abide by the rules like true professionals.

REFERENCES

1. Roth, A.E. The origins, history, and design of the resident match. *JAMA.* 2003;289(7):909–912.

2. Anderson, K.D., Jacobs, D.M., et al. Is 'match ethics' an oxymoron? *Am J Surg.* 1999;177(3):237–239.

3. National Resident Matching Program. NRMP policy change: All positions in the match. http://www.nrmp.org/all-in.pdf. Accessed December 27, 2011.

4. Fisher, C.E. Manipulation and the match. *JAMA.* 2009;302(12):1266–1267.

5. Carek, P.J., Anderson, K.D. The residency selection process and the match: Does anyone believe anybody? *JAMA.* 2001;285(21):2784–2785.

6. Carek, P.J., Anderson, K.D., et al. Recruitment behavior and program directors: How ethical are their perspectives about the match process? *Fam Med.* 2000;32(4): 258–260.

7. National Resident Matching Program. Impact of length of rank order list on match results: 2002–2011. http://www.nrmp.org/res_match/about_res/impact.html. Accessed December 27, 2011.

8. Roth, A.E., Peranson, E. The effects of the change in the NRMP matching algorithm. *JAMA*. 1997;278:729–732.

9. Mangan, K.S. Keeping 'the match' honest. *Chron Higher Educ*. 2001;48(15): A31.

10

LOVE AND MEDICINE: THE COUPLES MATCH

F or those who subscribe to the belief that love conquers all, you will be happy to know that love can even triumph over the dreaded residency Match. During 4 years of education, medical students who are single often have more on their minds than memorizing drugs and bugs and reading good old Harrison's from cover to cover. After all, many physicians meet their life partners while in medical school. The sparks of love and lasting bonds could happen at any time, whether during first-year orientation or surgery clerkship. Today, nearly every graduating class has its share of student couples, and marriages in which both partners are practicing physicians are on the rise.

TWO DOCTORS, ONE MATCH

Just like their fellow classmates, medical student couples have to cope with the confusion, frustration, and uncertainty involved in choosing a specialty. But, for graduating seniors involved in a relationship, an additional hurdle awaits: the Couples Match. In this process, every couple has the same two goals: (1) to secure a residency position in the desired specialty of choice and (2) to match at a program in the same hospital, city, or general geographic region.

The Couples Match is a special arrangement within the main residency matching system. In response to the increasing number of student couples as more women entered medical school, the National Resident Matching Program (NRMP) introduced the first Couples Match in 1984. It eliminated the chaotic behind-the-scenes negotiations couples used to secure residency appointments. The Match system now easily accommodates the additional flexibility medical student couples require to achieve their goals. According to NRMP data from the

2011 Match, 809 couples (the highest number to date) participated in the Couples Match, representing 5.3% of the total applicant pool of 30,589. However, there are also couples—such as those who participated in an early match like ophthalmology or urology—who coordinated a successful outcome without entering the Couples Match. Because NRMP data do not take into account these unofficial couples, the actual number of medical student couples is slightly higher.

In an official sense (meaning, for NRMP purposes), a couple is simply defined as two partners who are both graduating US seniors and entering the Match process at the same time. They can be from the same or different medical schools. Traditionally, most couples are engaged fiancés or married spouses. However, all types of couples can enter the Couples Match—boyfriends, girlfriends, newlyweds, gays, lesbians, or even close friends simply wishing to remain together during residency. Residency programs do not know which of their applicants are matching as couples, nor do they require couples to reveal the nature of their relationship. Technically, no romantic linkage is necessary. But before you and your best friend decide to Couples Match, remember that both partners in the relationship should be strongly committed to each other. After all, your futures (at least for the next 3 or more years) are intimately tied together. Based on recent Match statistics, the chances of matching together at the same hospital or in the same city are quite good (Table 10–1).

As described in Chapter 9, picking a specialty and then coping with the application and matching process as an individual applicant is hard enough. For

TABLE 10–1

STATISTICS FROM RECENT COUPLES MATCHES

YEAR	NUMBER OF COUPLES	MATCH RATE (%)
2011	809	94.6
2010	808	93.4
2009	788	93.1
2008	738	93.6
2007	621	91.9
2006	610	93.4
2005	606	94.3
2004	641	93.9
2003	570	94.7

Data from National Resident Matching Program.

couples, who have even more stressful challenges, the problems only multiply. In the residency application process, couples are usually limited to applying only to those programs with overlapping geography. If you are both applying in less competitive specialties, more flexibility exists due to the abundance of good residency programs within every major city. If one or both spouses are seeking extremely competitive specialties, the intense competition for a small number of positions will necessitate much more careful planning.

Because of the extraordinary amount of compromise and commitment involved, the Couples Match can cause much tension and anxiety throughout the fourth year of medical school. You should think long and hard and be sure that your relationship is ready for the stressful planning and possible outcomes. Read this chapter, talk with other successful resident couples, and consult with advisors and deans to discuss different strategies. By doing so, medical students who are planning lives together can prevent the unfortunate painful outcome of matching into programs that are thousands of miles apart (or even in a least preferred specialty!).

HOW THE COUPLES MATCH ACTUALLY WORKS

The residency application paperwork is the same for a couple as it is for an individual candidate. Both partners must separately fill out an online application

	BRIAN (PEDIATRICS)	REBECCA (INTERNAL MEDICINE)
1.	University of California—Los Angeles (UCLA)	University of California—Los Angeles
2.	Columbia Presbyterian	Cornell Medical Center
3.	New York University (NYU)	New York University
4.	Cornell Medical Center	New York University
5.	University of Chicago	University of Chicago
6.	University of Chicago	Northwestern Memorial Hospital
7.	Children's Memorial—Chicago	Northwestern Memorial Hospital
8.	Boston Children's Hospital	Massachusetts General Hospital
9.	Boston Children's Hospital	Brigham and Women's Hospital
10.	Boston Children's Hospital	No match

through the Electronic Residency Application Service (ERAS), collect letters of recommendation, and arrange for the transmission of transcripts and Dean's Letters. The only point at which you are officially considered a couple occurs at the submission of the final rank-order list (ROL) in February. When each partner registers for the Match on the NRMP Web site, the system allows the applicant to indicate his or her intention to match as a couple. This process requires both students to enter each other's name and social security number into the system (and to pay an additional $15 per person for the privilege of using the Couples Match). Remember, the decision to match as a couple is not binding until the final submission of the rank list. You may uncouple yourselves at any point during the application and interview season.

Through the Couples Match, two applicants who are seeking residency positions actually pair together their individual ROLs. For every program on one partner's list, there is a linked residency program on the other partner's list. These entries must, of course, be placed in the exact same ranking position: meaning, the program placed in rank position no. 1 on partner A's list is considered paired with an active program placed in the same rank position (no. 1) on partner B's list. Both lists, therefore, must contain an equal number of rankings.

After submitting the final lists (which may or may not be identical), the NRMP computer performs its magic. The matching algorithm of the Couples Match works the same way as it does for placing individual applicants into program slots. The couple will match to the most highly ranked paired set of programs on the list at which both partners have been offered a position. Because of the coupling involved, each partner receives the exact same choice on the ranking positions. If you fail to obtain matches as a couple, you will both be unmatched. The computer does not rerun the lists separately to generate individual matches.

Are you confused yet? Do not worry. Until you actually enter the programs into the online ranking system, the process may seem overly complicated. Take a look at the accompanying ROL of a fictional couple. It is a good illustration of the rules of the Couples Match and it demonstrates a few of the possible outcomes.

Note that these lists are not identical. At first glance, you may wonder why the ranking preferences of this couple are different. On closer inspection, the geographical overlap of their choices becomes apparent. Both Brian and Rebecca clearly decided that UCLA was their first choice for their respective specialties. Their second, third, and fourth choices indicate that they both wanted to be in New York City if they were unable to match at their top ranking. Although this couple grouped their programs by city (Los Angeles, New York, Chicago, and Boston), an applicant can certainly mix and match different locations, as long as both partners' paired programs are in the same city. If a couple applies in the same specialty, each student does not have to rank the same programs.

On Match Day, both partners receive appointments only to those programs at the same ranking position. For instance, Brian and Rebecca could possibly each receive their first choice, fourth choice, ninth choice, or none at all. Because of the pairing, the computer does not perform individual matches. Consequently, several outcomes are never possible, such as Brian matching to his third choice and Rebecca matching to her first choice.

In addition, the computer system allows an applicant to rank a particular program multiple times to generate as many permutations as the couple pleases. This is the reason why Rebecca listed NYU twice in rankings no. 3 and no. 4, and why Brian listed Boston Children's Hospital three times in rankings no. 8, no. 9, and no. 10. With more options in a given location, this feature allows for greater flexibility to accommodate one of the partner's preferences. You should also note that this fictional couple submitted a rank list with ten-paired programs. The NRMP allows for a maximum of 15 rankings, above which each program incurs an additional $30 fee. This policy is identical for individual applicants as well.

Take a closer look at position no. 10 in this fictional couple's rank list. Their choices here illustrate another important feature of the Couples Match. To allow for additional flexibility in decision making, the NRMP provides the option of selecting No Match in any of the pairings. If one partner matches with the program in that ranking position, the other partner willingly chooses to go unmatched on Match Day. This selection ensures that the couple can remain together in the same city. The unmatched partner then has to scramble for an unfilled position or apply again the following year. In the 2011 Match, about 40 couples (5.4%) found themselves in this situation. If our made-up couple receives their tenth choice, Brian becomes a pediatrics resident at Boston Children's Hospital and Rebecca scrambles for any open residency positions in the metropolitan Boston area (whether in internal medicine or any other specialty). This outcome is a small risk that some couples are willing to take to remain together.

OTHER ISSUES SURROUNDING THE COUPLES MATCH

One concern that medical student couples often raise is whether their couple status will place them at a disadvantage during the application process. In the 2011 Match, 94.6% of couples obtained a successful match, and a remarkably similar percentage (94.1%) of individual US seniors also received a first-year residency position on Match Day. Based on these numbers, it seems that most couples perform exactly the same in the Match as if they had applied and matched separately. This generalization, however, may not necessarily apply to couples in which one partner is a very strong candidate in a less-competitive specialty. For example, one successful couple, who applied in medicine-psychiatry and pediatrics, found the odds very much tilted in their favor. Program directors of medicine-psychiatry wanted the stellar candidate so badly that they called up the pediatrics residency director to improve the final ranking position of the partner. This situation only happens, of course, within the same institution. Medical student couples generally do not fit nicely into the formulas that program directors use for granting interviews and ranking candidates. Many times, departments often make exceptions for one another. On the other hand, if one or both partners are applying in extremely competitive fields, such as dermatology, there is less of an opportunity to use their couple status to increase their chances.

Regardless of specialty choice, applying as a couple should never decrease an applicant's chances of matching at his or her highest choices. Instead, the Couples Match usually has no effect on final candidate rankings, or, as illustrated above, yields an improved chance of matching. In general, residency programs look favorably on couples, no matter the level of commitment between the partners. Couples tend to be more stable applicants who are less likely to drop out of the program. In addition, couples who are residents in different departments, such as internal medicine and surgery, can foster better working relationships between two sets of housestaff. Thus, both departments gain something from accepting a couple into their institution.

If one or both members of the couple are applying to very competitive specialties, particularly outside the NRMP Match, they must be more strategic. In this complicated situation, one partner may be interested in an early Match specialty, such as otolaryngology, while the other plans to apply to orthopedic surgery. Non-NRMP matches, such as the San Francisco Match or the Urology Match, have no similar provisions for couples within their computer algorithms. Both organizations also do not coordinate matches with the NRMP. In these cases, your initial strategy should simply be to apply, interview, and rank as many programs as possible within the same cities or geographic regions. Candidates participating in the San Francisco Match will find out their results 1 month before rank lists are due for the NRMP. In this case, by knowing where one partner has already matched, coordination within couples becomes much easier.

If a couple consists of two stellar, highly desirable applicants both applying to extremely competitive specialties, another strategy is to negotiate with one of the programs for an out-of-Match contract. For example, one couple from the same medical school, John and Andrea, sought positions in urology and radiation oncology, respectively. John, an Alpha Omega Alpha (AOA) applicant who was highly sought after by his top choice residency, informed the program director of their situation. The urologist then contacted the director of radiation oncology at the same institution and encouraged him to sign Andrea, also an outstanding candidate, through an out-of-Match contract. By working together, both departments ensured that the couple ended up together at their hospital.

By having so many different specialties and matching systems, there are scores of possible scenarios for the Couples Match. There is, however, one other important and common possibility to mention. What if one or both partners of a couple apply to advanced specialties, such as anesthesiology or radiology, which require a separate PGY-1 rank list? Unfortunately, the Supplemental ROL, which is used only for these internship positions, is not part of the Couples Match algorithm. As such, both partners must prepare this list separately. Because the goal is simply to remain in the same city during that year, you should only rank those PGY-1 programs on the supplemental list that are geographically acceptable. Otherwise, the hopeful medical student couple may find themselves in a long-distance relationship for this rather difficult year.

WORDS OF WISDOM: SIX TIPS FROM MATCHED-AND-MARRIED COUPLES

1. Good Communication Is the Key for Surviving the Couples Match Intact

After assessing your relative competitiveness in the application process, you should have an honest discussion with your partner about career goals and professional needs. Both partners should talk about what they are looking for in a residency program. The couple must decide together which desires are open to negotiation and which cannot be compromised. These needs may range from location to program size, or from the call schedule to research opportunities. Most likely, both partners will not fall in love with same programs or hospitals. As such, you should seize this opportunity in your relationship to be open and honest and to get to know your partner even better.

For new medical student couples, the decision about where to attend residency training may be the first significant compromise they have had to reach. Whether the issue is location, program, hospital, or even specialty, both partners must be flexible and open to negotiation. Without excellent communication throughout the entire process, the outcome on Match Day may elicit feelings of disappointment or resentment. But participating in the Couples Match can be a stress-free, even enjoyable, experience. Remember, the final decision on the ranked list of paired programs does not occur until February. Every couple can allay much anxiety by pushing the strategizing and compromising until the end. By doing so, medical student couples will prevent the Match process from creating any rifts in their relationship.

2. When Deciding Where to Apply, Geographic Location Is the First and Most Important Consideration

The purpose of the Couples Match is to ensure that both partners obtain residency positions in the same city, not thousands of miles apart. Thus, the first step in the application process is to decide together on the list of programs to which you are submitting applications. If a couple applies for the same specialty, they do not have to interview at all the same programs. Instead, simply apply to a large enough number of hospitals within the same city. Strong candidates in less-competitive specialties often have more freedom in interviewing at programs in smaller cities and towns. If one or both partners seek very competitive specialties, they usually focus their efforts on larger metropolitan regions, such as New York City, Los Angeles, and Chicago. Because these areas have many hospitals with multiple programs in a given specialty, the odds of matching together are significantly higher.

3. Apply Early to as Many Programs as You Can

Because most medical student couples are typically constrained by geography, they submit more applications to increase their chances at matching in the same city. If one or both partners are seeking very competitive specialties, such as dermatology, it is even more important to apply early to the longest possible list of programs.

4. Always Inform Your Interviewers and the Program Director That You Are Matching as a Couple

Although not all applicants mentioned their partners in their personal statements, nearly all agreed on identifying themselves as a couple during the interview and postinterview stages. The NRMP does not reveal this information to residency program directors. At this point in the process, honesty serves you better than secrecy. Couples should be specific in mentioning the name of their partner and the specialty for which they are also interviewing. One successful couple, who sought positions in anesthesiology and radiology, felt that "we would not have matched if we had not told them we were couples matching."

5. Be Assertive and Aggressive as a Couple

The NRMP only knows that two applicants intend to match as a couple when the final paired ROL is submitted. As such, there may be times during the application and interview season when your status as a couple can help your chances at certain programs or hospitals. For couples applying in the same specialty, one partner may receive an interview at a desired program while the other does not. Instead of expressing jealousy or resentment, be forceful and confident. Inform the residency program director of your intent to match as a couple.

For example, one couple from the same medical school, Julie and Ken, applied together to similar programs in internal medicine. At one competitive California program, Julie received an interview and Ken did not. When they explained their situation to the program director, Ken was promptly granted an interview. The moral of the story: Couples should not allow their egos to prevent them from doing what it takes to make the Couples Match a successful reality.

6. The Perfect Couples ROL Involves Both Compromise and Strategy

Before entering the official rank list into the computer, both partners should first sit down and order their preferences alone. Ignore your partner or spouse, and disregard what you think the other would want. Instead, each of you must figure out your own rankings and only then compare lists. At this point, couples should discuss, negotiate, and compromise on specific factors (such as location, size of program, call schedule, and research opportunities). The only required common factor, of course, should be the same city. Otherwise, what was the point of entering the Couples Match?

In preparing the final rank list, refer to the guidelines in Chapter 9 on how to make a good ROL. In general, couples often rank two to three times more paired programs than an individual applicant does. As you assemble the preferences in order, remember that you do not necessarily have to match at the same program (if applying in the same specialty) or at the same hospital (if applying in different specialties). The rank-order system allows all applicants, whether individual or couples, to enter many possible combinations, such as different program types, specialties, hospitals, and locations. The end result is a list of mutually acceptable programs in the same city where both partners are content to begin their training.

11

TOP SECRET! THE ULTIMATE GUIDE TO A SUCCESSFUL MATCH

For students currently in medical school, those tough premedical years may seem like a distant unpleasant memory. As a doctor-in-training, you have become accustomed to the competitive nature of medicine. Beginning in high school—and progressing all the way through college, medical school, residency, and fellowship—all aspiring physicians learned that they had to be the best. This is the only way to achieve one's career aspirations in medicine successfully.

To become a pediatrician, radiologist, or any other specialist, every medical student must earn a training position in a residency program. The competition for certain specialties and residency programs, however, can be rather intense. While trying to figure out which specialty is best for them, medical students still have to work very hard academically during these 4 years.

Unfortunately, many students rule out some specialty choices for fear of not being accepted. Everyone knows that some fields of medicine have only a limited number of coveted residency spots and an overwhelmingly large number of applicants. Other specialties are not as tough to match in. Instead, the fierce competition exists for the most highly regarded hospitals and institutions within that specialty.

RISING ABOVE THE COMPETITION

The residency application and matching process has become a discouraging series of obstacles. Regardless of specialty choice, planning for residency is a 4-year process. It takes a great deal of strategy (and luck) to make yourself the most marketable candidate. Why is all this advanced preparation necessary? For each field of medicine, there are many myths and rumors regarding the criteria necessary to obtain a particular residency. There are subtle and hidden requirements that students must meet to match into the specialty, such as board score cutoffs, personal statement topics, published clinical research, and more.

Due to the increasing competition for certain specialties, there is less latitude for mistakes. Whether you are a first-year student wondering what type of doctor you will become, or a fourth-year veteran starting the residency application process, careful planning is a must to enhance your credentials and ensure success. This chapter will prevent any career-related regrets by showing what it really takes to match into each specialty and into the residency program of your choice. For each specialty, I have summarized the advice provided by a number of medical school seniors, residents, faculty members, and residency program directors. For medical students interested in the extremely competitive specialties, this inside information will allow you to plan far in advance. There should be no excuse for not doing all the right things and being the strongest candidate possible. Pay close attention, and heed the advice of those who have come before you: successfully matched residents from all the major medical specialties.

Based on statistical information from the 2011 NRMP, San Francisco, and Urology Matches, I have ranked the 20 medical specialties into four tiers of competitiveness (see Table 11-1). The unmatched rate (percentage of US seniors who fail to match into their desired field of medicine) serves as an excellent indicator of the difficulty of obtaining residency in a given specialty. The numbers represent those US seniors who applied to that particular specialty only—without any backup choices on their rank-order list. The 20 major fields of medicine are categorized in order according to these data.

You should, however, interpret these rankings with a grain of salt. Many aspects of medicine are cyclical. The relative popularity (and therefore competitiveness) of any field of medicine can change over time. While assessing their level of academic achievement, medical students go through a great deal of self-selection before committing to a specialty. Ultimately, only the most highly competitive students apply to the ultracompetitive specialties, which can skew the final unmatched rates. Also, the difficulty of matching to a specific residency program may differ significantly from the overall competitiveness of the specialty. Remember, even in the less-competitive fields of medicine such as family practice, the few positions in the top programs can be incredibly difficult to obtain. Competition, therefore, exists for all residency applicants, no matter the specialty of choice.

TABLE 11–1

SPECIALTY RANKINGS BASED ON 2011 UNMATCHED RATES FOR US SENIORS

	Unmatched Rate (%)
Extremely competitive	
Plastic surgery	24.6
Orthopedic surgery	20.6
General surgery	14.9
Dermatology	14.8
Radiation oncology	14.1
Very competitive	
Urology	14.0
Ophthalmology	12.0
Neurosurgery	11.8
Otolaryngology	11.8
Physical medicine and rehabilitation	8.2
Competitive	
Emergency medicine	7.3
Obstetrics–gynecology	5.5
Psychiatry	3.7
Pathology	3.4
Anesthesiology	2.8
Less competitive	
Internal medicine	2.7
Pediatrics	2.5
Family medicine	2.4
Neurology	2.3
Radiology	2.1

Data from National Resident Matching Program; San Francisco Matching Program; American Urological Association.

CONSIDERATIONS FOR OSTEOPATHIC MEDICAL STUDENTS

The same principles of choosing a medical specialty also apply to osteopathic physicians. Like the American Council on Graduate Medical Education (ACGME), the American Osteopathic Association (AOA) is the accreditation

TABLE 11–2

OSTEOPATHIC GRADUATES MATCHED BY SPECIALTY (2011)

Specialty	% of Total
Internal medicine	22.8
Family medicine	18.6
Pediatrics	14.5
Emergency medicine	11.3
Obstetrics and gynecology	7.7
Psychiatry	7.3
Anesthesiology	4.6
Surgery	3.0
Pathology	2.2
Neurology	1.9
Internal medicine—pediatrics	1.3
Physical medicine and rehabilitation	1.2
Radiology	0.7

Data from National Resident Matching Program.

body for osteopathic residency programs. There are many AOA-approved residencies for the major primary care specialties, in which most osteopaths obtain training. DO students interested in certain fields—such as neurology, anesthesiology, and pathology—will find fewer options, so they typically pursue an ACGME-approved allopathic residency.

Although the number of MD students in ACGME programs has decreased as an overall percentage, allopaths continue to dominate the most competitive specialties such as otolaryngology, dermatology, radiology, and urology. For instance, in 2011, of the 668 matches in orthopedic surgery, 658 were US seniors or graduates; only 2 osteopathic students matched. Instead, the largest number of osteopathic students matched into allopathic programs in internal medicine, family medicine, and pediatrics (see Table 11–2). These results are not surprising since fewer MDs entered primary care over the past two decades. However, DOs have had much less success in obtaining positions in the competitive surgical ACGME programs.

Keep in mind that the competition for ACGME residency slots is only going to get stiffer. More and more MD and DO students are graduating from expanded and newly opened medical schools. But the number of ACGME residency programs will likely remain stagnant due to lack of federal funding. Osteopathic students, therefore, should anticipate increased difficulty in obtaining ACGME positions in the more competitive medical specialties.[1] Regardless of specialty choice, osteopathic medical students who want to match with an allopathic residency program will have to place greater attention to their academic competitiveness. That is where this chapter comes in.

ADVICE FOR MEDICAL STUDENTS—BY SPECIALTY, A TO Z

Anesthesiology

Although the number of American medical graduates entering anesthesiology reached a low point in 1995, interest has steadily increased again. Program directors seek candidates who demonstrate excellence in one or two areas of interest— an extracurricular activity, research, hobby, or academic achievement. Do something that makes you stand out from the rest. The pursuit of research is neither a requirement nor a prerequisite for matching at a top residency program.

During your preclinical years, strive to earn high grades in physiology and pharmacology. Several years ago, most residency programs did not consider board scores when evaluating applicants. Today, do your best to earn higher than 210 on the United States Medical Licensing Examination (USMLE) Step I to obtain an interview at the most competitive programs. During the clinical years, audition rotations at other hospitals are generally discouraged; they do little to improve your chances of matching at that program. Instead, spend your senior year learning medicine other than anesthesiology, such as cardiology or critical care. Of course, you should take, at the minimum, one rotation in anesthesiology to confirm your interest and to collect letters of recommendation. Among your three to four letters, submit no more than two from an anesthesiologist; the rest should come from faculty in internal medicine or surgery. As always, a little name who knows you well is better than a big name who does not.

In your application, the personal statement should be a good read that clearly outlines your understanding of and interest in anesthesiology. Remember that poor grammar and spelling reflect on attention to detail, which is extremely important for this specialty.

Dermatology

In this extremely competitive specialty, most programs interview about 30 or so candidates (out of hundreds of applicants) for only two or three spots. Because of the stiff competition, future dermatologists must identify their interest very early in medical school. Because many students go into dermatology for the wrong reasons (lifestyle, money, etc), interviewers screen for those who are passionate and truly committed to this challenging specialty. Get involved with the department as early as possible. Clinical research and publications in journals are extremely important for your candidacy; therefore, find a research mentor during the preclinical years.

Board scores are also critical; earn the highest Step I score possible or else you may not make the cut. Nearly all programs heavily emphasize membership in Alpha Omega Alpha (the medical school honor society). In the clinical years, you will have to get lots of honors grades in your third-year clerkships to have the right numbers for interview selection. Take several electives in dermatology early in your senior year. Scheduling audition rotations at programs of highest interest can improve your chances of matching. During these rotations, work hard to portray yourself in the best possible light to the faculty and, in particular, the program director. Remember, connections are important in this specialty. Often, who you know will provide the greatest chance of matching dermatology.

Most candidates submit applications to nearly every program in the country (upward of 40 applications!). Three strong letters of recommendation from dermatologists are preferred, particularly with words such as outstanding, exceptional, and the best I have ever seen. In the personal statement, explain how you arrived at the decision to enter dermatology and why your personality attributes are a good fit with this specialty. Be articulate and engaging, tell a compelling story, and use this opportunity to stand out from the crowd in a positive way. Above all, do your best to get into dermatology at the first shot. Candidates who are rejected and reapply the next year (retreads) are rarely successful.

Emergency Medicine

Selection committees like to see evidence that you are a healthy, well-adjusted person with interesting hobbies. During the preclinical years, it is highly advantageous to pursue research. Any specialty of clinical medicine is fine; program directors give bonus points for emergency medicine-related research. Immerse yourself in medical school and community activities, such as serving on committees, exploring emergency medicine interest groups, and volunteering Mother Theresa-style at local clinics. One successful candidate at a top program emphasized the importance of extracurriculars, especially "things that are outdoorsy, wild, crazy, or can kill you."

For this very competitive specialty, strive for USMLE Step I scores above 220. If your results are low, program directors recommend taking Step II early during senior year and earning higher scores. During the clinical years, earn high grades in medicine and surgery. Competitive candidates should then complete at least two rotations in emergency medicine—one at their home institution, the other at an audition hospital. The most desirable away rotations fill up quickly; therefore, plan these fourth-year electives very early.

Because emergency medicine is a small community, obtain two letters of recommendation from emergency medicine faculty physicians. A strong letter from a community preceptor carries less weight than one from a program director or departmental chair. Most programs also prefer to see letters from every emergency medicine clerkship completed. Otherwise, their absence will raise concerns over your performance in those rotations. Finally, program directors place less emphasis on the personal statement, but it still should be well written. The essay should convey how you selected emergency medicine, why your personality and temperament are well suited for this specialty, and what you plan to do with your training.

Family Practice

Although family practice is a relatively noncompetitive specialty—with plenty of residency positions nationally for everyone—the most desirable and highly ranked programs are intensely competitive and still get their share of stellar applicants. Program directors like students who are heavily involved in extracurricular activities, particularly clinically related pursuits in which they interact with members of their community (volunteering at local clinics, education in schools, etc). Make sure to work hard and obtain leadership roles in these organizations.

Although research projects look nice on paper, it is not essential to publish an article or present an abstract to match into family practice. You should study hard for the USMLE Step I, but stellar scores are not necessary. Aiming for the mean is perfectly adequate for success in the match. In the clinical years, complete a community-based family practice elective, in addition to your medical school's core clerkship. Work hard to impress your attendings. If you are interested in a particularly competitive residency program, it is advantageous to complete an audition elective there. Because family practice is such a broad specialty, the remainder of the senior year should be spent in a variety of medical fields, from obstetrics to critical care.

After grades earned in third-year clerkships, program directors place the greatest emphasis on your three (or four) letters of recommendation. At least one should be from a family practitioner, but the remainder can be written by virtually any other specialist—internist, surgeon, or obstetrician. (Some programs may specify certain departments from which the letters should originate; therefore, make sure to check carefully ahead of time.) Above all, pick references from physician who know you very well, particularly when it comes to your clinical abilities.

Selection committees also highly value the personal statement, second only to letters of recommendation. The essay should be very well written, personal, and engaging. Appropriate topics include a description of your involvement in significant extracurricular activities or other relevant personal experiences, the reasons for choosing a career in family practice, and the specific aspects of a training program you are most seeking. A good personal statement allows the program director to have a good sense of your character, values, and goals. Overall, there is little specific preparation for a successful match in family practice; therefore, enjoy your medical school years and make an effort to become a very well-rounded physician.

General Surgery

Over the past several years, there has been a steady turnaround in the decline in the number of applicants (particularly US seniors) to general surgery programs. Competition has increased significantly and remains fierce for the most prestigious academic programs. Your academic credentials are most important. At some point during medical school, students should get involved with surgical research that could lead to a publication. If you want to be competitive for any program in the country, make it your personal goal to earn high clerkship grades (especially in the core surgery rotation—this is crucial!), election to AOA, and ranking in the top quarter of your class. Strive for Step I board scores well above the mean (>215). It is also very helpful to take the Step II examination early and score well—it reflects your application of clinical knowledge.

In your senior year, work hard during a month-long subinternship at your own institution. If you are interested in a particular program, sign up for a senior audition elective there (a maximum of two) and work hard to impress them on-site with a stellar performance. If you do, you will improve your credentials and look better than your fellow applicants, which could help you match. From all of your surgical experiences, choose three senior surgery attendings to ask for strong letters of recommendation. Ideally, they should be people who have worked directly with you and know you well, especially if they know your personal strengths in addition to your surgical skills. Letters from basic scientists or residents carry much less weight than those from the chairperson or program director at your medical school.

After applying, it can be helpful to use contacts to increase your chances of matching, and therefore have your departmental chairperson make some phone calls on your behalf. Selection committees are looking for candidates with desire, work ethic, and the ability to get the job done. For this reason, some programs may be more open to review your complete record and overlook any academic deficiencies by valuing any other accomplishments, such as volunteer and community work or other significant extracurricular activities.

Internal Medicine

Because there are hundreds of internal medicine programs, your chances of matching into this specialty are quite high. The stellar candidates all apply to the most prestigious hospitals; here, the competition is quite stiff. If aiming for these top-ranked academic programs, you need to strive for the strongest academic record possible. Earn high scores on the Step I boards and honors grades in your medicine rotations. Research is not essential, but can be helpful. Passion for nonmedical activities and interests are also important; therefore, get involved in your community through leadership positions or other commitments.

In the senior year, audition rotations are unnecessary and sometimes risky. After all, simply getting stuck with a bad attending could ruin your chances of matching at that program. The selection committees read your letters of recommendation closely; therefore, make sure to request references from physicians who know you well. For the most academic programs, it is imperative to obtain a recommendation letter from the departmental chairperson at your school. You should also submit two other letters from senior medical faculty (either third- or fourth-year rotation attendings).

Although the personal statement is less important, an excellent essay could clinch an interview for a borderline candidate, and a poorly written one could exclude a superior applicant. Successful residents in internal medicine recommend all candidates to be honest and enthusiastic throughout the entire process, complete their applications early, and notify their first choice program about their genuine interest.

Neurology

This specialty is becoming more popular among medical students. During medical school, research experience in neurology (either clinical or basic science) is very helpful, though not required. Your extracurricular activities are less influential factors, but you should try to score well on the USMLE Step I. In the clinical years, honors grades in neurology clerkships and subinternships are essential for matching at your top choice program. To prove your interest and commitment to neurology, get as much clinical experience as possible.

Away rotations are helpful in checking out any highly desired programs. When evaluating applicants, however, the three letters of recommendation carry the greatest weight among program directors. Two should be written by neurologists. The more renowned or senior the faculty member, the better. Additionally, the letter writers may have personal contacts at hospitals where they completed their residency or fellowship, which could increase your chances of matching. But make sure that you have worked with them enough to elicit a good letter; a lukewarm one may actually hurt your application. Although the personal statement is less important, a poorly written essay—especially if filled with bad humor or philosophical diatribes—would undermine an otherwise stellar opinion of your candidacy.

Neurosurgery

Historically, this extremely competitive specialty has always attracted the very best and brightest medical students. Get involved with the department at your medical school early on. During the preclinical years, study hard so that you will be prepared for the USMLE Step I examination. Neurosurgery residency programs often have cutoffs for academic credentials. Although earning a top score of 270 does not necessarily guarantee a Match, it will certainly keep you in the pool of highly sought after candidates. You should aim for a score in the mid-240s.

Extracurricular activities only matter if they are significant. It is much more impressive to have a few outside interests to which you are truly dedicated or in which you had a leadership role. Life experience and achievement in research, however, are more valuable than extracurricular activities. The highly competitive programs basically require some form of research. After all, everyone loves students who have published a lot. At many places, you will interview not only with neurosurgeons but also with neuroscientists associated with the department. In the clinical years, work hard to get stellar grades in your surgery and medicine clerkships, as well as the neurosurgery subinternship. AOA membership is helpful, but not necessarily a prerequisite for matching.

Audition rotations at other hospitals are generally not helpful. No matter how many physicians you may impress, it only takes one faculty member or resident whom you may have rubbed the wrong way to keep you out of the program. If you are a strong applicant, complete rotations only at your home institution. Program directors generally value letters of recommendation only from neurosurgeons. Obtain at least three of them, particularly from the chairperson of the department at your medical school. Because the personal statement is more likely to hurt you than to help, keep it neutral (unless you have something really amazing to say). At application time, apply to as many programs as possible. Your best chances of matching are often at your own institution—where people know you, like you (hopefully), and want you to remain there for residency. Because neurosurgery is a very small community, the interview ends up being an extremely important factor for selling yourself to selection committees.

Obstetrics–Gynecology

Although fewer medical students are entering obstetrics–gynecology, it is still a moderately competitive specialty (especially for the most highly ranked programs). During the preclinical years, spend time getting familiar with the field. You should find a mentor within the department, go to grand rounds, and attend national meetings if possible. Extracurricular activities are important credentials; therefore, make sure to do some volunteer work related to women's health in underserved settings (such as STD clinics). Research is not necessary for matching, but it looks great—especially as an ongoing interest rather than an isolated project.

To be most competitive, students should earn a score of 215 or higher on the USMLE Step I. Work hard during the required obstetrics–gynecology clerkship for an honors grade. During your senior year, you should take additional electives in the specialty. For the most competitive programs, audition rotations can be very helpful (but only if you make a good first impression). Applicants must obtain at least two letters of recommendation from prominent and well-respected obstetricians–gynecologists. The ideal references are upper-level faculty members and the departmental chairperson. After all, connections are important. Additionally, your personal statement should concisely explain your interest in obstetrics–gynecology and how your community service experiences will lead to better patient care. Although the numbers are important, selection committees ultimately look at the bigger picture. They want residents who are personable team leaders, go the extra mile, and have positive attitudes.

Ophthalmology

Stellar grades, high Step-I board scores (average was 225), and AOA membership are very important for matching into this second most competitive specialty. Although high academic achievement is a prerequisite, most program directors place the greatest emphasis on a candidate's letters of recommendation, clinical evaluations, and interview. Many are willing to consider the applicant as an individual with unique abilities and talents and look past any minor academic deficiencies — but only if compensated for by other outstanding qualities. Demonstrate your interest and commitment to ophthalmology by getting involved in clinical research projects, spending time shadowing residents and faculty in clinic, and scrubbing in on lots of surgeries.

Depending on your school's policy, complete electives in ophthalmology as early as possible. To improve your chances of matching, it is advantageous to do a few away rotations at programs of highest interest. (Just make sure to work hard and impress them with your superior knowledge base.) Obtain at least one glowing letter of recommendation from an ophthalmologist who knows you well, especially if he or she is the chairperson or program director. Mediocre references — ones that do not give any insight into your performance — from well-known names can actually be detrimental.

Inundated with topnotch candidates, selection committees often use the personal statement as a deciding factor for interview invitations. Your essay must be more than interesting, informative, and readable; it should differentiate you from other applicants by showing the intangibles that make you a good doctor. Because most programs grant interviews on a rolling basis, aspiring ophthalmologists should submit their applications as early as possible.

Orthopedic Surgery

This very competitive specialty requires a great deal of planning for success in the Match. Medical students need to work hard throughout all 4 years to achieve the best academic record possible. Earn stellar grades in all of your classes and rotations (especially the surgical ones!), because many competitive programs screen out candidates who have not been elected to AOA. Meaningful research projects, especially in orthopedics, can look very good on your application and will boost your credentials. Programs really put a lot of emphasis on having high board scores; therefore, it is important to do well on the USMLE Step I. Although there is no magic number for making the cut for an interview, aim for a ballpark range around 230.

Orthopedic surgery is one specialty in which it is almost mandatory for students to complete as many well-planned audition rotations at other hospitals as possible. You must work your butt off and shine (without being annoying). Many applicants with less-than-stellar credentials can maximize their chances of matching by impressing the program director with hard work during a subinternship.

Most students send out upward of 40 applications. Candidates should submit three to four letters of recommendation, which are typically the most important part of the application. At the minimum, two should be from orthopedic surgeons who know you well, especially if he or she happens to be the program director or departmental chairperson at your medical school. Avoid sending letters from nonsurgical specialties such as pediatrics, psychiatry, or internal medicine.

The personal statement should be brief, concise, and honest. Discuss what makes you unique and how you came to choose orthopedic surgery, but leave out any poetry or quotations and do not mention your parents if they are also orthopedic surgeons. Avoid listing personal inquiries as a reason for career choice. Around the time of assembling rank lists, have your advisor or chairperson make calls on your behalf if possible. After all, being proactive and using connections may sometimes make or break your chances at matching at a first-choice program.

Otolaryngology

Like other surgical subspecialties, otolaryngology (or ENT) is very competitive to match. You have to excel at many areas to stand above the rest of the competition. First, from the beginning of medical school, get to know the faculty at your institution so that they can guide you and help you. Nearly all programs seek applicants with extensive research experience, particularly in ENT. Early in the preclinical years, make an effort to seek out an otolaryngologist and get involved in some small basic science projects or case reports. Although it is still possible to match into ENT without research, having your name on a published paper or presenting a poster at a national conference will only further enhance your credentials.

When it comes to take the Step I board examination, you should aim for breaking at least 220. (If you score below 210, it might be wise to have a backup plan, such as applying for general surgery as well). During the clinical years, an outstanding performance in surgery is the bare minimum. Future otolaryngologists should also earn honors grades in medicine and other clerkships. With top grades, membership in AOA gives an applicant an advantage. However, it is important to know that many students without AOA match at top academic institutions and others with AOA status can find themselves unmatched. This is why letters of recommendation are very important in otolaryngology. You should obtain references from at least two otolaryngologists, particularly from someone well known in the field. In the small ENT community, everyone knows each other; therefore, connections can make a big difference. To obtain stellar letters, complete at least one audition subinternship at a large academic hospital with a well-known department. Work hard on these rotations and impress the faculty members. When it comes to apply, students should submit as many applications as financially feasible. In the personal statement, make sure you clearly state your reasons for entering a career in otolaryngology. At rank list time, applicants should have as many programs as possible in order to ensure a match.

Pathology

As more American medical graduates discover pathology, this unassuming specialty has become competitive again. In fact, the top-ranked programs like to see candidates with Step I board scores of about 220 or higher. In your preclinical years, learn all the basic sciences well. Research projects, publications, and presentations at national meetings are important credentials for matching at the most academic programs. A few of these institutions even do not consider granting interviews to anyone without a PhD in a basic science discipline. All students should demonstrate a committed interest in pathology, primarily by completing a month-long rotation. After the second year of medical school, some apply for competitive postsophomore fellowships—1-year positions in which they function at the level of a pathology resident.

Although pathology is developing more interest among medical students, some applicants come to it later in their training. The absence of specialty clerkships, therefore, is not viewed as an absolute negative for matching in this specialty. During the senior year, audition rotations (which are generally unnecessary) could substitute for not having a PhD when applying to the most competitive programs. To impress the program director, you should always take the initiative, help out the residents, and conduct many literature searches during these rotations. At application time, letters of recommendation from any type of clinical faculty are acceptable; make sure at least one comes from a pathologist who knows you well. Most important, in the personal statement and interview, never say that you chose pathology because of "lifestyle reasons." Doing so will instantly drop you to the bottom of every director's rank lists.

Pediatrics

The fun-loving nature of pediatricians makes applying for this specialty a much more enjoyable process. There are excellent programs all over the country at both university and community hospitals. If you are seeking a position at top programs in pediatrics, the competition is stiff. You will need higher board scores and stronger clinical grades than your peers. During medical school, it is not necessary to pursue research to enhance your credentials. Instead, take the time to immerse yourself in outside interests and other extracurricular activities, particularly those that involve kids. Become involved in substantial leadership, volunteer, or research projects. There are no unofficial board score cutoffs for pediatrics. Earn an honors grade in your required pediatrics clerkship, and follow this up with a stellar performance in a subinternship.

If you are interested in exploring a particular program, away rotations are helpful but not necessary. Most candidates submit about ten applications. Obtain letters of recommendation from one or two pediatricians who know you well. The rest can come from any specialty. If you are set on a particular program, do an outside rotation there, work hard to impress them, and obtain a letter of recommendation. The personal statement, an important part of the application, should be honest and straightforward and discuss how you decided on a career in pediatrics. Do not simply say "I love kids"—prove it with examples of what you have done. Pediatricians are easy-going folks in general. They are mainly interested in whether they will be able to work with you for 3 years, so relax!

Physical Medicine and Rehabilitation

This specialty has been largely undiscovered by most medical students. Positions in physical medicine and rehabilitation (PM&R) are available for nearly any interested student. Like most specialties, however, competition for the most highly ranked programs is intense. In the preclinical years, pursue outside interests that relate to the practice of physiatry, such as working with disabled people, athletic events, or public health issues. Research experience will definitely provide a distinct advantage when attempting to attract the interest of the top academic-based training programs. But just because applicants to PM&R do not have publications or presentations listed on their resumes does not mean that they are locked out of this specialty. It is certainly by no means a requirement. This specialty is, after all, broad enough to attract physicians with a wide variety of talents, education, and personal backgrounds. So go ahead and pursue your own interests and extracurricular activities. Just make sure to study enough to earn an above average score on the Step I board examination. This will place you in a comfortable position to be competitive during the application process.

In the clinical years, solid performances in the internal medicine, neurology, pediatrics, and surgery core clerkships are important. Complete a PM&R subinternship or elective early in the fourth year to make sure that it is the right specialty for you. Depending on the specific institution, audition rotations may have some benefit. If you want to enhance your chances of matching at a certain hospital, make sure to work hard during an away elective because selection committees will keep a close eye on you. You will need three letters of recommendation, with at least two of them from PM&R physicians and the remainder from other core fields. Obviously, if you are interested in pediatric rehabilitation, a reference letter from a pediatrician with whom you have worked is logical. Likewise, if someone has an interest in sports medicine, a letter from an orthopedic surgeon who practices sports medicine would be suitable as well. Just be sure, however, that the accompanying personal statement is truly personal, honest, and well written. Make sure to explain genuinely how you became interested in this field of medicine. Be creative, but avoid gimmicks.

Depending on their credentials, most candidates apply to around ten programs to ensure a match. If possible, have a well-placed connection make a tactful phone call on your behalf to a program director. Most important, never say that you chose this field because of the lifestyle, or that PM&R is a backup specialty after orthopedic surgery. It will be doing yourself and that residency program a huge disfavor.

Plastic Surgery

It takes a lot of preparation and achievement to match into plastic surgery—the most competitive specialty among all areas of medicine. Hundreds of impressive candidates are seeking one of the few spots in the integrated, or categorical, plastic surgery programs (5 to 6 years long). During the preclinical years, students should link up with an academic plastic surgeon and find out more about what the specialty involves. Hang out in the clinic and operating room to gain more exposure. Immerse yourself in extracurricular activities and outside interests. Program directors look for students who are great at what they are expected to do, but the candidate with outstanding unexpected achievement is looked upon very highly (eg, organizing a mission to an underserved area, training for the Olympics, writing a book).

Almost all selection committees look for achievement in clinical research (and most expect it); therefore, make sure to plan some kind of plastic surgery project and get yourself a publication. If you are graduating from a mid-level school, work hard in your courses and rotations to earn membership in AOA. For everyone, it is imperative to score high on the Step I boards, because most programs look for scores around the 90th percentile. In the clinical years, get top grades in your core surgery and plastic surgery rotations. By exposing your limited knowledge of plastic surgery, audition rotations at other hospitals can be disadvantageous—particularly when other programs see that you have gone somewhere else for a subinternship.

Applicants must submit letters of recommendation from the surgery departmental chairperson, the plastic surgery divisional chairperson, and one other plastic surgery attending. (If you apply to general surgery as a backup, make sure you have two sets of letters that refer to the correct specialty.) In the personal statement, discuss your motivations and experience in plastic surgery and highlight any outstanding achievements. Selection committees look closely at academic achievement and reference letters to determine if you are a dependable, honest, smart, and hardworking team player.

Psychiatry

A solid performance in medical school can land you a position in nearly any psychiatry program. The top programs, however, only accept the most stellar of candidates. If you are aiming for these hospitals, high board scores on Steps I and II are helpful. Your clinical performance in the psychiatry clerkship is key to success in matching. In addition, above-average evaluations in other rotations and a thoughtful, complete application are sufficient to garner interviews at some of the best hospitals in the country. Audition subinternships can be helpful for specific programs, but are not completely necessary and may even work against you if your rotation performance goes awry.

Letters of recommendation should come from at least two psychiatrists who know you well in addition to one other clinical faculty member. The personal statement is an extremely important part of the application. It should address your reasons for entering a career in psychiatry and the type of residency program sought. The style must demonstrate maturity, empathy, and honesty.

Radiation Oncology

Over the last several years, this specialty has become ultracompetitive. Nearly all applicants are US seniors at the top of their medical school classes. Many even have a PhD in engineering, physics, or other basic sciences. Because radiation oncology is a very academic field, you should engage in as many scholarly endeavors as possible. Clinical or basic science research—particularly with publications—looks very impressive to selection committees. Find a mentor in radiation oncology and spend time with him or her on a research project or at least in the clinic. You should strive for the best possible scores on the USMLE Step I (at least 220 or above). Membership in AOA is helpful, but not essential. Regardless, try to earn high grades in third-year clerkships. Early in the senior year, take a month-long elective in radiation oncology and work hard to impress your attendings.

Rotations at outside programs are particularly worthwhile for enthusiastic students with less strong academic records. Try to convey your excitement for delving into the scientific literature of the field. Because of the stiff competition, all candidates should submit as many applications as financially possible. You will need three letters of recommendation with at least one from a radiation oncologist who knows you well (even better if he or she is a big name, well-connected, or departmental chairperson). Although the personal statement varies in importance between programs, it should succinctly convince the reader of your passion for radiation oncology (not just for the decent hours and good pay). Program directors look for applicants with intellectual curiosity, competent clinical skills, and a friendly demeanor. If you meet this description, your chances of matching are quite good.

Radiology

As many stellar applicants discover the attractions of diagnostic radiology, this specialty has now become competitive. If you are interested in this specialty, you should immerse yourself in the radiology department at your medical school, particularly during the preclinical years. Clinical research in radiology will improve your chances in matching, particularly at the powerhouse programs with lots of grant money. By starting early, it may be possible to publish papers in radiology journals.

You should, of course, strive for high grades in gross anatomy. Program directors also widely use the USMLE Step I score to screen out applicants. The average score for matching in radiology is reportedly around 220 to 230, with scores higher than 240 necessary for the higher caliber programs. During the clinical years, you should try to earn stellar grades in all of your clinical rotations. Many programs eliminate candidates who have not achieved AOA status. In general, audition rotations do little to improve your chances at matching at that particular program. Unlike in other specialties, as a student, it is difficult to impress radiology attendings and residents with your knowledge and work ethic. At application time, apply to as many programs as you can possibly afford. Most candidates submit between 30 and 50 applications.

The personal statement is the appropriate place to convey that you are smart, hard working, and easy to get along with. Letters of recommendation are helpful from physicians from any number of specialties, as long as they particularly emphasize your ability to work well in a team. In theory, radiology letters do not mean much unless coming from a big name. Due to the extremely competitive nature of this specialty, nearly all program directors recommend ranking preliminary medicine programs at the end of the primary rank list. This way the unsuccessful candidate can reapply while completing the required medicine internship year.

Urology

This specialty is at the top of the list when it comes to being one of the most competitive. Future urologists should immerse themselves in extracurricular activities to distinguish themselves in some way. Clinical research in urology is extremely valuable and can make you shine in the eyes of program directors, especially if it leads to publications or presentations. Many high-powered academic programs even go so far as to require research experience without divulging this to applicants. Basically, you need to excel at everything—particularly in academic achievement. AOA membership is helpful, but not a strict requirement. Study hard during the preclinical years and earn a high score on the USMLE Step I—at least around 220 to 230. (Because urology is an early Match, most programs do not require Step II scores.) Honors grades in the surgery core clerkship and fourth-year urology electives are essential.

Away rotations at other programs are only necessary if there are no well-known urologists at your own institution from whom to request letters of recommendation. You should, however, consider doing a subinternship at one or two of your top-ranked programs. Urology is a very small medical community; therefore, connections are important. Your letters of reference from well-known physicians could make or break your candidacy. Applicants should obtain three to four letters from faculty members who know them well, especially one from the chairperson of urology at their medical school. They are perhaps the most important part of your application. Submit as many applications as financially feasible. The personal statement is relatively important and should be unique and engaging. Make sure to outline clearly the reasons for your interest in urology and to convey that you are diligent, honest, and do not have a large ego. To avoid being unmatched, all candidates should list all acceptable programs that they would be willing to attend (preferable to not training at all in urology) in their desired order.

REFERENCE

1. Cummings, M., Sefcik, D.J. The impact of osteopathic physicians' participation in ACGME-accredited postdoctoral programs, 1985–2006. *Acad Med.* 2009;84(6):733–736.

12

YOUR MEDICAL CAREER BEYOND RESIDENCY

After selecting a specialty, medical students usually postpone thinking about practice options until the residency years. "Why bother worrying about how I will practice until the time gets closer?" most of them insist. Students should remember, however, that it is these two challenging decisions that define every doctor's medical career. The different choices and opportunities that lie ahead for every young physician-in-training range from being a professor of medicine at a university medical center to working on cruise ships all over the world.

Thinking about future practice options does not imply that now is the time to commit to one, especially because your energy should be focused on the more immediate problem at hand—choosing a medical specialty. But it is important to ponder exactly how you might use your specialty training throughout your career. Most medical students find it difficult to map out their long-term career goals and aspirations. To better organize your thinking, ask the following questions with your chosen specialty in mind:

- What do you want to get out of your medical career?
- For whom do you want to work?
- Do you want to be a leader in your specialty?
- How much time do you want to devote to research, teaching, or administrative work?

Planning the medical career you want is just as challenging as choosing the ideal specialty. For both, you must identify your personal and professional goals and find the right match with your personality and work ethic.

145

TO SUBSPECIALIZE OR NOT: THE FELLOWSHIP DECISION

Before considering their practice options, residents in every specialty have to decide whether or not to subspecialize. The additional time spent in fellowship training gives them advanced knowledge and skills—both of which are essential for practicing as an expert in a focused variety of specialty medicine. Depending on the subspecialty, fellowships can last anywhere from 1 year (eg, interventional radiology, obstetric anesthesiology, clinical neurophysiology) to 3 years (eg, gastroenterology, rheumatology, pediatric cardiology). Applying for these fellowship programs (which typically begin about 1 year before the anticipated completion of residency) is much less rigorous and complicated than applying for residency positions. Although some competitive fellowships use a computerized matching system, selection committees look primarily at letters of recommendation, the residency program's reputation, and personal contacts.

Every specialty has its own set of fellowships; however, not all are alike. Most training programs are officially approved by the Accreditation Council of Graduate Medical Education (ACGME). Successful completion makes you eligible to sit for the subspecialty examination, and a passing score leads to full board certification status. Some accredited fellowships, like those in adolescent medicine and geriatric psychiatry, do not yet have board certification examinations and instead bestow a certificate of special achievement as the formal recognition. Another large group of subspecialties—such as cardiac anesthesiology, neuroimmunology, and hyperbaric/undersea medicine—are neither ACGME approved nor lead to board certification. In these cases, the lack of accreditation simply reflects a lack of uniformity across programs. But these fellowships still provide the same clinical experiences and advanced training as their ACGME-approved counterparts. So choose a subspecialty based on your sincere interest and enthusiasm for the subject matter. Your future employers will care about your clinical aptitude, your skills as an excellent subspecialist, and your ability to connect with patients— not about the accreditation of your fellowship program or board certification status.

By adding another layer of medical expertise, fellowship training changes the nature of how a future physician will practice medicine. In fact, many subspecialists have vastly different lifestyles, work schedules, incomes, and patient populations than those practicing in their parent specialty. Internal medicine is a perfect example. General internists spend long hours in clinic evaluating dozens of patients, practicing preventive medicine, and treating common problems such as diabetes, hypertension, and osteoarthritis. They rely on drug therapy as their primary form of intervention. Their colleagues who completed fellowships in cardiology, gastroenterology, and critical care have quite different practices. These subspecialists are usually at the hospital at all hours of the day and night, placing stents in coronary arteries, looking at colons and stomachs through scopes, and manipulating respiratory ventilators. They perform more procedures, earn more money, and practice solely in that one narrow area of medicine.

On the other hand, for some medical fields, subspecializing does not have as much impact on practice style. For example, perhaps because of smaller patient volume, neurologists specializing in headaches or radiologists specializing in abdominal CT have essentially the same professional lives that their colleagues do, with minimal differences in work hours, income, and lifestyle. In fact, these subspecialists usually still practice general neurology and radiology, for instance, more so than their subspecialty area.

Residents who become inspired by a particular organ system or a complex problem within their specialty should seriously consider pursuing a fellowship. The training provides sophisticated knowledge and skills, making you an expert to whom colleagues look for advice and teaching. Knowing one narrow area very well can enhance your career satisfaction and build your professional confidence. With an emphasis on research and scholarly endeavors, fellowships are also great preparation for careers in academic medicine.

Are there any disadvantages to pursuing a fellowship? Just one—the temporary financial sacrifice. You will have to wait several more years before paying off all those big educational debts hanging over your head.

CONVENTIONAL PRACTICE OPTIONS

Private Practice: Delivering the Best Patient Care

Most of you will enter private practice after completing residency or fellowship. In the private sector, physicians either work by themselves or with others, providing high-quality medical care to all types of patients. Because they are not tied strictly to the large academic medical centers, private practitioners have the flexibility to set up shop anywhere in the country—urban, suburban, or rural. Depending on the specialty, you may be working in the office clinic (dermatology, rheumatology, allergy medicine), the hospital (anesthesiology, radiology, pathology), or both (internal medicine, surgery, pediatrics). Some private practitioners also make rounds at other places, such as nursing homes (geriatricians, internists), state facilities (psychiatrists), and prisons (internists, family practitioners).

Although it is generally true that private practitioners earn a great deal of money, they work hard for their salary. With income directly proportional to the number of patients seen or procedures performed, their focus is on patient volume, turnover, and productivity. In return for the higher salary, private practitioners generally sacrifice the opportunity to take care of interesting, complicated cases. Unlike their colleagues in academic medicine, private practice doctors take on a greater proportion of routine bread-and-butter cases. The rare, complex diseases (zebras) are typically referred to specialists at university medical centers.

If you are interested in private practice, the two most common options are going it alone with your own practice or joining a group.

1. *Solo Practice*: With the increasing domination of managed care, fewer physicians undertake solo practice. Those who do can either start their own practice or purchase an existing one (with its fully equipped office and established patient base). Because solo practitioners have complete financial responsibility for their operating expenses, the economic risks are substantial. Many take additional loans to cover their initial start-up and overhead costs until the practice becomes profitable. Until word of mouth increases their case volume, solo physicians have to work long hours building a solid patient base. So why practice on your own? For doctors with an entrepreneurial or administrative side, solo practice provides freedom and autonomy. You can create your own schedule and run your practice any way that you see fit. Without the problem of less-productive partners who could hamper profits, solo practice has a greater potential for a higher income.

2. *Group Practice*: Most residents sign on with group practices at some point during their final year of training. In this form of private practice, two options exist: single-specialty or multispecialty groups. By sharing patient care with colleagues, you have more flexibility for scheduling issues, such as on-call coverage. Being a member of a group provides an established patient base without the overhead cost of starting your own practice. Once you become a full partner in the practice and start sharing in its profits, your salary increases greatly. However, there are shortcomings to group practice. Working in a team means having less autonomy and control over one's work schedule. In fact, because senior doctors prepare the schedules, junior physicians often perform a disproportionate share of the work.

No matter what type of practice you end up having, all private physicians have to deal with many hassles. You will spend hours on the phone with managed care and third-party insurance companies. You will learn more than you ever wanted to know about securing proper reimbursement and coding diagnoses, office visits, and procedures. You will be frustrated by the high premiums for malpractice liability insurance. Additionally, private practitioners need to arrange privileges at local hospitals for either admitting or surgical purposes. Part of every day will be spent driving to different hospitals to round on patients, deliver babies, perform surgery, or administer anesthesia.

Academic Medicine: Shaping the Future of Your Specialty

Medical students who want to be leaders in their specialty should consider a career in academic medicine. A much smaller percentage of physicians work at university hospitals than in the private sector. Academicians serve as medical school faculty members in their specialty's department and also provide patient care at their affiliated teaching hospital. With less emphasis on patient volume and turnover, the pace of academic medicine is more relaxed than that of private practice. Although the job market for new faculty physicians is quite strong, the tertiary care medical centers are usually in major metropolitan areas. This limitation means that academic physicians—whether pediatricians or interventional radiologists— have less geographic flexibility than their counterparts in the private sector.

Although private practitioners deliver patient care to the masses, academic physicians in every specialty and subspecialty have a set of three universal—and equally important—responsibilities.

1. *Teaching*: Every doctor receives residency training in a teaching hospital. By staying there to practice, academic physicians instruct generation after generation of specialists. Much of this time is spent supervising and teaching fellows, residents, and medical students. Through hours of mentorship, academic physicians can make a meaningful difference in their charges professional lives by shaping their formative years of clinical training. These inexperienced young doctors will pepper you with lots of probing questions, keeping you sharp in your specialty. Most faculty members recruited out of residency or fellowship start teaching at the level of assistant professor. Promotion and tenure—just like in nonmedical fields—are directly related to your ability to teach and conduct groundbreaking research.

2. *Research*: Through cutting-edge clinical and basic science research, academic physicians are responsible for advancing their specialty. They generate new knowledge, develop procedures and drugs, and evaluate the efficacy of

different types of treatment. For instance, a general surgeon might conduct a study looking at the best time to take out a chest tube, and an internist investigates the outcomes of treating diabetic and renal failure patients with angiotensin-converting enzyme (ACE) inhibitors. Academic physicians also have to teach their colleagues in private practice about the latest advances in their specialty. They do so by writing up their findings in medical journals and giving lectures at national conferences. To carry out any research project, academic physicians have to obtain the necessary funding—by submitting grants themselves or by receiving money from their department. In the world of academia, the number of papers published and amount of federal research grants received confer prestige on a university medical center. (In a certain weekly news magazine, the formula used to rank US hospitals and medical schools gives the greatest weight to research awards from the National Institutes of Health.)

3. *Patient Care*: In every specialty, academic physicians provide the latest and most innovative medical care. Tertiary medical centers draw a diverse mix of patients, from the indigent (most teaching hospitals are historically located in underserved city neighborhoods) to the very wealthy (eg, Saudi princes who fly in for the most advanced treatment). Most patients receive care directly from residents and fellows, who are supervised by their attending physicians, of course. Compared with private practitioners, full-time faculty members generally take less call, devote fewer hours to patient care, and earn less money. All revenue generated from clinical practice goes directly to the medical center instead of counting as personal income. In turn, the hospital pays each faculty physician a fixed salary that is directly proportional to the type and volume of medicine he or she practices. This is why academic pediatricians earn less than an academic cardiothoracic surgeon.

Academic medicine is perfect for doctors inspired by working with some of medicine's greatest minds—the authors of well-known textbooks, the renowned researchers who develop new drugs and vaccines, the innovators who figured out how to surgically separate two newborns sharing the same brain. Because teaching hospitals are part of major referral centers, academic physicians are the ones who manage most of the rare and complicated cases. You will take care of diseases and conditions on a level that few physicians ever surpass. This career path, therefore, gives you the autonomy to become a true leader in your specialty.

Locum Tenens: The Fill-in Physician

Do you love to travel? Want to avoid all the mundane administrative tasks involved in a typical medical practice? If the answer is yes to both, you might consider practicing medicine locum tenens style for a couple of years. Like independent contractors, locum tenens (Latin for place holder) physicians only work short-term medical jobs. These nomadic doctors are hired to take the place of a physician who is temporarily absent. Hospitals turn to locum tenens to solve any type of staffing shortage: a need for more doctors because of increased patient demand, difficulty attracting newly graduated residents, or simply too many physicians on vacation. Although these options used to be limited to rural hospitals, now even cities and suburbs need their share of temporary doctors. All types of physicians are welcome, but today there is a greater demand for specialists and subspecialists.

Many new doctors fresh out of residency training are taking a closer look at locum tenens practice. They are joining the traditional locum tenens workforce: older doctors who have recently retired or who are just sick of the hassles of their full-time practice. It is quite easy to acquire a locum tenens position right away. You can go to Web sites such as www.locumtenens.com or sign on with national agencies that will find you that ideal short-term job. For a fee, these agencies take care of all the headache-inducing paperwork, such as arranging for malpractice insurance, state licensure, and accommodations. Many hospital employers even pay your travel and living expenses.

What accounts for this newfound interest in locum tenens? This type of practice offers a great deal of flexibility. With most assignments being 2 to 6 weeks long, you can design a month-to-month schedule (including vacation), choosing only the jobs that have hours that suit you. Working a series of temporary jobs in different systems—hospitals, clinics, managed care, group practice—is invaluable experience. It gives a new physician time to figure out what to incorporate in a future practice. It adds a new layer of medical expertise by presenting diseases and clinical problems you might not encounter in other places. Locum tenens also gives you the opportunity to check out different parts of the country, which can help a new physician decide where to set up a practice. At the end of the assignment, it is not uncommon for the employer to offer a full-time position to the stellar locum tenens physician.

There are some less rosy aspects to life roaming the country as a locum tenens physician. They often get their assignments at the last minute, earn less income than a permanent doctor, and face a great deal of pressure to prove their medical skills to their new colleagues. Moreover, life on the road can be hard on your personal life. Most physicians do not make a long-term career out of locum tenens practice. Instead, they pursue it for a couple of years at various points in their careers—beginning, middle, or end—to break the monotony of full-time private practice.

ALTERNATIVE MEDICAL CAREERS

If none of these practice options sounds appealing, there are always the alternative medical careers. Physicians can integrate their highly specialized training into careers outside of traditional medicine. And there is no reason to feel guilty about pursuing a medically related occupation that does not involve direct patient care. Everyone looks at their MD degree in a different light. For some, it could be the foundation for careers in business, law, industry, or even the entertainment world. Instead of worrying about being viewed as an outsider, you should spend your energy drawing on your creativity and resourcefulness to carve out an alternative niche within the medical profession. Let us take a closer look at some of the more popular choices.

Pharmaceutical Industry

Some doctors choose to work as physician-scientists for large pharmaceutical companies. Pharmaceuticals are a multibillion-dollar business, and so they only hire the best and brightest candidates. Physicians are unique, indispensable employees because they have lots of direct experience taking care of patients and they have an in-depth understanding of human pathophysiology. In these companies, physicians from all different specialties come together and apply their collective medical knowledge for a common goal: the development of new drug therapies. Specialists currently in high demand include neurologists, geriatricians, pain specialists, pulmonologists, oncologists, cardiologists, and infectious disease specialists.

Physicians working in the pharmaceutical industry help get new medications approved by the US Food and Drug Administration. They participate in this highly regulated process in many ways, such as administering large-scale double-blind randomized clinical trials or conducting bench laboratory work in pharmacology. By working on a drug that can be delivered to everyone, pharmaceutical physicians can leave a much greater mark on health care than those in traditional practice. They have special insight into what it is like for patients to take the kinds of medications that are being developed. Knowing how drugs can affect a patient's life is essential for figuring out the best way to test a new compound in human clinical trials.

Like their colleagues in academia, doctors working in the pharmaceutical industry have careers in applied medical research involving experimental medications. They spend much of their time designing large-scale clinical trials, interpreting the data through statistical analysis, and presenting reports to the approving authorities. They also travel around the country attending scientific and clinical meetings. As members of multidisciplinary teams, they sacrifice autonomy for the chance to work with other professionals, like those in statistics, product development, and marketing. But industry doctors do not have to worry about securing grant funds, administrative hassles, or promotions—issues that academic physicians face every day. They also have regular hours, good lifestyles, and high incomes with lucrative stock options and bonuses. Clinical activities, however, are kept to a bare minimum (usually only 1 day per week at most).

Federal Government

Millions of Americans live in rural communities without primary health care. If you are committed to a primary care specialty (general internal medicine, family practice, obstetrics–gynecology, general pediatrics, or psychiatry), consider joining the National Health Service Corps (NHSC). This government agency recruits primary care physicians to serve in medically underserved areas—rural and inner city—where adults and children have the greatest need for primary health services. The NHSC offers competitive scholarships for medical students who are committed to this endeavor. They will pay for all 4 years of medical school tuition, fees, and educational expenses (books, etc), as well as provide a monthly stipend for personal use. After residency, the NHSC assigns physicians to practice sites in a federally designated area with a shortage of health professionals. You must serve 1 year for every year of financial support (for a 2-year minimum commitment). Breach of contract results in immediate payback of the entire scholarship. You can also sign on with the NHSC after medical school. They offer a range of loan repayment public-service programs (such as the Indian Health Service Loan Repayment Program) in exchange for a minimum 2-year commitment.

International Medicine

Many physicians volunteer abroad to practice international medicine at some point in their careers. Most are either retired doctors or those who just want to take a break from the grind of day-by-day private practice. Surgeons, anesthesiologists, and primary care physicians are especially needed in countries seeking medical relief. By donating their time and skills, they give themselves selflessly to others who are in desperate need of medical care to ease their suffering. Few experiences can match this level of personal dedication and fulfillment.

There are millions of people in the world today who need this kind of self-sacrificing care. They are refugees, displaced people, or victims of war, epidemics, starvation, disaster, neglect, and widespread infection (particularly tuberculosis, malaria, and AIDS). In regions such as Africa, India, and Central America, volunteer doctors have many responsibilities. They deliver emergency medical care, perform surgery, administer vaccines, and help to construct new hospitals and clinics. They also train the local doctors about the latest medical care and educate the community about basic public hygiene. If this sounds appealing, it is easy to get involved as a volunteer physician. Organizations such as Health Volunteers International, Doctors Without Borders, World Medical Missions, and many religious groups all sponsor short-term medical missions to third-world countries. International medicine gives every physician the opportunity to develop cultural sensitivity and to learn how to deliver medical care in the most rudimentary conditions.

Cruise Ship Medicine

Every large cruise ship needs a doctor on board, holding regular office hours and being on call for emergencies. Like mini-ambulatory centers, these fully equipped medical offices have basic laboratory and x-ray capabilities. To handle the variety of clinical problems that may occur during a cruise, ships usually hire generalist physicians with broad-based skills, such as those in primary care. Specialists in emergency medicine are among the most experienced and sought-after doctors. (In fact, the American College of Emergency Physicians has its own Section of Cruise Ship and Maritime Medicine, which oversees academic fellowships in cruise ship medicine.)

Just like practicing in an emergency room or urgent care center, cruise ship medicine is full of the unexpected. You have to be ready to treat all types of minor or severe medical and surgical problems, from traveler's diarrhea and seasickness to passengers who fall overboard or have encounters with marine creatures. Younger patients come in with injuries related to sports or alcohol use. Most passengers, however, are older men and women with chronic medical conditions (like heart failure or emphysema) who can present with complications while traveling. Cruise ship doctors have to know how to handle emergencies such as heart attacks, strokes, arrhythmias, respiratory failure, blood clots, and fractures. They need to be skilled in cardiopulmonary resuscitation, intubation, and rapid evacuation. It can be an exciting clinical practice on the high seas!

Special Fortes

There are dozens of other ways for a physician to diversify his or her career opportunities. After all, a medical degree is a unique and invaluable asset to other professions as well. For the creative physician, lots of possibilities exist. Here are just a few more examples

- If you have an interest in broadcasting and media, you could sign on as a correspondent for local news channels, helping them with their nightly health segments.
- For the writers and budding authors out there, the field of medical writing is a great option for any specialist. Check out the American Medical Writers Association for examples of opportunities in continuing medical education, fiction, marketing, promotion, and patient education.
- Doctors who like a university setting often work at student health centers.
- Interested in medical informatics? When it comes to patient care documentation, all physicians will have to get accustomed to Electronic Health Records (EHR). Companies who develop the software interface need doctors who are familiar with coding and computer science.
- Some orthopedic surgeons become personal physicians for major athletic teams.
- If you have a penchant for business, consider going for an MBA and then entering a career in health care, market research, venture capital, or even investment banking.
- Physicians who hold a Juris Doctor (JD) can sign on with law firms, become expert witnesses, and defend (or prosecute) other doctors, hospitals, or managed care organizations.
- Careers in public health are great alternatives for physicians who have obtained a Masters in Public Health (MPH) degree. You could work in areas such as epidemiology for organizations such as the National Institutes of Health or the Centers for Disease Control and Prevention.
- MDs with an interest in medical education are often hired by commercial test preparation companies to prepare test questions and teach courses.
- Doctors with a burning desire to initiate legislative change in the US health care system can enter political careers. Several prominent members of Congress are current or former physicians.
- Have a knack for human resources? You can become an executive recruiter (also known as a "headhunter") and earn a hefty commission-based salary for a recruitment firm.

Is there any relationship between a physician's specialty and his or her choice of an alternative medical career? One study sought to answer this question by asking senior medical students what alternate career they would have pursued had they not entered the medical profession.[1] Students who were entering anesthesiology, radiology, surgery, and internal medicine were more likely to choose substitute careers in more highly technical fields—science, research, engineering, business, architecture, or law. Future pediatricians, family practitioners, psychiatrists, pathologists, obstetricians–gynecologists, and emergency medicine specialists were more likely to consider alternate careers in a helping/humanities category—teaching, journalism, writing, the arts, other health professions (such as dentistry), and nonprofessional careers (such as airplane pilot). These findings suggest that all physicians enter medical school with certain personality traits that not only influence their specialty choice but also their desired career path (whether alternative or traditional).

The options for careers outside the traditional realm of clinical medicine are basically unlimited. If you are imaginative, resourceful, determined, and assertive, you can find your own niche within the professional world and have a long, satisfying career—in any specialty.

REFERENCE

1. Rabinowitz, H.K., Rosenthal, M.P., et al. Alternate career choices of medical students: Their relationship to choice of specialty. *Fam Med*. 1993;25:665–667.

2
SPECIALTY PROFILES

13

ANESTHESIOLOGY

Brian S. Freeman

E ther. Chloroform. Nitrous oxide. Because they are widely popularized in popular culture, you are probably well aware of the first universally accepted general anesthetics. The anesthesiologist's domain, however, extends far beyond these drugs. It is unfortunate that many medical schools do not require a rotation in anesthesiology, sedation/analgesia, and pain management. Most students do not come to medical school intending to become anesthesiologists. Instead, they likely share the common misperception that anesthesiologists are scientific technicians who just "put people to sleep." Nothing could be farther from the truth. They are doctors whose lives are dedicated toward a noble goal: the relief of pain. They thrive on the fast pace of acute medical care. They are often the unsung heroes of the operating room (OR).

THE SPECIALTY OF PERIOPERATIVE MEDICINE

Anesthesiology is dedicated to the complete medical and anesthetic care of the surgical patient. It is a precise, technical, and intellectual specialty that requires high standards and attention to detail. Anesthesiologists care for the whole patient— before, during, and after the operation. They administer powerful anesthetics, render patients insensible to pain and stress, provide respiratory support, and manage every medical need of the patient throughout the surgical experience. To do so, anesthesiologists closely monitor and treat the acute pathophysiology of multiple organ systems: cardiac, pulmonary, renal, endocrine, hematologic, and neurologic. It is a specialty that ties together the cerebral nature of internal medicine with the procedural interventions and life-support of critical care medicine.

But anesthesiologists are more than just "operating room internists." In ORs across the country, they often end up saving lives. Every anesthetic administered

WHAT MAKES A GOOD ANESTHESIOLOGIST?

✓ Can pay attention to detail for long periods of time.
✓ Likes working with his or her hands.
✓ Can make fast decisions during stressful, rapidly changing situations.
✓ Is a congenial, confident, easy-going person.
✓ Likes to see immediate results of his or her efforts.

THE INSIDE SCOOP

involves some element of "resuscitation" — even for simple cases or healthy patients. But when sick patients truly crash on the table, the anesthesiologist comes to their rescue. Remember the ABCs (airway, breathing, circulation)? These concepts are essential to safe perioperative care. As such, anesthesiologists have contributed immensely to advances in cardiopulmonary resuscitation and airway management.

The role of anesthesiologists as perioperative physicians has become increasingly diverse and complex. Although anesthesiologists are primarily involved in the action of the OR, they also offer anesthetic consultations in many other settings. In fact, the anesthesiologist is probably the only physician who is comfortable with the entire spectrum of clinical medicine. They provide care in every single component of the hospital: ORs, intensive care units, labor and delivery, patient wards, emergency departments, radiology suites, and outpatient clinics (preoperative testing and pain medicine). They interact with a diverse set of colleagues, from neurosurgeons and obstetricians to interventional radiologists and gastroenterologists. Many physicians will call upon an anesthesiologist for advice on pre- and postoperative medical management or for assistance in managing cardiopulmonary or airway problems.

It may surprise you that anesthesiology is both a highly focused specialty and a field of medicine that, in a way, is quite broad. Like their colleagues in family practice and emergency medicine, anesthesiologists care for patients of all ages, ranging from neonates to geriatrics. Within this spectrum, the surgical patient can also present with any number of complex diseases, from systemic lupus erythematosus to coronary artery disease. Thus, the practice of anesthesiology requires knowledge of all aspects of clinical medicine, whether from pediatrics, internal medicine, obstetrics, or surgery. Intraoperative medical consultations do not exist in the world of anesthesiology. In the OR, the anesthesiologist also becomes the patient's cardiologist, pulmonologist, endocrinologist, etc, and treats problems such as myocardial ischemia, bronchospasm, and soaring potassium levels. Every patient requires a different strategy to match anesthetic needs with his or her underlying medical conditions and procedural requirements. Because of extensive progress in anesthesiology, critically ill patients can now undergo even more complicated operations and surgical procedures.

ESSENTIALS OF ANESTHESIA

Anesthesiology is a specialty in which the clinical application of many basic sciences becomes most palpable. Your fundamental knowledge base draws heavily on the key principles of physiology, pathophysiology, and pharmacology. This is why anesthesiologists are different from "traditional" doctors. Typically, they neither diagnose nor treat disease. Instead, anesthesiologists must have an intimate understanding of their patient's altered physiology, such as mitral regurgitation, hyperthyroidism, or end-stage renal disease. Good patient care in this specialty requires maintaining physiologic homeostasis in the face of three potent stressors: an invasive surgical procedure, powerful anesthetic agents, and the patient's underlying disease states (which may not be treated or optimized). The art of differential diagnosis, therefore, is much different in anesthesiology than in, for example, internal medicine. You will become *the* expert on diagnosing and treating acute, life-threatening physiologic derangements: airway obstruction, high (and low) blood pressure, cyanosis, abnormal cardiac rhythms, massive hemorrhage, catecholamine surges, acidosis, low urine output, and much more. For sick patients undergoing the stress of major surgery and anesthesia, treating vital sign aberrations in the OR can be quite challenging!

To maintain physiologic homeostasis, anesthesiologists are experts on the latest advances in clinical pharmacology and drug delivery systems. Every day, they use an impressive arsenal of drugs: potent inhalational and intravenous anesthetics, local anesthetics, opioids, sedatives, cardioactive agents, neuromuscular paralytics, and many more. And what could be more fascinating than altering someone's level of consciousness? Be forewarned, however—this responsibility is great. Anesthesiologists use powerful drugs that can kill people. They are the only physicians who bypass pharmacists and nurses to dose, prepare, and administer the drugs themselves. These agents cause immediate physiologic outcomes that, for an anesthesiologist, provide instant gratification. In a way, each surgical case offers the opportunity to test a physiologic hypothesis with a pharmacologic intervention. Most medical students are attracted to this specialty because of the pace of acute care in the OR. "You get to use powerful drugs to correct problems in physiology—and the solutions come to life right in front of your eyes," one physician commented. "Unlike the slow pace of other specialties, I never have to wait months to see if my manipulations work."

The seal of the American Society of Anesthesiologists (a lighthouse inscribed with the motto "vigilance") symbolizes the importance of good patient monitoring. You will always focus on one patient at a time. If you want to become an anesthesiologist, you should feel comfortable manipulating monitors, pumps, ventilators, and other high-tech equipment. Anesthesiologists communicate with their unconscious patients by monitoring their physiology. Although they are the guardians of patients' lives during surgery, anesthesiologists do not simply stare at monitors all day long. These doctors keep a close eye on the patient and the case itself, which is equally as important, and watch for potential problems such as acute blood loss or compromised airways. As attentive observers of physiologic parameters, anesthesiologists become adept at multitasking. While listening to the beeping pulse oximeter and the sounds of suction, they monitor the patient's electrocardiographic rhythm, follow alterations in blood pressure, and integrate changes in urine output in their management.

To achieve such crucial goals on a minute-by-minute basis, anesthesiologists make use of a wide array of complex monitoring equipment. These include end-tidal CO_2 monitors, pulse oximetry, invasive cardiovascular pressure monitors, Swan-Ganz catheters, arterial blood gas analysis, neuromuscular monitors, and electrocardiography—plus more sophisticated tools such as real-time transesophageal echocardiography. Anesthesiology is therefore a great specialty for medical students who wish to incorporate the latest advances in biomedical engineering into their careers. Because of their skills in patient monitoring, anesthesiologists have greatly improved patient safety and allowed for the development of more advanced and invasive procedures.

From beginning to end, the practice of anesthesiology for each patient is similar to flying an airplane. As captain, the anesthesiologist first conducts a complete preoperative history and physical examination. Induction of anesthesia, using powerful drugs such as sevoflurane or propofol, represents the "take-off" into the flight of the procedure. This part is more than just pushing medications— anesthesiologists have to set up the appropriate monitoring equipment and then secure the patient's airway. Once the patient is fully anesthetized, paralyzed, and breathing by a ventilator, maintenance has been achieved. Like a pilot, the anesthesiologist keeps careful watch over the patient, always adjusting physiologic parameters with pharmacologic agents as the case proceeds. Any OR crises ("turbulence") require rapid interventions and quick thinking. The captain then lands the "anesthesia plane" by reversing neuromuscular paralysis, assessing cardiopulmonary stability, discontinuing the anesthetic, and safely extubating the patient. This basic process applies to the five major types of anesthesia: general, epidural, spinal, peripheral nerve block, and monitored anesthesia care (MAC).

COPING WITH INTRAOPERATIVE EMERGENCIES

Once the surgical patient becomes successfully anesthetized with a secure airway, the operation is off and running. In a routine case, such as an appendectomy in a healthy young man, most of the anesthesiologist's time is spent monitoring the patient and his vital signs. The anesthesiologist, not the surgeon, is responsible for making sure that the unconscious patient wakes up at the end of the case alive, well, and breathing spontaneously.

Performing anesthesia can be much more dangerous than it looks, however. For all types of operations, anesthesiologists perform difficult tasks in a life-threatening environment. Always concerned that something may go wrong, anesthesiologists mentally prepare for any potential disasters during every case. Many describe their job as being "90% routine care, 10% sheer terror." Complications can arise due to the patient's pathophysiology or from anesthetic (such as an airway or nerve block complication) or surgical misadventures. When patients deteriorate during surgery, they can crash fast. Whether the problem involves massive acute hemorrhaging, intraoperative myocardial infarction, or dropping oxygen saturation, anesthesiologists must think fast, act quickly, and draw on their vast medical knowledge to make on-the-spot decisions.

Today, many surgical patients are quite sick with multiple medical problems, leading to rather complicated intraoperative courses. For example, under general anesthesia, even a patient with "only" a history of high blood pressure can create problems for the anesthesiologist. Maintaining the patient's blood pressure within normal limits is quite challenging in the face of faulty sympathetic responses and other homeostatic mechanisms. Moreover, bad things typically happen all at once. While dealing with a plummeting blood pressure, the pulse oximeter alarm will probably start beeping (indicating rapid oxygen desaturation) and the patient will likely start twitching and moving.

Rapid decision making, therefore, is extremely important. Working with the surgeon, anesthesiologists guard the line between life and death for the unconscious surgical patient. Medical students interested in this field should be aware that anesthesiology requires one to react well to nerve-wracking situations. You will transfuse more blood than any other physician. A patient can die very fast

RESIDENCY TRAINING

Residency in anesthesiology requires 4 years of postgraduate training. It requires an internship year (PGY-1), plus 3 years of clinical anesthesiology (CA-1 to CA-3). There are currently 131 accredited programs. The PGY-1 internship year can be internal medicine, surgery, or transitional. The first 2 months of residency usually include a tutorial, in which new residents work alongside a single attending. Residents are also responsible for emergency intubations when respiratory failure or cardiac arrests occur on the medical wards. Due to implications for patient safety, the American Board of Anesthesiology does not allow residents to work more than 24 consecutive hours in a shift. As a result, all programs permit residents to leave the hospital at 7:00 AM after their night on call. Residents average about 60 hours on duty per week. The typical monthly rotations include general OR, obstetrics, cardiothoracic, vascular, orthopedics, pain service and clinic, gynecology, urology, ambulatory/regional, critical care, and pediatrics. Based on case volume, the strength of any anesthesiology department correlates with the strength of the surgical department. Board certification involves both written and oral examinations after completion of residency.

THE INSIDE SCOOP

under your hands, making anesthesiology a more stressful field of medicine than most.

MASTERS OF THE AIRWAY

Anesthesiology is, without a doubt, a highly procedure-oriented, hands-on specialty. You will place intravenous and arterial lines, administer ultrasound-guided peripheral nerve blocks, perform direct laryngoscopy, and mask ventilate patients left and right. This is where the science of anesthesiology becomes an art form. After all, smooth anesthesia is equally as important as secure anesthesia. An anesthesiologist in academics believes that "anyone can inject someone with thiopental, but being able to smoothly do fiberoptic intubation and ventilating only one lung, now that is an art!"

Anesthesiologists' manual dexterity and expertise in the art of intubation make them masters of the airway. Both in and out of the OR, they perform thousands of these procedures throughout their career. Craving an adrenaline rush? Anesthesiologists are often called to the emergency room, intensive care unit, or patient floors to deal with the emergency management of a difficult airway.

Like all practical skills in medicine, the relative ease of endotracheal intubation reflects the technical dexterity of the anesthesiologist. During the preoperative clinic visits, the anesthesiologist conducts a thorough history and physical examination to identify potential airway problems in the patient, then prepares the proper instruments needed for intubation. The choices are many: different endotracheal tube styles, multiple laryngoscope blades, fiberoptic bronchoscopes, laryngeal mask airways, light wands, and nasal airways. It is kind of like having your own fancy toolset. During residency training, many hospitals offer simulated instruction on computerized mannequins to practice intubating patients with difficult airways. For medical students who enjoy a good mix of technical skill and intellectual challenge, anesthesiology may be the ideal specialty.

THE DOCTOR–PATIENT RELATIONSHIP

Most surgery patients feel reassured after spending time with the anesthesiologist, whose face is the last they see before losing consciousness. This specialty offers more than an intellectual challenge and a good lifestyle; it allows physicians to make a profound impact on their patients' lives. Anesthesiologists' contact with patients may be limited in duration but extremely intense and rewarding in scope.

The preoperative consultation, a key interaction, involves more than taking medical histories and performing physical examinations. This quality time is spent answering questions about the planned anesthetic care and allaying patients' anxiety. Anesthesiologists need excellent interpersonal skills to comfort patients who are terrified of surrendering control of their lives under general anesthesia. They help patients emotionally who are undergoing one of the most stressful episodes in their lives. The best anesthesiologists are compassionate, sensitive, and supportive. Because of the specialty's emphasis on procedures, they must recognize that often one has to hurt somebody a little to help a lot. At all times, anesthesiologists are quick with a smile or a hand on the shoulder to foster comfort with their nervous patients. In most cases, empathy and compassion have a more lasting effect than premedication. Patient interactions, therefore, are always positive.

Although the relationships between anesthesiologists and their patients can be extremely rewarding, these physicians remain largely anonymous to health care consumers. Most anesthesiologists do not have their own group of patients, nor do patients undergoing surgery choose their anesthesiologist. As a result, the general public has never completely understood the critical role of the anesthesiologist in surgical care. Many patients are unaware that these physicians have received the same length of training as most other doctors. Thus, medical students should know that this specialty, unlike more glamorous ones, rarely brings a lifestyle of fame, fortune, and glory.

"After surgery, most patients only remember the name of their surgeon, not their anesthesiologist. We never hand out business cards, and we never get interviewed on television for helping to save a trauma victim," said a university-based anesthesiologist. "A patient who never mentions their anesthesia experience is the one who is the satisfied customer. It means that the patient made it safely through surgery without pain. That is when I can go home feeling gratified I did a good job for the day."

If you want to become a world-renowned expert to whom patients come from all over the world, anesthesiology is probably not for you. Like other hospital-based specialists, such as those in radiology and emergency medicine, anesthesiologists do not depend on recognition from their patients for ego gratification. Instead, these behind-the-scenes doctors simply derive their personal satisfaction from within. Subspecializing in pain management or critical care can provide a more traditional doctor–patient relationship. A few institutions also offer combined 5-year programs with internal medicine or pediatrics. By earning additional board certification in either internal medicine or pediatrics, you can also establish a traditional long-term medical practice outside of the operating room.

BELOW THE BLOOD–BRAIN BARRIER: RELATIONSHIPS WITH SURGEONS AND STAFF

One medical student who completed a rotation in this specialty commented that "anesthesiologists seem like mellow and easy-going people." Lacking huge egos, they are collegial physicians who communicate well with others. Although they are a diverse group not dominated by any particular personality type, all anesthesiologists have a high degree of intellectual curiosity.

Because of their relaxed disposition, anesthesiologists usually have excellent working relationships with OR personnel, particularly surgeons. After all, many medical students interested in this specialty shudder at the thought of working with the stereotypical surgeon who curses, throws instruments, and yells at the entire OR staff, including the anesthesiologist. In most hospitals, however, the days when the surgeon was the captain of the ship are over. Instead, anesthesiologists now share leadership responsibility. As directors of the OR, anesthesiologists inform the surgeons when they should start, stop, and continue operating. As a consultant in perioperative medicine to the surgeon, this relationship is quite unique.

Unfortunately, relationships with OR staff in academic teaching hospitals are sometimes more problematic. In this setting (where anesthesiology slowly developed as a rigorous academic discipline but under the control of surgery departments), many attending surgeons neither understand nor appreciate the important role of the anesthesiologist. They prefer, instead, to boost their egos by attempting to exert power in the OR in front of their residents, students, and nurses. Here, OR nurses tend to jump for the surgeons first, anesthesiologists second. These ancillary staff members, who watch the anesthesiologist transporting patients and starting intravenous lines, sometimes continue to buy into the old captain of the ship mentality. A good academic anesthesiologist, therefore, knows both when and how to assert leadership and to take charge as the primary physician during times of crisis.

In community hospitals and private practice, the relationship is quite different. Here, one hand feeds the other. The surgeon relies on the anesthesiologist to keep the patient alive, safe, and pain free during the perioperative experience. By controlling turnover time between patients, anesthesiologists dictate the pace of the OR and, consequently, its profits. Like the host at a busy restaurant, they coordinate the OR schedule. In return, the anesthesiologist depends on the surgeon to provide case volume. In private practice, surgeons who upset their anesthesiologist with disrespectful comments may find them slowing down preoperative assessments and inductions, delaying or even canceling cases, and hampering profitability. You can see that this relationship is mutual. In most private practice settings, anesthesiologists and surgeons work together as a team, with respect and affability.

ANESTHESIOLOGISTS AND DRUG ADDICTION

The problem of chemical dependency is particularly prevalent in anesthesiology. Among physicians, anesthesiologists, who primarily abuse major opioids, reportedly have the highest incidence of drug addiction.[1] They comprise approximately 4% of all US physicians but make up about 12% to 15% of all doctors currently in addiction treatment programs.[2] However, the significance of the prevalence of drug addiction in anesthesiology, as compared with other specialties, is somewhat controversial. Anesthesia departments are better trained than others to detect early signs of addiction. Increased awareness of drug abuse, rather than greater frequency, may lead to an unusually high statistical representation of drug-abusing anesthesiologists. Moreover, another study found the highest levels of self-reported drug dependence not among anesthesiologists but among psychiatrists (who abuse benzodiazepines) and emergency room doctors (who take illicit drugs).[3]

Regardless of drug or practice environment, physician substance abuse is a serious and universal problem.

There are several reasons why anesthesiologists are three times more likely than other physicians to start abusing drugs. They regularly administer highly addictive drugs (such as fentanyl and sufentanil) that most physicians never prescribe. They are among the few specialists that actually prepare and dose intravenous narcotics themselves (usually done by a pharmacist). As a result, they have easy access to controlled substances, whether by blatant stealing, falsifying records, or switching syringes. They may become especially curious about the effects of the drugs they administer and want to experience what the patient feels. Finally, anesthesiologists are often under a great deal of stress. They have to cope with responsibility for a patient's life, pressure for rapid turnover time, anxiety that a minor error can cause a patient to die, and fatigue. The sheer strain of this specialty may cause an anesthesiologist to be susceptible to chemical dependency.

Because physician drug addiction is a concern in every specialty, this issue should not discourage medical students from considering anesthesiology. But medical students who have a personal history of substance abuse, whether of alcohol or illicit drugs, should be wary of the possible occupational hazard in anesthesiology. Because of the daily temptation, recovery and reentry into the OR environment can be exceptionally difficult. Most departments of anesthesiology have developed excellent mechanisms to identify individuals who may be susceptible to addiction. After all, the consequences are quite damaging. Depending on the point of their career, addicted anesthesiologists can lose their medical license, job, residency program position, or, at the worst, their life. A recent mortality study found that anesthesiologists are, compared with internists, at twice the risk of drug-related suicide and three times the risk of any drug-related death.[4] Although anesthesiologists are recognized as leaders in patient safety, their occupation can, at times, place their own lives at risk.

LIFESTYLE CONSIDERATIONS AND PRACTICE OPTIONS

Although all anesthesiologists must become morning people due to the early start times of surgery, their lifestyle is rather enjoyable. The hours of patient care are predictable and scheduled. This means that your time spent out of the hospital is nicely protected. Unless you are on call, do not expect to be bothered by middle-of-the-night pages. The frequency of call depends on the size and type of practice and whether the hospital offers trauma and obstetric services. Recent surveys of lifestyle differences among various specialists show that anesthesiologists are the biggest news and stock market junkies, tend to listen to rock music, are highly satisfied with their marriages and sex lives, spend a lot of time surfing the Internet, and avidly attend films and rent videos.[5,6]

As an anesthesiologist, your career can follow many different directions. The practice environments are as diverse as the patient population. Most choose the traditional role of personally administering anesthesia in the OR and taking care of patients perioperatively. Practice modes also vary from physician-delivered anesthesia in busy ambulatory surgicenters to leadership of an anesthesia care team (residents, Certified Registered Nurse Anesthetists [CRNAs], and anesthesia assistants). Others draw on their business and administrative skills to become medical directors of ORs or intensive care units. Academic anesthesiologists spend their time teaching new residents and conducting innovative research on topics ranging from clinical pharmacology to improvements in patient safety. For those seeking longer patient interactions and continuity of care, the subspecialty of pain management has become very popular. Many anesthesiologists are joining freestanding pain clinics where they perform interventional pain management procedures. No matter the role, anesthesiologists remain the experts on determining perioperative risk and the safest way to care for critically ill patients.

A PRIMER ON THE ANESTHESIOLOGIST–CRNA DEBATE

Many medical students considering a career in anesthesiology often wonder about job security due to the presence of CRNAs. Today, many groups of non-MD mid-level health care providers are seeking more autonomy to increase their scope of practice. Primary care doctors, for instance, work with both physician assistants and nurse practitioners. Yet, when medical students gossip about "doctors being replaced by nurses," the CRNA issue seems to surface more than any other. The notion of anesthesiology as a threatened specialty destined for take over by nurse anesthetists is erroneous. By helping to set up and monitor patients, CRNAs reduce the overall physical work in the OR and allow the anesthesiologist to oversee multiple cases at once, thus increasing efficiency.

The differences between the two providers are significant. Although anesthesiologists are true perioperative physicians, CRNAs, like other nurses, have a knowledge base that is primarily experiential and practical. During their short training, they learn the basics of administering anesthesia, especially the necessary procedural skills. After all, most technical abilities in medicine—such as taking history and physicals, delivering uncomplicated pregnancies, and suturing—can be taught to capable mid-level providers, whether nurse practitioners, midwives, or physician assistants. But when life-threatening emergencies arise, nurse anesthetists need the supervising anesthesiologist to come to their aid. This is why they are the principal providers of anesthesia care (under physician supervision) in rural hospitals, where routine bread-and-butter surgical cases abound. The tertiary medical centers of metropolitan regions, with its sophisticated care and disproportionately sickest patients, rarely rely on only nurse anesthetists for their anesthesia services. A study of Medicare patients found a higher mortality rate during surgery and failure to rescue from complications when an anesthesiologist was not either directing or significantly involved in care.[7]

Anesthesiologists' depth of training and breadth of knowledge allow them to make rapid decisions and exercise clinical judgment. Their understanding of pathophysiology and pharmacology far surpasses that of nurse anesthetists. Critically ill patients undergoing complicated surgery, whether they have underlying scleroderma or develop a malignant arrhythmia, require anesthesiologists to make life-saving cognitive judgments in addition to technical interventions. They are the ones who can capably perform regional anesthesia, invasive monitoring techniques, and other procedures that require skill and judgment. They also oversee interventional pain management and are heavily engaged in research to advance the field as a whole. Anesthesiologists conducting basic science and clinical research have made many significant innovations, such as improved anesthetic agents, advanced patient monitoring, and new pharmacologic therapy.

Since 1966, the federal government has required that a physician must oversee the delivery of anesthesia care in Medicare cases because of safety issues. The debate over whether to eliminate the physician supervision requirement was a key element of the Clinton administration's health care reform plans. In January 2001, 2 days before leaving office, President Clinton signed the bill that would have allowed CRNAs to give anesthetics to patients without being supervised by a doctor. But in recent national polls, an overwhelming majority of Medicare beneficiaries and aging baby boomers opposed eliminating the physician supervision requirement.[8]

Upon arrival in office, therefore, the Bush administration suspended the bill for further review by the Center for Medicare and Medicaid Services. The final federal rule, published in November 2001, stipulates that every Medicare- and Medicaid-approved health care facilities require physician supervision of nurse anesthetists. On the state level, governors can petition for an exemption after consulting with state boards of medicine and nursing and determining that this change is consistent with state law and in the best interest of its citizens. As expected, the only states considering an opt out from the physician supervision requirement are those with large rural and underserved areas that cannot attract anesthesiologists (or other specialists). Moreover, many patients undergoing surgery today have multiple and complex medical problems. If a hospital requires physician supervision of nurse anesthesia services, the surgeon would be held legally accountable for the nurses' actions.[9] Would any surgeon really want to take on this additional responsibility and liability? Regardless of resolutions made at state level, the final decision over these scopes of practice issues lies with the hospitals and operating facilities themselves. They are the entities ultimately responsible for patient safety in the OR.

Although the political lobbying continues today, this bureaucratic debate should in no way discourage medical students from considering a career in anesthesiology. As discussed in Chapter 2, the current and projected shortage of anesthesiologists has created a robust job market with lucrative offers and high salaries. Anesthesiology departments at many academic medical centers are recruiting new faculty. It is also well known that the nursing profession has experienced a significant decline in recruitment for the past several years. Within this shrinking group of health providers, CRNAs make up a very small minority of nurses, especially compared with the much larger group of nurse practitioners. In one recent workforce study, CRNAs, the majority of whom are close to retirement age, are the only nonphysician providers among ten groups that are projected to decline further in the next two decades.[10]

Because CRNAs will always have a role in dispensing health care, the practice of anesthesiology has morphed into the anesthesia care team model. Its members may include anesthesiology residents, nurse anesthetists, anesthesiology assistants (AAs), respiratory therapists, and recovery-room nurses. As the senior expert, the anesthesiologist medically directs and delegates responsibility to team members for the technical aspects of anesthesia care. The anesthesiologist is responsible for preoperative medical evaluations, the creation and implementation of anesthetic plans, and personal participation in the most challenging procedures (such as those involved in induction and emergence). The final responsibility and direction lies with the anesthesiologist. Therefore, future anesthesiologists will have multiple responsibilities: managing the ORs, taking care of sick patients undergoing complicated surgery, and supervising mid-level anesthesia providers.

FELLOWSHIPS AND SUBSPECIALTY TRAINING

Pain Management

The multidisciplinary field of pain medicine applies the principles of anesthesiology outside of the OR. Both acute and chronic pain is an extremely common complaint of patients. As such, there is a rapidly growing demand for specialists who can manage different pain syndromes. A typical patient is often an injured employee on workers' compensation. Anesthesiologists who specialize in pain management see patients in a clinic setting, such as a freestanding pain center. Here, the continuity of care lends itself to a more traditional doctor–patient relationship. They diagnose the etiology of pain syndromes and treat these problems with medication or procedural therapy (injections of local anesthetics, peripheral and central nerve blocks under fluoroscopy, implantation of spinal cord stimulators and intrathecal pumps, and transcutaneous nerve stimulation). In pain management, you can also earn certification in performing acupuncture.

Because of the emphasis on procedures, pain medicine has become a lucrative area of expertise. However, you must be able to handle drug-seeking patients, chronic problems that sometimes fail to respond to treatment, and increasing competition from neurologists and physiatrists. In the academic setting, pain specialists often conduct research on the pathophysiologic mechanisms of pain. Regardless of the practice model, most patients consider you their personal hero for having alleviated their pain and suffering. A fellowship in pain management typically lasts 1 to 2 years following residency. The American Board of Anesthesiology (ABA) offers a specialty examination for board certification.

Critical Care Medicine

Anesthesiologists are natural and highly sought-after intensivists. By specializing in critical care medicine, they apply their ability to make rapid clinical assessments, treat acute pathophysiologic problems, and perform a variety of procedures. Anesthesiologist–intensivists serve as medical directors of surgical and cardiac intensive care units, where they manage the complicated postoperative care of critically ill patients. Because anesthesiologists care for very sick patients during surgery, their domain logically extends into the sophisticated medical care of intensive care units. Critical care specialists with training in anesthesiology bring unsurpassed airway management skills, as well as expertise in monitoring, mechanical ventilation, fluid resuscitation, and other forms of high-tech life support.

Because pulmonary medicine physicians are the most prevalent specialists in intensive care, most medical students are unaware that anesthesiologists also practice as intensivists. The numbers, though, are small: anesthesiology-trained intensivists in the United States make up 4% of all anesthesiologists and provide 6% of critical care.[11] In contrast, their colleagues in Europe, who provide the majority of intensive care, have a much more dominant role. Despite the low interest, the aging US population will greatly

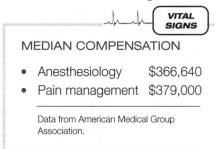

VITAL SIGNS

MEDIAN COMPENSATION

- Anesthesiology $366,640
- Pain management $379,000

Data from American Medical Group Association.

increase the demand for critical care services, particularly access to a full-time intensivist. Critical care fellowships typically require 1 year of additional training, after which you are qualified to take the ABA specialty board examination for certification.

Subspecialties

Several subspecialty areas of anesthesiology have evolved to meet the needs of increasingly advanced operations. Currently, these areas include cardiac, pediatric, obstetric, regional, ambulatory, and neuroanesthesia. By receiving special training in one of these subspecialties, an anesthesiologist can better manage the pathophysiology of intricate surgical cases, create more complicated anesthetic strategies, and, of course, optimize job opportunities. Cardiac anesthesia, a popular option, allows an anesthesiologist to gain expertise in sophisticated intraoperative techniques, such as hemodynamic monitoring and cardiopulmonary bypass, and earn certification in transesophageal echocardiography. Most of these fellowships require 1 additional year of training. At this time, pediatric anesthesiology will be the next subspecialty fellowship to offer a board examination.

WHY CONSIDER A CAREER IN ANESTHESIOLOGY?

The discovery of anesthesia and the ability to perform surgery without the sensation of pain remains one of the greatest accomplishments of medicine. October 16, 1846—the first public demonstration of anesthesia—was an important date for all anesthesiologists. In the now-famous Ether Dome of the Massachusetts General Hospital, Dr William Morton administered the first anesthetic (ether) to a patient undergoing neck surgery. To the amazement of the skeptical surgeon

~~~~~ **VITAL SIGNS**

ANESTHESIOLOGY 2011 MATCH STATISTICS

- Number of positions available: 1404
- 1079 US seniors and 359 independent applicants ranked at least one anesthesiology program
- 96.4% of all positions were filled in the initial Match
- The successful applicants: 78.5% US seniors, 7.4% foreign-trained physicians, and 8.4% osteopathic graduates
- Mean United States Medical Licensing Examination (USMLE) Step I score: 226
- Unmatched rate for US seniors applying only to anesthesiology: 2.8%

Data from National Resident Matching Program.

and observers, the patient did not scream at the moment of first incision near his tumor. Since that time, more and more anesthetics followed: cyclopropane, halothane, sevoflurane, propofol, and many others. Today, the field of anesthesiology has made incredible progress in patient care, safety, and quality. Yet, in spite of these achievements, the mechanism of how general anesthetics actually work continues to remain largely a mystery.

If you are considering a career in anesthesiology, the future looks very bright. The current data project a significant shortage of anesthesiologists for the next 10 years.[12] Anesthesiology was one of the most competitive specialties to match in the 1980s and early 1990s. After a substantial drop in applicants in the 1990s, it is poised for a remarkable comeback, as the specialty's popularity has skyrocketed today among top graduates from US medical schools. In 2002, while only 6% of all US seniors entered the field of anesthesiology, there was a 27% increase in applicants, which led to the lowest number of unfilled residency positions in the history of the anesthesia match.[13]

Anesthesiology is a challenging, fast-paced field that combines many aspects of medicine: on-the-spot differential diagnoses, the use of advanced pharmacology to correct problems in physiology, rewarding patient contact, and hands-on procedures. Every day, you are given the inspiring, yet humbling, responsibility of keeping patients safe during surgery. After all, anesthesiologists "are doctors who keep patients alive while surgeons do things that would otherwise kill them."[14] As their guardian and advocate, you protect their lives during a time when they cannot do so themselves. Some might consider anesthesiology the best kept secret in medicine.

ABOUT THE CONTRIBUTOR

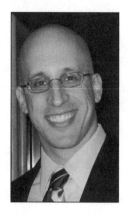

Dr Brian Freeman, the author of this book, is an attending physician in the Department of Anesthesiology at Georgetown University Hospital in Washington, DC. He is also the director of the department's residency program. His clinical interests include regional, ambulatory, and obstetric anesthesia. After growing up in the suburbs of Boston, Dr Freeman graduated from Brown University and then went on to attend medical school and complete residency training at the University of Chicago—Pritzker School of Medicine. When not in the operating room, he enjoys relaxing with his wife Rebecca, playing ice hockey, working on his house, and traveling. He can be reached by e-mail at *nerveblock1@yahoo.com*.

REFERENCES

1. Angres, D.H., Bettinardi-Angres, K., et al. *Healing the healer: The addicted physician.* Madison, CT: Psychosocial Press; 1998.

2. Talbott, G.D., Gallegos, K.V., et al. The medical association of Georgia's impaired physicians program review of the first 1,000 physicians: Analysis of specialty. *JAMA.* 1987;257:2927–2930.

3. Hughes, P.H., Storr, C.L., et al. Physician substance use by medical specialty. *J Addictive Dis.* 1999;18:1–7.

4. Alexander, B.H., Checkoway, H., et al. Cause-specific mortality risks of anesthesiologists. *Anesthesiology.* 2000;93:922–930.

5. Crane, M. Pop culture: No fluff, please, we're doctors. *Med Econ.* 2000;19:121.

6. Grandinetti, D. Sex and the satisfied doctor. *Med Econ.* 2000;19:62.

7. Silber, J.H., Kennedy, S.K., et al. Anesthesiologist direction and patient outcomes. *Anesthesiology.* 2000;93:152–163.

8. Stewart, W., Tringali, B. *Key Findings from a Nationwide Survey of Attitudes Among Medicare Beneficiaries About Anesthesia Services in the U.S.* The Tarrance Group, National Anesthesia Study; 1999.

9. Semo, J.J. Surgeon liability for nurse anesthetists: Fact or fiction? *Am Soc Anesthesiol Newsletter.* 2000;64(12):7.

10. Cooper, R.A., Laud, P., et al. Current and project workforce of nonphysician clinicians. *JAMA.* 1998;280:788–794.

11. Hanson, C.W., Durbin, C.D., et al. The anesthesiologist in critical care medicine: Past, present, and future. *Anesthesiology.* 2001;95:781–788.

12. Eckhourt, G., Schubert, A. Where have all the anesthesiologists gone? Analysis of the national anesthesia worker shortage. *Am Soc Anesthesiol Newsletter*. 2001;65(4):16–19.

13. *Data and Results—2002 Match*. Washington, DC: National Resident Matching Program;

14. Cottrell, J.E. View from the head of the table: Against putting people to sleep. *Surg Rounds*. 1989;12:81–88.

14

DERMATOLOGY

Amy J. Derick

The integumentary system, comprising skin and related structures, is the largest of all organ systems and can present with a vast number of diseases and conditions ranging from benign skin disorders and cosmetic issues to the surgical treatment of skin cancers. Dermatology intertwines with principles of internal medicine because many diseases of the skin are indications of systemic problems. One of the most competitive residencies to obtain, dermatology provides a rewarding and intellectually satisfying medical career. Dermatologists become expert diagnosticians of complex skin problems (integrating both medical and surgical treatment options) and provide patients with emotional and psychological support, as well.

MELANOMAS, MOLES, AND MORE

Dermatology is the branch of medicine concerned with skin and skin-related diseases and disorders. Skin physically protects our bodies from being harmed by the outside world, and skin also helps regulate body temperature and synthesizes vitamins.

Dermatologists see people of all ages who present with skin diseases (benign or malignant) involving the mouth, hair, nails, sweat glands, sebaceous glands, external genitalia, and mucous membranes. Typical patients might include a teenager with severe acne vulgaris, a middle-aged woman with dermatomyositis, a sunburned farmer with squamous cell carcinoma, a young woman suffering from psoriasis, or a baby with irritant dermatitis from her diaper. Common skin problems include infections, benign growths, rosacea, shingles, seborrheic dermatitis, scabies, vascular birthmarks, warts, and many rashes, usually either infectious or autoimmune in origin. Similar to the types of problems evaluated

WHAT MAKES A GOOD DERMATOLOGIST?

✓ Is an intellectual, practical, and empathic physician.

✓ Enjoys being an expert in a very specialized area of medicine.

✓ Likes working with a variety of patients.

✓ Likes seeing the results of treatment.

✓ Listens well to patients' concerns.

THE INSIDE SCOOP

by internists, many dermatologic conditions are chronic and require long-term treatment.

Although dermatologists are specialists in skin disorders, they also understand disease processes associated with internal medicine because many skin conditions are external manifestations of pathologic processes happening inside the body. For instance, the secondary stage of syphilis (a sexually transmitted disease) presents with a distinctive rash. Cancers of visceral organs such as the stomach or colon can promote the development of dark, thickened areas of the skin, commonly in the axillary region (acanthosis nigricans). Endocrine disorders (such as Cushing syndrome and hyper/hypothyroidism) and rheumatologic disorders (such as dermatomyositis, rheumatoid arthritis, and lupus erythematosus) all have cutaneous presentations. Because skin signs can and should motivate an investigation for an underlying systemic problems, dermatologists help their patients' overall health by understanding the pathophysiology and treatment of diseases that may cause certain skin abnormalities.

Being a good dermatologist starts with collecting thorough patient histories. For example, skin lesions can change over time, and thus lesion location, duration, course, details of spread, and associated symptoms of itching, pain, burning, or oozing should be documented. Because dermatologists also think beyond the skin to make proper diagnoses, they also ask questions about the patient's general health, medical history, family history (patients who suffer from psoriasis, for example, often have a family history of psoriasis), prior usage of medications, and a complete history of allergies.

In addition to collecting patient histories, dermatology emphasizes thorough physical examination skills, with clinical precision being critical. Under proper lighting, dermatologists examine patients' skin, hair, nails, and mucous membranes. Dermatologists must be able to look at a skin lesion and describe its physical attributes and implications. Dermatologists must master precise terminology, for example, whether a skin characteristic is a papule, macule, bulla, or plaque. The physical dermatologic examination differs from other areas of medicine. Dermatologists do not use stethoscopes or reflex hammers in their physical examinations. Rather, they inspect the patient with their eyes or with the aid of a technique called dermoscopy, which allows for the physician to see beneath the superficial layers of skin. Good dermatologists know what to look for, understand what they are seeing and feeling, and communicate precisely to patients and relevant others. The distribution of lesions in dermatology is important for proper diagnosis, with herpes zoster (shingles) being a good example.

DERMATOLOGY IS BOTH MEDICINE AND SURGERY

Medical students are usually attracted to dermatology because they like the mix of medical and surgical therapy, that is, treatments range from lotions to lasers to surgery. A generalized knowledge of medicine is critical, for instance, when administering medicines with systemic toxicity such as biologic therapy for inflammatory skin conditions. Dermatologists treat patients with a range of topical ointments, especially steroids and topical antifungals. At the bedside or in the office, dermatologists conduct simple tests to confirm suspected clinical diagnoses. This includes skin biopsies of suspicious lesions, potassium hydroxide stains of fungal infections, Gram stains for identifying bacterial causes of skin infections such as cellulitis or impetigo, Tzanck preparation smears for isolating herpes infections, and oil preparations to rule out scabies in patients presenting with itchy rashes.

According to the American Society of Dermatologic Surgery (ASDS) in its 2010 Procedure survey, the number of skin surgeries and procedures performed in 2010 was nearly 8 million. The most common procedure was treatment of skin cancer. One of the most demanding forms of skin cancer surgery is Mohs micrographic surgery. This advanced treatment for skin cancer involves the removal of cancer from certain areas, such as the face or ears, where skin-sparing excisions are important. Mohs offers the highest potential for cure. Historically, skin cancers were removed with a standard margin that would ensure the removal of the entire cancer. However, a certain portion of skin removed would be cancer free, therefore taking unnecessary skin. In order to spare normal tissue, Mohs surgeons remove serial slices of skin and evaluate them under a microscope, ensuring clear margin free of cancer, minimizing removal of normal skin. Mohs procedures allow the dermatologist to see beyond the disease and remove the entire tumor while leaving the healthy cells alone. After completely removing the skin lesion, the Mohs surgeon repairs the wound with complex closures.

More surgically oriented dermatologists can perform Mohs surgery with complicated flaps and grafts. Surgical dermatologists also perform procedures (typically performed by plastic surgeons) such as liposuction, blepharoplasties (eyelid surgery), and even rhytidectomy (face lifts). Dr Jeffrey Klein, a dermatologist, developed a technique called tumescent anesthesia, which is now the standard anesthesia for liposuction. Surgical treatments also include procedures such as excisions, electrodessication and curettage, cryotherapy, sclerotherapy, laser surgery, hair transplants, and tissue augmentation therapies. In the 2010 survey of dermatologic procedures, neurotoxin injections ranked second to skin cancer treatment as the most common procedure performed by dermatologists, followed by laser/light therapy, soft tissue fillers, and laser hair removal.

Cosmetic dermatologists also perform medical and surgical skin rejuvenation procedures. Medical rejuvenation involves the use of tretinoin, alpha-hydroxy acids, and topical antioxidants for the treatment of age-related skin changes. Surgical rejuvenation procedures include botulinum toxin injection, soft tissue augmentation, chemical peels, dermabrasion, sclerotherapy, and laser skin resurfacing. Many cosmetic dermatologists also perform laser surgery, which involves the use of a laser (light amplification by the simulated emission of radiation) to treat wrinkles, pigmented lesions (such as birthmarks), scars, tattoos, warts, and unwanted hair.

The field of cosmetic dermatology has grown rapidly. According to a 2005 ASDS Procedures survey, there was a 32% increase in minimally invasive cosmetic procedures compared with 2003 and a 58% increase compared with 2001. In 2010, an estimated 4.8 million cosmetic procedures were performed by an increased number of dermatologists. These practitioners cite the perceived threat in the 1980s and 1990s that managed care would find ways to depress the earning potential of dermatologists practicing classical procedures. Furthermore, a recent study suggests that medical students who incur large educational debts in medical school believe that practicing surgical dermatology will be more lucrative than practicing classical dermatology.[1] Medical students should keep in mind, though, that dermatology is a major branch of the tree of internal medicine. This is why many academic dermatologists believe the core of dermatology comes from those diseases most often treated with medical, not surgical, therapy.

THE DOCTOR–PATIENT RELATIONSHIP

Dermatologists engage in long-term relationships with their patients whose chronic skin conditions require multiple follow-up appointments over the course of their lives. Patients appreciate their dermatologists for advice on preventive medicine as well as treatment of acute skin diseases. Dermatologists also educate patients about the importance of skin cancer prevention: staying out of the sun, using sunscreen, and self-inspecting for suspicious moles. Many patients do not realize that mole self-checks are just as important as monthly breast self-examinations.

A dermatologist must have excellent listening skills. Dermatologists are a combination of physician and counselor. Because of the public-facing nature of skin disease and skin disorders, mental well-being of patients should not go unnoticed. Dermatologists must take the time to know how patients feel about their skin disease. Patient attitudes will influence choice of treatment.

MISPERCEPTIONS ABOUT DERMATOLOGY

Medical students interested in dermatology often feel physicians, in general, do not understand or appreciate the complexity of dermatology, and some primary care physicians believe they can practice dermatology. Some people view dermatology an expensive and superfluous luxury. If we allow misperceptions to prevail, the number of dermatologists in this country will decrease, and the quality and availability of dermatologic care (often live-saving care) for patients with skin diseases will erode. It also does not help when dermatology is lampooned in popular culture. You may recall, for example, the episode of *Seinfeld* in which a dermatologist is mocked as an "aloe pusher" and "pimple popper, MD."

Dermatologists are lifesavers when it comes to the treatment of deadly skin cancers. Although most skin diseases are benign, skin cancer is the most common cancer in this country. According to the American Cancer Society, one person dies of melanoma almost every hour, and among people between the ages of 25 and 29, melanoma is more common than any nonskin cancer. Dermatologists are uniquely trained to screen, diagnose, and treat patients for life-threatening diseases.

The recent surge of media attention about dermatologists who provide botulinum toxin injections and cosmeceuticals in their practices has left the general public with additional misperceptions. Cosmetic dermatology actually plays a small role in the whole field of dermatology, with the majority of dermatologists' time being spent on medical and noncosmetic surgical procedures. Little known to the public, dermatologists specialize in the diagnosis and treatment of the more than 3000 diseases that plague the human skin.

LIFESTYLE CONSIDERATIONS AND PRACTICE OPTIONS

Regular work hours, flexible employment opportunities, lack of overnight calls, and attractive compensation give dermatology its reputation as a field associated with a good lifestyle. According to Medscape Physician Compensation Report 2011, dermatologists are indeed ranked highest in overall satisfaction in a recent study of physicians representing 22 medical specialties. Unlike other medical fields, dermatology has few life-threatening emergencies; therefore, overnight calls in the hospital are rare. Most of the delivery of dermatologic services happens in an outpatient setting during regular business hours. In addition, almost all surgical interventions are in an outpatient setting.

Dermatologists practice in either academic or private settings. Private dermatologists build practices to treat their clients' skin-related ailments. Some private dermatologists teach residents in academic centers. In academic dermatology, physicians typically choose between the following types of practices: serving as faculty in academic hospitals, seeing patients at Veteran's Administration centers, or conducting research, either funded by the government or by pharmaceutical companies. For academic dermatologists, government-sponsored funding is more difficult to obtain, because typical dermatology research is translational (applying basic science research on patients and their illnesses). Government sponsorship traditionally favors basic science research over translational research. Because of the scarcity of federal grants, academic dermatologists may have to explore private settings and/or funding.

Like other fields of medicine, the practice of dermatology can be tailored to accommodate individual interests. Some dermatologists enjoy working with a microscope, focusing on diagnosing pathologic slides, and/or seeing patients in the clinic on a part-time basis. Other dermatologists prefer performing procedures such as Mohs surgery. Regardless of preference, nearly all dermatologists love the combination of outpatient medicine, procedures, pathology-based

---

VITAL SIGNS

MEDIAN COMPENSATION

Dermatology $350,627

Data from American Medical Group Association.

clinical medicine, regular hours, patient calls, and serving as a point person in a patient's general medical care.

DERMATOLOGY'S ORIGINS AND FUTURE DIRECTIONS

More than 200 years ago, in 1798, Robert Willan, a British physician, published his masterpiece, *On Cutaneous Diseases*, which organized and categorized skin lesions by small differences in morphology. Sorting out the definitions of the various lesions has been called "one of the great achievements of the dermatology of the nineteenth century."[2] In 1799, the first hospital devoted to dermatology opened in France. In the United States, the first dermatologic hospital ward opened in Massachusetts General Hospital in 1870. At this time, dermatology was actually an inpatient-based specialty with patients who were managed for prolonged periods of time in the hospital. Now, only 2% of patients admitted to the hospital for dermatologic diseases are managed by dermatologists.[3]

Much has occurred since Willan's time to expand professional knowledge about the morphology and distribution of skin lesions. Today's body of dermatologic knowledge is both wide and deep. In addition to the study of the morphology and distribution of skin lesions, the histopathology of skin lesions has become of paramount importance in understanding these diseases. The nature of dermatology has also changed dramatically over the past couple of decades. What was once a male-dominated field, at least 50% of today's would-be dermatologists, if not more, are women.

Despite the growth of dermatologic specialization, primary care physicians are playing an increasing role in the treatment of dermatologic maladies. More than one quarter of Americans seen by their primary care physicians have a skin-related complaint, and dermatologic disorders account for 6% of all chief complaints.[3] Primary care physicians are becoming more comfortable in treating basic and uncomplicated dermatologic diseases such as acne and fungal infections. (The use of isotretinoin, which can cause birth defects, for the treatment of acne remains within the control of the dermatologists.) Many patients prefer dermatologists for these problems because they can offer patients advice on general skin care as well as prescribe medicine. Some dermatologists welcome the involvement of primary care physicians for basic needs and have consequently shifted their practices to focus on more special needs such as oncological, surgical, and cosmetic procedures.

The accuracy of nondermatologists diagnosing dermatologic diseases has been called into question. In a study designed to quiz physicians on dermatologic

RESIDENCY TRAINING

Residency in dermatology requires 4 years of postgraduate training. There are currently 112 accredited programs. A select number of integrated programs allow residents to earn combined certification in both dermatology and internal medicine. In either case, dermatology training does not begin until the second postgraduate year after completing a general internship (internal medicine, surgery, pediatrics, or transitional year). Because dermatology is an outpatient specialty, work hours during residency are generally benign but also include a significant amount of outside reading and self-study. During the advanced years of training, on-call requirements are limited to call from home. Residents spend time on different rotations including dermatopathology, pediatrics, Mohs surgery, VA clinic, inpatient consultation service, and general inpatient service. The majority of time during residency is spent in a hospital outpatient clinic with fewer weeks in a nonhospital ambulatory care setting.

THE INSIDE SCOOP

diagnoses using slides and high-quality transparencies, dermatologists performed better than nondermatologists (93% vs 52% correct).[4] However, family practice physicians did perform better than internal medicine specialists (70% vs 52%). This study suggests that when something goes wrong with the skin, a consultation with a dermatologist is in order.

In the twentieth century, the microscope revolutionized the practice of dermatology. For today's medical student, the digital camera may change the practice of dermatologists in the twenty-first century. *Teledermatology*, or the practice of dermatology using digital cameras, is a hot topic. This type of dermatology can be practiced in two ways: (1) the patient and the dermatologist have a real-time conversation via camera or (2) the patient's skin is photographed and viewed at a later time (store and forward method) in conjunction with a clinical history. Proponents of teledermatology argue that these services allow for equitable service to those patients in remote areas who may not have access to centers of excellence in dermatology. Also, studies have shown that teledermatology is an accurate and reliable way of diagnosing disease. Although teledermatology has been seen as a useful mode of communication for patients, the greatest concern has been the lack of relationship between physician and patient.[5]

While dermatologists must master the basics of medicine, they also must understand the interactions of various cells and the interplay between disease processes in the skin, for example, inflammation, immunology, oncology, and infection. The diagnostic process is fascinatingly rich—with an infinite arrangement of colors, patterns, and textures. It is this complexity that defines the field.

FELLOWSHIPS AND SUBSPECIALTY TRAINING

There are many choices for specialized training within dermatology after the completion of basic residency training. Only two fellowships (Dermatopathology and Clinical and Laboratory Dermatological Immunology [CLDI]) lead to certificates of added qualifications. Practice in a dermatology subspecialty requires 1 or 2 additional years of training. The following are the four most common fellowships, but other nonaccredited fellowships exist in areas such as contact dermatitis and cutaneous allergy, cosmetic dermatology, and dermatologic research.

Mohs Surgery

For dermatologists with a knack for surgical procedures, this fellowship provides additional experience in the rigorous technique of Mohs micrographic surgery. The focus of practice becomes the surgical treatment of skin cancer.

Dermatopathology

For those with a passion for the basic sciences, this fellowship creates experts in the pathologic diagnosis of skin diseases, including those of infectious, immunologic, degenerative, and neoplastic origin. You will spend much of your time in the pathology department poring over slides through microscopes.

Clinical and Laboratory Dermatological Immunology

This fellowship trains subspecialists in the use of specialized laboratory procedures

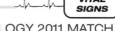

VITAL SIGNS

DERMATOLOGY 2011 MATCH STATISTICS

- Number of positions available: 372
- 407 US seniors and 135 independent applicants ranked at least one dermatology program
- 98.1% of all positions were filled in the initial Match
- The successful applicants: 83.1% US seniors, 2.42% foreign-trained physicians, and 0% osteopathic graduates
- Mean USMLE Step I score: 244
- Unmatched rate for US seniors applying only to dermatology: 14.8%

Data from National Resident Matching Program.

to diagnose disorders characterized by defective responses of the body's immune system.

Pediatric Dermatology

This fellowship provides additional expertise in the treatment of skin disorders more commonly found in children. You will become adept at treating genetic skin disorders—such as ichthyosis, epidermolysis bullosa, and pigmentary diseases—as well as a variety of vascular malformations, including birthmarks.

WHY CONSIDER A CAREER IN DERMATOLOGY?

Medical students interested in this specialty should not let the extremely competitive nature of the field discourage them. It is a specialty that can lead to a rewarding career in medicine. From the wide variety of skin problems to the different types of patients, dermatology is a diverse field. If you seek a high-pressured specialty with critically ill patients, then look elsewhere. In dermatology, the results of treatment are visible and apparent to both the doctor and the patient. Unlike lowering blood pressure or treating diabetes, the effects of treating a skin disorder are noticeable to the patient. Many medical students like this clearly defined aspect of dermatology, which applies to each step in the diagnosis, treatment, and prevention of skin diseases.

ABOUT THE CONTRIBUTOR

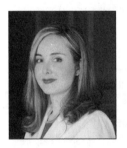

Dr Amy Derick is the founder and director of Derick Dermatology, LLC in Barrington, Illinois, which serves the medical and cosmetic dermatology needs of nearly 22,000 patients in the region. She is an instructor of Clinical Dermatology at Northwestern University's Feinberg School of Medicine. Dr Derick completed her dermatology residency at the University of Chicago Hospitals in 2006 and served as chief resident during her senior year. She attended medical school at the University of Chicago—Pritzker School of Medicine, where she graduated in the top 10% of her class. She earned her undergraduate degree *summa cum laude* from the University of Notre Dame. Dr Derick is particularly interested in medical and cosmetic dermatology, patient/public education, as well as tattoos and body art. She contributes as a media resource for the American Academy of Dermatology, the American Society for Dermatologic Surgery, and the Women's Dermatologic Society, where she also serves on the Board of Directors. Dr Derick can be reached by e-mail at contact@derickdermatology.com.

REFERENCES

1. Werth, V.P., Voorhees, J., et al. Preserving medical dermatology: A colleague lost, a call to arms, and a plan for battle. *Dermatol Clin.* 2001;19(4):583–592.

2. Crissey, J.T., Parish, L.C. Two hundred years of dermatology. *J Am Acad Dermatol.* 1998;39(6):1002–1006.

3. Prodanovich, S., Kirsner, R.S., et al. Inpatient dermatology: A prescription for survival. *Dermatol Clin.* 2001;19(4):593–601.

4. Federeman, D.G., Concato, J., et al. Comparison of dermatologic diagnoses by primary care practitioners and dermatologists. *Arch Fam Med.* 1999;8(2):170–172.

5. Weinstock, M.A., Nguyen, F.O., et al. Patient and referring provider satisfaction with teledermatology. *J Am Acad Derm.* 2002;47(1):68–72.

15

EMERGENCY MEDICINE

Jeremy Graff

N early all medical students have watched emergency room physicians save lives and cure disease on *E.R.*, the popular television series. They witness the high drama, witty banter, cool procedures, diagnostic coups, and romance. Life (and medicine), though, is usually nothing like the TV show. Does the specialty of emergency medicine (EM) really live up to its glamorous image?

Fast-paced and unpredictable, EM is one of the newest specialties in medicine. It has grown to meet the challenge of 100 million emergency room visits per year. As you know, the emergency room is always open and easily accessible. Emergency physicians (EPs) must be prepared for any type of medical problem that arrives at the door, whether by foot, car, ambulance, or helicopter. It is never boring. They take care of a wide cross-section of Americans of all ages and races, rich and poor, insured and uninsured. These specialists like to work fast and think on their feet while serving on the front lines of medicine.

WHAT IS EMERGENCY MEDICINE?

Emergency medicine involves the immediate care of urgent and life-threatening conditions found in the critically ill and injured. These physicians are really specialists in breadth—their broad-based training encompasses acute problems that span several clinical disciplines. No other specialty can match the astounding variety of patients found within the emergency room. You will see, hear, and smell things that most doctors will not. In just one shift, an EP may care for patients presenting with asthma attacks, atrial fibrillation, gunshot wounds, dislocated

189

WHAT MAKES A GOOD EMERGENCY PHYSICIAN?

✓ Likes working with his or her hands.

✓ Is an adventurous, action-oriented leader and team player.

✓ Can make logical decisions during rapidly changing situations.

✓ Likes variety and the unexpected.

✓ Is capable of juggling multiple tasks at once.

THE INSIDE SCOOP

shoulders, and even cockroaches stuck in their ears. Every now and then, the EP will discover a zebra, such as a pheochromocytoma (adrenal gland tumor) in a young woman with high blood pressure and headaches.

Emergency medicine became a specialty only about 30 years ago. Until then, most doctors who covered acute, emergent, and traumatic illnesses were actually board certified in other fields, such as internal medicine or surgery. In smaller hospitals, just about anyone (including psychiatrists) could provide coverage in the emergency department (ED) for anything from a minor cut to an inflamed appendix. Some of these doctors left their original specialty to work full-time in EDs and grandfathered their way into becoming EM specialists.

During the 1960s, physicians began to realize that patients would have better clinical outcomes if they received prompt and appropriate care from the moment they entered the hospital. This small group of physicians recognized the need for formal study and training in EM and subsequently founded the American College of Emergency Physicians in 1968. Over the next 5 years, they worked to establish the first residency program at the University of Cincinnati and lobbied Congress to pass the Emergency Medical Services Act. As a result, EM began to expand rapidly, using federal funds to develop prehospital emergency systems and to expand EDs. In 1979, the American Board of Medical Specialties recognized EM as an official clinical specialty.

Today, only physicians who have completed an EM residency are hired in the nation's emergency rooms. All across the country, EPs provide immediate recognition, evaluation, care, and disposition of a diverse adult and pediatric population. When dealing with acute problems, whether nonurgent or life threatening, their primary role is to stabilize the patient. They evaluate the ABCs (airway, breathing, circulation), take quick histories, perform focused physical examinations, order relevant laboratory and radiology tests, and contact consultants. In the contemporary ED, these specialists must be completely sure that all life-threatening causes of particular symptoms are completely worked up and ruled out. Despite being such a young arm of medical practice, EM has matured into a rigorous clinical specialty. You will receive formal training to handle just about anything that may walk through that door.

A typical shift in the ED is full of variety, drama, and excitement. As you greet the frequent fliers, who often come for both food and medical care, the chart boxes begin filling up with new patients to be seen. First might be a man clutching his stomach due to abdominal pain caused by pancreatitis. The next patient may be a pregnant woman who presents with vaginal bleeding and cramping abdominal pain—possible signs of an ectopic pregnancy. In this case, you take on the role of gynecologist, conducting a pelvic examination to see if the cervix is open or closed. You may even, depending on your training, take on the role of radiologist in such a case, using a handheld ultrasound device to determine if the patient has a viable intrauterine pregnancy. Obviously, the EM physician has to love juggling dozens of different problems, situations, and treatments while teaching and interacting with patients at the same time. At any time, a code blue (cardiac arrest) or trauma could bring this somewhat orderly environment crashing down. You are generally the first doctor to arrive in the resuscitation room, a place where patients in respiratory distress—with dropping oxygen saturation and pink frothy liquid coming out of their mouths—need immediate endotracheal intubation.

The practice of modern EM does not formally include any continuity of patient care. Because EPs work in shifts and only focus on acute medical problems, there is no patient follow-up. (Unless, of course, the patient returns to your emergency room a few days later.) After admitting or discharging a patient, the EP moves on to the next one sitting in the waiting room or being flown in by helicopter. Thus, medical students interested in this specialty should carefully consider whether having their own group of long-term patients is important. Unlike world-renowned experts in other specialties, EPs—and other hospital-based specialists such as radiologists and anesthesiologists—are behind-the-scenes doctors who may remain largely anonymous to health care consumers.

Working in an ED does not necessarily mean that all patient interactions are curtailed by shift work and acute care. Although EPs do not develop long-standing ties with their patients, they often establish a strong relationship with the community in which they practice. Plenty of patients, especially uninsured indigent persons looking for warmth, food, a place to sleep, and regular medical care, visit the emergency room often and form bonds with its staff. "Do I get to have a primary care-type relationship with all patients? Of course not, but I do get to know my community and many of the people in it," commented an EM specialist at an inner-city hospital. "This is 'their' hospital and for many of them I, or one of my colleagues, actually end up taking the role of the family doc. It's hard to do in a busy ED, but building good rapport and relating with some of our most challenging patients is one of the more rewarding aspects of emergency medicine."

GENERALIST OR SPECIALIST?

Despite their specialized focus, EPs are, in a way, true generalists. Although some may categorize these physicians as "jack of all trades, master of none," EPs do have their own area of expertise: knowing the most important (ie, acute or life-threatening) presentations of problems across the entire medical spectrum. They must be as comfortable with a gynecologic emergency as with a pediatric trauma patient. In a single work shift, an EP can deliver a baby, stabilize an accident victim, evaluate a possible case of appendicitis, manage a traumatic airway, treat an asthma attack, and diagnose congestive heart failure. No other specialty of medicine, not even EM's closest cousin—family practice—matches the breadth of acute problems that these physicians must be prepared for. Because EM physicians really get to do it all, students who enter this specialty like the fact that they will be real doctors. You will know what to do if someone has a heart attack on an airplane or when a child gets hurt at the playground.

Although the spectrum of disease varies depending on practice location and community, EPs are trained to handle anything, including patients, usually indigent or uninsured, who use the emergency room as their primary care clinic. This is why some describe the ED as "the world's largest family practice clinic." As an EP, you will not necessarily see true emergencies all the time. In fact, about half of your patients will present with problems that are more appropriate for a primary care doctor—the common cold, musculoskeletal pains, rashes, and other nonurgent complaints. It is kind of like being a family doctor but without the long-term continuity, practice of preventive medicine, and clinic setting. Your goal, instead, is to treat the acute problem at hand and then direct patients to the next appropriate step for their medical follow-up.

EMERGENCY MEDICINE REQUIRES MANY SKILLS

For most patients who seek urgent medical care, the EP is usually the first doctor on the case. This initial evaluation is both a privilege and a challenge. Patients do not arrive in the emergency room with their medical chart or old records. They may answer your questions poorly. As such, EPs often have to piece the clinical history together from fragments provided by unresponsive sick patients, family members, emergency medical technicians (EMTs), police officers, and other sources. Being the first person to ask the appropriate questions in a limited amount of time can be frustrating. You must act like a sleuth. You must have the confidence to make fast medical decisions based on limited, incomplete information. For an EM doctor, nothing is more satisfying than taking a few bits and pieces of history (and abnormal physical findings), ordering some lab tests, and coming up with a working diagnosis and treatment plan.

While one case is being stabilized, many more are waiting patiently (and often impatiently) for evaluation, treatment, discharge, or admission. The EP constantly juggles many tasks at once, whether acquiring data, making decisions, or performing procedures. Patients, lab results, nurses, chest x-rays, family members, and other physicians all vie simultaneously for your immediate attention. Because you are doing so many things at once, emergency care sometimes requires knee-jerk action, after which additional thinking is necessary. In a short amount of time, you coordinate a wide range of treatment plans, from readjusting an asthma patient's medications to suturing wounds of another patient who also just received a chest tube. With recent advances in medicine, more and more patients are coming to the emergency room with complex problems, such as unusual drug interactions, or complications from procedures that did not exist before, such as organ transplants. Now, EM specialists find themselves with even more responsibilities to manage at once.

With many stressful events occurring at the same time, the ability of an EP to triage patients becomes even more important. Based on the French word trier, meaning "to sort," triage involves allocating treatment to patients based on a priority system that assigns resources to where they are most needed. As patient advocates, these doctors must recognize the difference between the truly sick and those with less urgent problems. After all, "some patients are not as sick as they think, and others are not as well as they wish."[1] This is where triaging comes in. Without it, many people desperately in need of medical care might not receive it while their physician's attention is focused elsewhere. All EPs learn to master this skill. After sorting patients correctly when many arrive at once, emergency doctors take care of them all the way through discharge or admission.

While triaging and examining patients, EPs apply lots of technical procedures in their diagnosis and treatment plans. Yes, these doctors really do get to perform much of that wild and crazy stuff seen on television. Remember, EM is a specialty in which urgently treating the very sick involves manipulations and hands-on procedures. You will insert nasogastric tubes, reduce joints, defibrillate hearts, suture lacerations, incise and drain abscesses, intubate with endotracheal tubes, and deliver babies. Like playing with needles? Every day, there are always opportunities to place intravenous, central, and occasionally intraosseous lines. Even more complicated procedures such as cricothyrotomies (inserting a needle through cartilage of the neck to create an airway) and thoracotomies (cracking the chest) are also possible. For medical students who like to work with their hands and think surgery is the only answer, take a closer look at this specialty. EM is a quicker route to being a broad-based doctor who also gets to play with scalpels, needles, and thread.

TREATING TRAUMA PATIENTS

The dramatic, cool procedures that attract medical students to the field of EM are often performed on trauma patients—people with knife and gunshot wounds, or those who have been critically injured in motor vehicle accidents, drownings, construction accidents, natural disasters, and more. They are quickly transported to trauma centers and met by eager, capable EM physicians waiting to perform miracles. The idea of saving lives every day excites many medical students and is the strong appeal of this specialty.

A multidisciplinary problem, trauma always involves an entire team of doctors, namely, EPs, trauma surgeons, and anesthesiologists. As an EP, do not expect to be the sole individual doing all the work. Typically, the trauma surgeon calls the shots during the resuscitation. After all, the appropriate management of internal injuries due to trauma falls within the realm of surgery. It is important for EPs to recognize the boundaries of their special knowledge and skills. You must learn to appreciate the presence of and guidance by the surgery team with whom you share space.

Furthermore, these divisions will depend a lot on the EP's practice environment. Working at a large university-affiliated trauma center is very different from working at a small community hospital ED. Some EPs are literally the only doctor in the hospital, and although one would not expect trauma patients to be taken to such a place by ambulance, the "walk-in" trauma—someone with a gunshot wound dumped at the hospital door by friends, or someone who gets to the ED on their own without activating the emergency medical services (EMS) system— is a reality. Such situations clearly require a lot more out of the EP since other vital staff (surgeons and anesthesiologists) may be several minutes away from the hospital.

In saving patients with traumatic injuries, the specific role of the EP depends on the type of trauma and the hospital. First and foremost, all EPs secure the patient's airway, which can often be surprisingly difficult. For those who thrive on adrenaline-inducing challenges, intubating trauma patients may involve suctioning blood, teeth, or even brain matter out of the way while keeping the patient immobile in a C-collar. Doing this while listening to the falling tones of the oxygen saturation monitor, indicating that the patient's blood oxygen level is reaching dangerously low levels, is not for the faint of heart!

Before the surgery team arrives, the emergency doctor continues the rest of the trauma assessment: evaluating the patient's breathing, circulation, disability, and exposing them. While stabilizing the patient, these roles can be quite fluid, depending on the patient's next outcome. To assess the need for surgery, one might use ultrasound imaging to locate free fluid in the belly of a patient with blunt trauma. A quick ultrasound that locates fluid around the heart or air in the chest cavity (pneumothorax) can lead to a life-saving procedure before the x-ray technician even gets to the trauma bay. EPs often place central lines and chest tubes. Once again, however, their most important role is to stabilize the patient until definitive treatment (surgery) arrives. As such, future EPs who want to go at it alone, or who become easily annoyed by orders from surgeons, may find their role in caring for trauma patients much more limited than they anticipated.

OCCUPATIONAL HAZARDS IN THE ED

For the next 20 to 30 years, your workplace will be a chaotic, messy, and tense environment. For some, the confines of the emergency room seem like a more dangerous work environment than the clinic, operating room, or ward. You will often be performing invasive procedures under time pressure, with blood splattering everywhere. Patients may not necessarily divulge any possible pathogens they may be carrying. And all sorts of nasty bugs and critters make the ED their very special home. Here, brave EPs are at an increased risk for exposure to everything from multidrug-resistant tuberculosis to hepatitis B and C, from HIV to potential biological warfare agents. The ED is, after all, one of the top locations where medical students have been exposed to accidental needlesticks.[2]

Although there is the potential of being exposed to an infectious agent, most modern EDs take all sorts of steps to minimize the risk. As a result of universal precautions, the rates of infection of the most concerning viruses (hepatitis B and C, HIV) are extremely low.[3] Regardless, emergency doctors realize that hazards exist every day on the job, including stray radiation from portable x-ray machines and the stress of shift work. They are willing to accept these challenges to practice in a challenging, dynamic, and fun environment.

The emergency room is also a place where everyone wants something from you immediately, and nine out of ten are angry with you. ED patients who can be unruly, impatient, difficult, rude, or outright violent are another kind of occupational hazard. All hospital EDs are required to care for every patient who comes through the doors, regardless of their ability to pay and how hostile or belligerent they are. Furthermore, as our population ages, health care coverage decreases, and ED visits increase, future EM doctors are bound to encounter more patients, sicker patients, and, most certainly, angrier patients. Hospital EDs certainly feel the greatest crunch due to a health care system that is stretched very thin. Rising medical care costs and the lack of universal health care have left almost 40 million Americans uninsured. With the shortage of health care professionals, fewer hospital beds are available, which leaves upset patients in emergency rooms waiting sometimes for days until a bed opens up.

The end result? Many patients hate the emergency room and often greet their EP with hostility and impatience. They are unhappy that it took 6 hours before their lacerated finger was sutured. They become agitated when you refuse to prescribe antibiotics for their viral-induced cough or narcotic painkillers for their sore backs. There will always be aggressive drunks and argumentative prisoners who will all want something from you, fast. Sometimes, the anger and hostility of unruly patients turns to violence. ED physicians, nurses, and prehospital providers attempting to care for intoxicated or emotionally disturbed patients can often become victims of assault. During a 9-month period in one ED, members of the staff were kicked, grabbed, pushed, punched, or spat upon nearly 20 times.[4] Future EM physicians should be aware of the threat of violent and dangerous encounters.

In a busy ED, pleasing all of the patients waiting for medical care is usually impossible. Thus, you must be very thick skinned while juggling the needs of these patients with the more pressing needs of trauma victims and other critically ill persons. Using woefully inadequate resources, you will become adept at pushing the flow of patients through the ED into hospital beds, back home, back to prison, back on the streets, or wherever they most appropriately need to go.

LIFESTYLE CONSIDERATIONS: WORKING IN SHIFTS

Today, the trends in specialty selection among medical students have shifted toward lifestyle specialties—ones with controllable hours and the possibility of a better social and family life. EM is at the top of this list. EPs typically show up at the hospital and work for 8 to 12 hours in a given shift. There is no such thing as being on call, and they never need to carry a beeper outside of the hospital. Once your shift is over, the noise, stress, and demands of the patients waiting in the ED are all left behind as you head out to the golf course, the rock climbing gym, or the beach. Because of the predictable

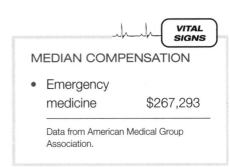

VITAL SIGNS

MEDIAN COMPENSATION

• Emergency
  medicine $267,293

Data from American Medical Group Association.

hours, EPs have the flexibility to plan family and relaxation time without having to worry about getting their patients covered. Unlike other physicians who are called at home, the illnesses and disasters that befall patients everywhere cannot tear you away from your picnic, night at the theater, or errands on a weekday morning.

However, the rotating shift schedule also has many drawbacks. The ED is open 24 hours a day, 365 days a year. Whether just out of residency or approaching retirement age, all EPs find themselves working nights, weekends, and holidays. If you cannot imagine practicing medicine on Christmas Day, Saturday night, or other inconvenient times, especially with a family at home, then you should perhaps consider another specialty. You may dislike having a weekday off when friends and family are working or at school. Moreover, shifts sometimes last longer than anticipated. EM doctors cannot simply walk away from a patient who presents with a possible heart attack 5 minutes before the scheduled end of the shift. They must also arrive a little early and stay a little later to help sign out patients, dictate charts, and tie up other loose ends from the previous shift.

Shift work quickly disrupts your circadian rhythms and normal sleeping and eating patterns, because the shifts typically alternate. In a given week, you may find yourself rotating through several blocks of tiring night shifts interspersed with day shifts or long weekend hours. Furthermore, your responsibilities do not always end after completing an overnight shift. Academic conferences, meetings, family duties, and errands often require your time during the day and prevent you from immediately going to sleep. As a result, EM doctors are always recuperating from their alternating shifts. This life of permanent jetlag can make a 40-hour workweek feel more like 80 hours' worth. Furthermore, constantly upsetting and resynching your body's internal clock can have adverse effects on your health. Studies have shown that rotating shift work contributes to higher rates of drug and alcohol abuse, hypertension, heart attacks, divorce rates, work-related accidents, and more.[5,6]

Basically, shift work is both a blessing and a curse. Most hospitals at least attempt to schedule shifts in a block format, rather than frequently alternating, for at least 1 week at time. Ostensibly, this format would allow your body and mind to readjust to a normal circadian rhythm again. By working the same type of shift for a large block of time, emergency doctors could better adapt their bodies and improve their cognitive performance. Despite the inevitable toll on body and mind, nearly all EPs love being able to sign out patients and go home completely free of patient and medical responsibility. There is ample time to spend with your family, to spend weekends at the beach, and so on.

STRESS, BURNOUT, AND CAREER SATISFACTION

EM has only existed as a specialty for 30 years. Yet, for some time, there have been discussions about the high attrition rates in this specialty. Many medical students contemplating a career in EM worry about the potential burnout factor and career dissatisfaction. Is this specialty really better for younger physicians rather than middle-aged doctors? Several studies refute this notion.

One study, which measured the degree of burnout among emergency doctors, found that although 60% registered in the moderate to high burnout ranges, the projected attrition rates were comparable with other medical specialties.[7] Another study, which measured the actual attrition instead of surveying EM doctors about their future career expectations, concurred with these conclusions.[8] These authors found that 15 years after graduating from residency, 86.8% of respondents were still practicing EM, which came to an annual attrition rate of less than 1% per year. They also found that the average percentage of time spent in clinical work decreases from 86% in the 1st year of practice to 60% by the 15th year of practice, while the amount of time spent in administration increases from 5% to 25% over the same time period. Physicians who left the specialty cited shift work as the most important reason, along with emotional stress, family considerations (especially working weekends and holidays), and physical stress.

Regardless of the actual attrition rate, EM does have inherent stressors, in addition to working shifts, that, over time, could lead to burnout: high patient volume, pressure, time constraints, and intensity. In a given shift, you might find yourself working for 8 or 12 hours straight without taking a break for food or rest. The lack of continuity of care, isolation from other physicians in the ED, abusive patients, and little positive feedback from either patients or consulting physicians all can exacerbate stress. EPs also experience a great deal of doubt over the pressured decisions they make while managing unfamiliar situations with little information. There is always the potential for every visit to be a missed diagnosis (with associated liability). They worry, for instance, about getting sued for discharging patients who should have been admitted.

A lack of respect from other medical colleagues can also contribute to career dissatisfaction and burnout among EM doctors. Due to the fishbowl nature of an emergency room, these clinicians often feel the pressure of their decisions being observed and criticized by other doctors, especially in hindsight. EPs without thick skins and manageable egos will find themselves burning out quickly. Many times you will not have the skills, specialized knowledge, time, or equipment to properly care for your patients, and you will have to call other extremely busy consultants and specialists (surgeons, private internists, etc) for assistance evaluating an acute abdomen or clearance for admission to the medical wards. Because the ED is perceived as the source of more work for already overburdened doctors, many consultants may question the urgency of an EP's request and wrongfully dismiss them as triage nurses who simply decide whether the patient should be admitted or discharged.

As EM has matured into a full-blown specialty, however, issues of fundamental distrust or disrespect from other physicians, though still present, have subsided. Many of the older medicine and surgery attendings, who never really trusted the abilities or judgment of emergency room physicians, are no longer practicing. Today most physicians, whether pediatricians or thoracic surgeons, agree that their colleagues in EM are well trained and appropriately call for help when the patient's condition warrants it.

PRACTICE OPTIONS: THE REAL WORLD

EPs can work pretty much anywhere. Such a variety of jobs should satisfy just about anyone's needs. Because of the shift work and lack of fixed office practice, EPs are somewhat nomadic — they frequently change jobs, move across the country, or work part-time in multiple hospitals. Most are based in suburban community hospitals, academic medical centers, inner-city county hospitals, or rural acute care centers. Some work internationally or even on cruise ships. Depending on the location, EPs can be salaried hospital employees, independent contractors, members of a practice group, or staff in a managed care organization. Regardless of the situation, part-time jobs abound in EM. Despite the obvious salary reduction, this possibility allows you to balance work, family, and other interests as you choose.

Urban EM offers constant excitement, high patient volume, trauma, and always engaging multicultural milieu. Although not every city ED serves as a Level I trauma center, the urban EP deals with a greater variety and abundance of sicker patients than their suburban or rural colleagues. Furthermore, a large city hospital usually means a greater availability of specialists for consultations. On the downside, as previously discussed, are the hazards that come with working in the emergency room of an overcrowded urban hospital (infectious disease, needlesticks, and hostile patients), as well as the possibility of violence.

How about rural practice? Because many people still live in the large rural areas of the country, being the small town EP is a truly rewarding experience. An isolated, rural setting allows the EP to draw on all their skills without having to consult another specialist. As the only physician for miles around, you are responsible for managing many problems yourself. While knife and gunshot wounds are rare, trauma is still inevitable in these locations. Farming accidents occur at a rate of roughly 10 accidents or injuries a year for every 100 full-time farm workers.[9] Because of the lack of tertiary care facilities in these regions, rural emergency room doctors become experts at stabilizing very sick patients and then transporting them elsewhere. The increasing use of telemedicine technology adds an exciting new twist to the practice of rural EM.

A smaller number of EPs choose careers in academic medicine. Teaching hospitals provide the greatest resources and access to a wide range of expert specialists. Clinically, academic EPs work fewer shifts than those in private practice. Instead, they receive protected time for teaching new residents (at times even paramedics and firefighters), attending academic conferences, and conducting research. EM physicians are immersed in a broad variety of basic science and clinical topics, from the molecular mechanisms of cardiopulmonary resuscitation to the clinical outcomes of novel treatments for asthma. In academics, you stay on the forefront of advances in this field.

Emergency medicine allows you have a great deal of control over your practice and working life. You can be mobile, choose your own hours, and not be bound to the business of setting up your own practice. For new graduates of residency programs, the job market remains wide open. Despite the closure of hundreds of EDs over the last decade due to cutbacks by health care systems, there still remains a shortage of EPs. Although the number of ED visits nationwide is increasing, the number of departments is decreasing, thus placing great stress on those that remain open. Under most of the scenarios tested, a significant deficit of board-certified EM specialists will remain for at least several decades.[10] Of the 32,000 EPs practicing in the United States, only little more than half (16,600) are certified by the American Board of Emergency Medicine (ABEM). As a result, most EDs are now hiring only board-certified or board-eligible physicians who are trained specifically in EM.

FELLOWSHIPS AND SUBSPECIALTY TRAINING

Medical Toxicology

A generation ago, a little green sticker called Mr Yuck helped to prevent countless poisoning accidents. In 2000, more than 2 million toxic ingestions or exposures, including 920 fatalities, were reported to poison control centers nationwide. Specialists in medical toxicology know all about the nasty substances that both kids and adults manage to get inside themselves, either accidentally or purposely. These poisons include medications, illicit drugs, chemicals, household toxins, industrial pollutants, hazardous materials, and environmental waste. In light of the growing awareness of biological and chemical terrorism, medical toxicologists provide an essential service. They apply their underlying knowledge of EM with sophisticated expertise in pharmacology. Many times, the treatment for one type of poison could exacerbate the situation if the wrong chemical exposure was diagnosed. The ABEM offers a board certification examination following this 1-year fellowship. If the idea of working in a city or regional poison control center sounds appealing, then you should consider this cool career choice!

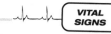

VITAL SIGNS

EMERGENCY MEDICINE 2011 MATCH STATISTICS

- Number of positions available: 1626
- 1484 US seniors and 762 independent applicants ranked at least one EM program
- 98.7% of all positions were filled in the initial Match
- The successful applicants: 78.5% US seniors, 5.6% foreign-trained physicians, and 11.2% osteopathic graduates
- Mean USMLE Step I score: 223
- Unmatched rate for US seniors applying only to EM: 7.3%

Data from National Resident Matching Program.

Emergency Medical Services

Were you one of those kids who chased fire engines on your tricycle? Many medical students have worked as paramedics and EMTs before becoming physicians. Specialists with fellowship training in EMS study the logistical, organizational, and medical aspects of delivering quality care to sick individuals outside the hospital. These services include paramedic training, new prehospital treatments, disaster preparation, community organization, and more. EPs with fellowship training in EMS typically serve as medical directors of city- or county-wide emergency medical systems.

Pediatric Emergency Medicine

Do you like working with kids in an acute setting? All ED physicians receive training in the acute care of infants, children, and teenagers. It is rare, however, to find a doctor who feels completely at ease treating these younger charges. "Can I stabilize a sick kid? Absolutely. But, I am much more comfortable working with adults," commented a resident at a large urban hospital. "Kids can fool you—sometimes you'll see a bunch with minor complaints and then out of nowhere one will really surprise you." With further training in pediatric EM, EM doctors can easily take on any acute pediatric problem—croup, seizures, earaches, child abuse, fevers of unknown origin, asthma attacks, and trauma. Pediatric EM is an exciting and very rewarding branch of medicine. You will typically work in the ED of a major children's hospital. After completing this 2-year fellowship, the ABEM offers a subspecialty examination for board certification.

Undersea and Hyperbaric Medicine

For physicians who love scuba diving, this is the perfect fellowship. These specialists are experts at the use of hyperbaric oxygen therapy—the delivery of 100% oxygen at pressures greater than atmospheric pressure. With proper training and use, oxygen becomes a form of treatment that enhances the physiologic oxygenation of the blood and tissues. Physicians who complete this fellowship can treat the harmful nitrogen bubbles of decompression sickness (the bends) and other diving accident cases. They also use this special therapy for patients suffering from carbon monoxide poisoning, gas gangrene of soft tissues, nonhealing wounds, bone infections, and tissue damage secondary to burns and radiation. If you have a special interest in diving, physiology, and gas mechanics, this interesting subspecialty provides an opportunity to apply novel approaches in EM to previously intractable treatment problems. Board certification is available.

Emergency Ultrasound

A single clinical specialty does not oversee the use of ultrasound. In the emergency room, physicians perform focused ultrasound examinations to seek a "yes/no" answer to a clinical question. At 3:00 AM, you will be responsible for evaluating the patient with excruciating abdominal pain. Is it pancreatitis, appendicitis, or cholecystitis? Emergency ultrasound is brief, interactive, and answers a limited number of discrete questions regarding one or two organ systems. For example, rapid ultrasound imaging can determine the presence of life-threatening ectopic pregnancies; diagnose pericardial tamponade (blood in the sac surrounding the heart); evaluate the abdomen for trauma, internal bleeding, or aneurysms; and even rule out lower-extremity blood clots without sending patients to the vascular lab. The modern emergency ultrasonographer is trained to perform at a comparable level with that of a radiologist. Because only a handful of 1-year fellowships exist, this new subspecialty has not achieved subspecialty board status.

Sports Medicine

Just like their colleagues in family practice, EM doctors are eligible for primary care type fellowships in sports medicine. Of course, they do not perform orthopedic surgeries. Instead, these sports medicine specialists evaluate the overall health of athletes in a clinic setting. Through continuous care, they are responsible for enhancing their patients' general physical health and fitness and treating injury and illness through medical management. They draw on their knowledge of exercise physiology, nutrition, and rehabilitation to promote a healthy lifestyle for all active individuals. The ABEM offers certification examinations after completion of this 1- or 2-year fellowship.

Critical Care Medicine

Patients presenting to EDs today are sicker than ever. People are now living with chronic medical conditions such as congestive heart failure, HIV, and transplants that would have been unimaginable a generation ago. A shift in the ED these days may involve managing a septic patient by titrating vasopressor agents and fluids while still taking care of sore throats and sprained ankles in the nearby hallway. These factors as well as recent research that shows early focused management of critical illnesses such as heart attack, stroke, and sepsis all contribute to better patient outcomes, combined to alert leaders in the fields of EM and Critical Care Medicine (CCM) that a pathway for EM-trained physicians to gain certification in CCM was needed. In September 2011, a joint program between the American Board of Internal Medicine and the ABEM was announced whereby EM-trained residency graduates will be able to attend CCM fellowships and become boarded in CCM. The exact specifics have yet to be announced at this date, but having a pathway available for EM-trained residents to become boarded in CCM is a very exciting development.

WHY CONSIDER A CAREER IN EMERGENCY MEDICINE?

Medical students who would thrive on a career in EM typically like the wide spectrum of clinical challenges and the multidisciplinary approach.[11] As the only specialty in which doctors are required by law to treat all patients seeking care, whether or not they have insurance, EM can be very challenging. These heroes juggle what seems like a thousand tasks at once, constantly readjusting moment-by-moment plans as events unfold. They also have the challenge of interacting with a dizzyingly varied group of people while caring for their patients, which sometimes involves fighting with the medical staff to make things happen. So, an EP must meet the challenge of being a diplomat and team player. EPs also thrive on the intellectual challenges. They must be astute clinicians with a solid knowledge of nearly every single organ system and ailment. They really are the only contemporary practitioners who are skilled in the truly broadest range of medicine.

Emergency medicine specialists must have compassion, empathy, and an open ear, because every shift involves many social and emotional issues. In 1 day, you might have to tell a family that their loved one has died, counsel a battered woman afraid to go home to her violent husband, manage angry patients, perform a sexual assault examination,

RESIDENCY TRAINING

Residency in EM requires either 3 or 4 years of postgraduate training. Unlike other specialties, there are actually three types of EM residency programs. The majority (90%) are 3-year programs that begin immediately after medical school. Some (14%) are full 4-year programs. Another small group (20%) require 3 years of EM residency after a separate internship year (transitional, medical surgical). During residency, the length and number of shifts worked per week varies per hospital. Regardless of type of program, EM residents also complete rotations in general medicine, critical care, anesthesiology, cardiology, and obstetrics–gynecology. The bulk of their training consists of monthly rotations in adult and pediatric EM, trauma, toxicology, emergency medical services, and aeronautical medicine. Many programs require a research project.

THE INSIDE SCOOP

address homelessness, and communicate with police and other community services. For many patients who come to the ED for care, the EP is the only doctor looking out for their best interests, whether medical, emotional, or social. You will feel especially proud to serve as their advocate to make sure they get more advanced, specialized treatment when needed. Because of the variety of patients (some with emergent problems, others who are not really sick), your treatment plans will be as wide ranging as their complaints. The primary role, however, of the EP is to stabilize patients, treat acute problems, and determine if they need to be admitted for further workup. EPs, in the end, are experts in rapid decision making. Over time, you will be amazed at how quickly and efficiently you can provide medical care to such a diverse group of patients.

ABOUT THE CONTRIBUTOR

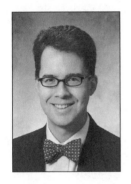

Dr Jeremy Graff completed his residency (and served as chief resident) at the Alameda County Medical Center—Highland Hospital in Oakland, California. After attending college at the University of Chicago, where he majored in psychology, Dr Graff spent 2 years as a PhD candidate in psychology at Stanford University. Medicine turned out to be his true calling; therefore, he returned to the University of Chicago for medical school. Dr Graff is currently the medical director of an emergency department at a community hospital in Hayward, California, serving 36,000 patients a year. He enjoys roaming the state's many redwood forests, restoring vintage stereo gear, raising chickens, and cooking gourmet meals. He can be reached by e-mail at freedom1095@yahoo.com.

REFERENCES

1. Kuhn, W.F. Emergency medicine: A unique opportunity for medical students. *Acad Med.* 1999;74(7):755–756.

2. Osborn, E.H.S., Papadakis, M.A., et al. Occupational exposures to body fluids among medical students: A seven-year longitudinal study. *Ann Intern Med.* 1999;130:45–51.

3. Henein, M.N., Lloyd, L. HIV, hepatitis B, and hepatitis C in the code one trauma population. *Am J Surgery.* 1997;63(7):657–659.

4. Foust D., Rhee K.J. The incidence of battery in an urban emergency department. *Ann Emerg Med.* 1993;22:583–585.

5. Gordon, N.P., et al. The prevalence and health impact of shift work. *Am J Public Health.* 1986;76:1225.

6. Steel, M., et al. The occupational risk of motor vehicle collisions for emergency medicine residents. *Acad Emerg Med.* 1999;6:1050.

7. Goldberg, R., Boss, R.W., et al. Burnout and its correlates in emergency physicians: Four years' experience with a wellness booth. *Acad Emerg Med.* 1996;3(12):1156–1164.

8. Hall, K.N., Wakeman, M.A. Residency-trained emergency physicians: Their demographics, practice evolution, and attrition from emergency medicine. *J Emerg Med.* 1999;17:7–15.

9. Runyon, J.L. A review of farm accident data sources and research: Review of data sources. U.S. Department of Agriculture National Safety Database. Retrieved April 15, 2003 from www.cdc.gov/nasd/docs/d001001-d001100/d001044/d001044.html.

10. Holliman, C.J., Wuerz, R.C., et al. Workforce projections for emergency medicine: How many emergency physicians does the United States need? *Acad Emerg Med.* 1997;4:725–730.

11. Stamoudis, C., Collings, J. Third year medical students' perceptions of emergency medicine as a career. *Acad Emerg Med.* 2000;7(5):545.

16

FAMILY MEDICINE

Michael Mendoza and Lisa Vargish

The specialty of family medicine encompasses such a wide range of clinical care that it is difficult to define a single scope of practice. Some physicians devote most of their time to high-risk obstetrics and operative deliveries, and others manage a harried clinic full of adults, children, and elderly in varying states of wellness and sickness. Many others are actively engaged in research, health policy, and community advocacy. In the tradition of this community-based specialty, family physicians are well integrated into their communities and actively address issues in their patients' lives other than medical problems. This is why family physicians serve as advocates—for patients, health care systems, and social change. No matter the role, these physicians emphasize health maintenance, disease prevention, and chronic illness management, always aware of the psychosocial dimensions of their patients' lives.

DEFINING THE SCOPE OF PRACTICE

The American Academy of Family Physicians (AAFP) defines family medicine as "the medical specialty [that] provides continuing and comprehensive health care for the individual and family . . . [and] integrates the biological, clinical, and behavioral sciences. It is a specialty in breadth that integrates the biological, clinical and behavioral sciences. The scope of family medicine encompasses all ages, both sexes, each organ system and every disease entity".[1] In essence, there are few limitations to what family physicians can do when it comes to practicing medicine.

It is no wonder that many medical students contemplating a calling in family medicine have some trepidation about assuming such a breadth of practice in a single specialty. For others, this very breadth of practice motivates them to select family medicine as their career. No other specialty can possibly match family medicine when it comes to its diverse practice environments, wide spectrum of patient demographics, and embrace of the entire breadth of clinical medicine. Being a family physician requires the ability to solve challenging problems of all organ systems, to take comfort in your scope of knowledge and practice, and to accept universally all factors (biological, clinical, and behavioral) that can affect your patients' physical, emotional, and mental state of wellness.

Because of the extreme diversity within this specialty, the specialty of family medicine is responsible for most of the health care delivered in the United States. In 2008, 62% of the 1.1 billion ambulatory care visits were made to primary care delivery sites.[2] About one-quarter of all visits were to general and family practice physicians and approximately one-third were to primary care physicians specializing in internal medicine, pediatrics, or OB/GYN.[3] Family physicians, who care for newborn infants to the elderly, see more patients daily than any other specialist.[4]

As a family physician, you will draw your knowledge base from, among other areas, internal medicine, obstetrics–gynecology, pediatrics, psychiatry, and surgery. You may wonder how these specialists in these specialties can require 3 to 7 years to master any one of these fields, while family physicians spend only 3 years on all of the above. The answer: as all residents discover upon entering the world of practice, completion of residency confers upon its graduates competency, not mastery, in their area of specialty. A physician who receives training in family medicine can competently manage patients presenting with diverse clinical and social complaints and also speak confidently about the nature of that complaint and how to diagnose and treat it. No properly trained graduate in family medicine or in any other specialty, however, will be able to say that he or she knows everything. The competent family physician needs to know what is outside the scope of his or her practice. Family physicians also need to commit to staying up-to-date with developments in primary care.

The ability to analyze and manage a variety of problems is the cornerstone of clinical family medicine. Unlike a specialty setting where patients arrive with a referral for a specific problem, patients often present to family physicians with what may seem to be vague symptoms—weakness, dizziness, lower back pain, abdominal pain. The competent family physician must elicit the correct information and obtain the proper clinical data to make the correct diagnosis, initiate the proper treatment, or make the appropriate consultation. If the problem at hand is beyond their experience or knowledge, they initiate a specialist referral. That said, only 5.1% of all visits to family physicians result in referrals to other physicians.[1] Clearly, family physicians not only diagnose but are also able to treat most clinical problems in the outpatient setting.

The academic challenge of family medicine is that you must be content knowing something about everything, but not everything about anything. It comes as no surprise that family physicians must be adept at approaching the widest variety of clinical complaints. According to the US Department of Health and Human Services, the most common reasons prompting a visit to any physician are for a general medical examination, cough, postoperative care, and prenatal care.[1] Family physicians receive training in all of these areas and encounter these problems routinely. Compared with all other specialties, patients identify family physicians most commonly as their usual source of care for artherosclerotic cardiovascular disease (56%), stroke (56%), hypertension (63%), diabetes (67%), cancer (60%), COPD (62%), asthma (58%), and depression (62%).[5] In addition to these chronic illnesses, family physicians provide health maintenance services that include pediatric anticipatory guidance, women's health, preventive screening, and end-of-life care.

Family physicians are most often identified as patients' primary care physician. In a recent survey, the majority (62%) of patients stated that they had a family physician as their individual source of care.[6] Among patients older than 65 years, family physicians outnumber general internists as the patient's source of primary care.[7] In addition, family physicians often see patients with a variety of symptoms but no preestablished diagnosis. Forty percent of patient visits to family physicians are for reasons not listed among the 25 most common complaints in primary care visits, reflecting the broad scope of family medicine and the diversity of its diagnostic challenges.[8] From the patient's point of view, one key advantage of having a family physician is that the patient can receive the vast majority of his or her preventive care, chronic illness care, and preventive services from one physician without having to visit with a variety of specialists who might provide a subset of these services independently.

Providing continuity of care often takes form in settings outside the traditional outpatient clinic setting. For family physicians, this means the opportunity to participate in a wide range of a patient's clinical care, including hands-on procedures and a variety of inpatient types of care. There are many office-based diagnostic tests that family physicians perform, such as electrocardiography, excision of suspicious moles, endometrial biopsy, spirometry, vasectomy, colposcopy, and obstetrical ultrasound. In addition to office-based minor surgical procedures, many family physicians are trained in and perform more involved operative procedures, either independently or with consultation with a surgeon. If you choose to include obstetrics as part of your practice, you will definitely have a lot of hands-on work delivering babies and even performing caesarean sections (depending on your training and experience). Family physicians receive training in intensive care and emergency care as well. In a recent survey of 1334 family physicians, half of the respondents reported regularly caring for patients in intensive care units. In addition, half of them care for patients in emergency room settings.[9] Many family physicians also provide care in home-based settings, nursing homes and long-term care facilities, and in mobile in community settings.

SPECIALIZING IN PRIMARY CARE AND GENERALIST MEDICINE

A common question that students ask is "How can one be a specialist in generalist medicine?" The answer to this is that providing comprehensive primary care to patients of all demographics requires specialized knowledge in the diagnosis and treatment of the breadth of undifferentiated clinical problems that occur in a primary care setting. A career in family medicine, however, goes far beyond understanding a breadth of clinical problems. Over a span of months or years, the emphasis during office visits is on continuity, prevention, and health maintenance (unlike specialty clinics or inpatient settings where visits are sporadic or single problem focused). For example, family medicine encourages you to think comprehensively about a patient's abdominal pain, not simply as a pathologic process that can be medical or surgical in etiology, but rather as a manifestation of an occurrence in a person's life. It may be acute or chronic and may have resulted from any number of medical, surgical, or social factors that greatly impact that person's ability to function in his or her job, family, or spiritual life. So the practice of family medicine, with its many dimensions of medical care, is as much a philosophy as it is a body of medical knowledge or clinical skill.

As generalists, family physicians have a special focus on disease prevention. They derive great satisfaction from preventing illness—just as much as they do in treating it. Routine physicals, well-child checkups, school and camp physicals, and cancer screenings are all important examples of this type of care. These physicians epitomize what primary care medicine is all about: preventing illness, maintaining health, managing a person's total care, and being the entry point into the health care system. They also practice cost-effective medical care, taking into account the scientific and clinical evidence, the patients' specific medical needs and preferences, and the values of the patients and their families. As generalists, the skills and knowledge they need differ according to the patient population of the particular community. For instance, family physicians working in the inner city have to address different types of problems than those working in rural geographic areas.

Inevitably, physicians responsible for family-centered primary care confront complex interpersonal social and behavioral issues. As such, all residency programs include family and individual therapy as part of training. For example, if a child presents with enuresis and encopresis (inability to control urination and defecation) at the age of 12, it would not be uncommon for other family members to feel some effect of their loved one's medical concerns. For instance, a parent may suffer from depression while attempting to cope with this situation. Other siblings may feel alienated if the focus of the family turns heavily toward one individual, perhaps further exacerbating the situation. Although pediatricians and internists are well trained to address the individual concerns of the children or adults, in this scenario the family physician is uniquely trained among primary care physicians to handle the behavioral and medical concerns of everyone involved. In addition to referring to an appropriate behavioral specialist, the family physician may have a family visit to explore the entire context of one family member's condition.

Due to their large numbers and broad medical focus, family physicians contribute immensely to public health and primary medical care. For instance, in areas of the country with a large supply of primary care providers, colon and breast cancers are more likely to be detected at earlier stages, leading to higher cure rates.[10,11] Furthermore, countries with the best health care systems (as measured by longevity, infant mortality, and patient satisfaction) have the highest percentage of family physicians.[12] Socioeconomic status, however, is the only powerful factor that surpasses access to a family physician as a predictor of a person's health.[13] Although the relationship between physician workforce composition and the state of health care is complex, there is clearly a positive association between access to quality primary care and improved health outcomes.

The United States relies on family physicians more than any other physician to supply primary health care to underserved areas. The federal government designates health personal shortage areas (HPSAs) based on the shortage of primary care physicians per capita, namely, a ratio of people per primary care physician greater than 3500 to 1. In 1995, 25.4% of all US counties were designated as HPSAs.[14] Of the remaining counties, 58% would actually qualify as HPSA without the contribution of family physicians, as opposed to 2% without general internists, 0.5% without general pediatricians, and 0.4% without obstetricians.[15] As you can see, family physicians provide the vast majority of primary care for these underserved populations.

THE DOCTOR–PATIENT RELATIONSHIP

The long-term relationship between family physicians and their patients is one of the core aspects of this specialty. The level of bonding can be intense. Family physicians typically spend every appointment discussing issues in their patients' lives that may not seem to have anything to do with their current complaint. Family physicians guide patients through illnesses, problems, and other landmarks of life, from delivering babies to controlling high blood pressure, from treating cancer to coping with the loss of loved ones. In these relationships, patients develop great trust in their family physicians. You learn about their hopes, dreams, and fears. You are with them through both good times and bad. This privilege is like none other in medicine and is not found in other specialties as it is in family medicine. Many patients consider you part of their family, especially if you are a family physician practicing in small, intimate communities where everyone knows each other.

Only in family medicine does continuity with patients span the entire life cycle and all the biological and social influences that bear upon it. It is not uncommon, for example, for a family physician to deliver and care for multiple generations of newborns in a single family. Even within the context of a single medical problem, the primary care physician is the one who integrates contributions from various specialists into a single treatment strategy. After establishing a plan and passing the acute phase of a disease, family physicians are able to manage most of these conditions. Specialists in different organ systems, although their contributions are invaluable, typically do not provide ongoing comprehensive care for patients with medical conditions outside their specialty.

As you can see, family physicians have the unique opportunity to care for all the members of a family simultaneously. It is common, in fact, for a family to present for care as a whole, with the family physician caring for all members in the clinic room at once. When emphasizing preventive measures, the family unit is a key consideration. A family with a long history of diabetes and high blood pressure, for example, will cue the family physician to emphasize proper nutrition and exercise as a means of primary prevention for all members of the family, not simply those who might currently have risk factors for cardiovascular disease. You cannot simply educate a teenager about exercising or avoiding an unhealthy diet without addressing the eating habits and psychosocial dynamics of the entire household.

Family physicians are also often called upon to initially manage complex medical problems in the context of "the family." If, for example, an adult family member is diagnosed with a condition thought to be hereditary, the family physician already has legitimate clinical relationships with other family members. They can easily encourage them to seek appropriate counseling and diagnostic testing. Although physicians in other specialties certainly participate in family-centered care, few other physicians share the same level of involvement with all family members.

Family physicians know that their relationships with patients are special because they take into account everything about the patient when making clinical diagnoses. Listening to their symptoms and examining for physical signs of diseases are just the beginning. Family doctors also listen to the patient's feelings, look at his or her behavior, and take into account the social and family history. If your patient presents with a chronic cough, you should still ask about his or her family, job, children, or anything else going on in his or her life. This is what good family medicine is all about.

Not all of your patients will require chronic medical care. Some just have problems that are bothering them and need someone to talk to and express their feelings. When it comes to caring for patients, a good family physician knows when to "wait and see" and is not overly aggressive with tests and treatment. In family medicine, medicine is not always about ordering blood tests, prescribing medications, scheduling procedures, and giving referrals. Many times you are simply there for your patient as a compassionate human being who can provide simple reassurance when it is appropriate to do so.

LIFESTYLE CONSIDERATIONS AND PRACTICE OPTIONS

Lifestyles in family medicine are as varied as the specialty itself. The practice of most family physicians centers on comprehensive ambulatory medicine. By seeing dozens of patients every day in the clinic, you will lead a very busy life. Work schedules of course depend on the type of group and practice setting. Most

RESIDENCY TRAINING

Residency in family practice requires 3 years of postgraduate training. There are currently 464 accredited programs. Unlike other specialties, nearly all programs are sponsored by community teaching hospitals that carry some kind of affiliation with a medical school. The curriculum is the broadest of all specialties. Integrating both inpatient and outpatient experiences, residents spend several months rotating through multiple specialties: family practice, internal medicine, obstetrics, gynecology, surgery, emergency medicine, critical care, psychiatry and behavioral health, and numerous medical and surgical subspecialties. Call schedules and work hours depend upon the specific rotation. In the first 2 years of training, there is a greater emphasis on inpatient rotations; the final year consists of more ambulatory experiences. Throughout the entire program, residents carry their own set of patients and provide ongoing care to the same patients in the family practice center.

THE INSIDE SCOOP

are flexible for part-time work, maternity leave, and shared practice arrangements. In group practice, you do not have to take call all the time after office hours. You will instead share call with the other members of your group and cover its entire patient base. Innovations in primary care, like the personal medical home, hold much promise for improving the delivery of outpatient primary care.[16] But the inpatient side of the practice is also important. Family physicians have to round on their patients who require admission to the hospital. If a patient is ready to deliver a baby, and your practice includes obstetrics, you have to leave what you are doing—whether seeing a patient in clinic or having dinner with your family—to deliver the baby at the hospital. Thus, the lifestyle is very dependent on how much inpatient and obstetrical responsibility you choose to carry.

Some family physicians choose comprehensive practices involving obstetric care and surgical activities, whereas others define their scope more narrowly. Some may be the only physician for a large population, whether it is a rural community, an underserved urban community, a nursing home, or a Native American reservation. Those who practice a narrower scope of medicine may work within a multiprovider arrangement with specialists from other fields. In the last decade, there has been a shift both toward solo practice arrangements, sometimes called the "Ideal Micro Practice," with 15.8% of FM graduates practicing in a solo setting in 2008. Family practice or multispecialty groups remain the most common arrangement, comprising two-thirds of all FM graduates.[17] In a larger group setting, a family physician's practice may focus on pediatric, adolescent, or adult populations while still emphasizing family care, prevention, and education.

VITAL
SIGNS

MEDIAN COMPENSATION

Family medicine
(with obstetrics) $197,655
Family medicine
(without obstetrics) $202,047

Data from American Medical Group Association.

Because the role of the family physician in health care today is as complex as the specialty's scope itself, family physicians are often faced with the question of having sufficient knowledge. Although many family physicians supplement their residency with additional training in medical subspecialties, public health, or business, it is certainly not a requirement to practice good family medicine. Many physicians discover on-going training comes from learning what is necessary to care for a particular population. Others simply choose to devote time to their families and extracurricular pursuits. Although the years of residency are rigorous, the life that follows for many is one of immense possibility, filled with the same complexity and life-long inquiry as in any other medical specialty. You can find family physicians heading local departments of public health, conducing health services research, leading national movements for universal health care, or seeing dozens of outpatients a week in a local clinic. Most enjoy a good degree of free time, autonomy, and financial compensation that allows them to successfully integrate their personal and professional goals.

For many family physicians, the broad education and emphasis on systems-based (rather than individual-based) delivery of care provides the ideal foundation for a career in public health. Although formal graduate-level training is not a prerequisite to such a career, a master's degree in public health affords one a certain level of legitimacy among public health professionals. Within this field, the possibilities for career development are endless. Family physicians often work as directors of public health in the same underserved areas where they developed their practice or were trained as a resident. Others become more involved in community-oriented primary care, effecting local changes to strengthen a particular group's capacity to access care and prevent illness. Yet others may find their calling in a joint academic appointment in a medical and public health school, helping to shape future health professionals' thinking about communities and society.

FUTURE CHALLENGES FOR FAMILY MEDICINE

Although today's health care system challenges all physicians to be flexible when caring for their patients, some challenges are unique to family medicine. The core-defining philosophies of family medicine—comprehensive, continuous, coordinated, and patient and family-centered care—are often inconsistent with the apparent goals of the current health care system. For instance, some patients and payers seem to value incidental medical interventions without continuity of provider over the relationship-based and more cost-effective care of family physicians.[18] Among its many provisions, the Patient Protection and Affordable Care Act of 2010 authorizes specific programs to expand the primary care physician workforce and provides an immediate 10% increase in primary care physician payment.[19]

Medical students who might be interested in family medicine encounter multiple challenges. Several academic medical centers continue to resist the promotion of family medicine and primary care. Most medical schools still emphasize the subspecialties in their curricula and encourage students to choose them for future careers. In these environments, family medicine remains a true counterculture. As a result, students may continue to face discouragement as they show interest in pursuing family medicine as a career. In addition, the structure of undergraduate medical education cannot fully capture the richness of family medicine or other primary care specialties. Because medical students frequently rotate from one rotation to the next, they are unable to experience longitudinal outpatient primary care with the same patient more than once or twice. Further, because much of the clerkship experience is hospital based, few students will ever fully appreciate community-based public health or many of the other practice settings in which family physicians work. Finally, participating in the intergenerational care that underlies family medicine is not possible in the course of medical school or even medical school and residency. Compared with other medical specialties, it is difficult to experience the scope of family medicine before deciding to enter it.

Because the scope of clinical research in family medicine is so broad, it may be difficult for students and other physicians view family medicine as the academic specialty it has now become. Although recent initiatives demonstrate a broad range of interests, there is currently a lack of experience in and funding for academic family medicine. As a result, academic inquiries that have fallen out of the traditional organ- or demographic-based scope have found their home in a broader scope: health systems, public health, and health policy research. As these areas of academic investigation develop, family medicine will further define its contribution to the practice of medicine.

A final challenge for medical students entering family medicine is the growing misperception that family physicians will become obsolete as physician assistants and nurse practitioners become more popular.[20] In actuality, however, there has been a steady decline in the number of physician assistants and nurse practitioners entering primary care specialties. Furthermore, as health care reform emphasizes team-based and population-focused care, health care delivery will grow increasingly dependent on primary care and family physicians whose training is naturally in family-centered and community-based health promotion.[21] The challenge facing family medicine, therefore, is preserving interest in and expanding primary care, not worrying about whether other health care professionals will replace them.

FELLOWSHIPS AND SUBSPECIALTY TRAINING

The majority of family physicians do not choose to subspecialize formally. However, some doctors develop specific interests within family medicine and choose to pursue a special area of competence through fellowship or other postgraduate training. Graduates of family medicine residency can complete fellowship training in any number of subspecialties. However, geriatrics and sports medicine are the only accredited fellowships that lead to a certificate of added qualifications. Depending on the fellowship, further training may consist of 1 to 3 years beyond residency.

Geriatrics

This fellowship is similar to the one offered to internal medicine residents. You will gain additional experience in the special medical issues relevant to the elderly. As the population continues to age, there will be a greater need for physicians with specialized training in geriatric medicine.

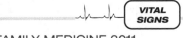

VITAL SIGNS

FAMILY MEDICINE 2011 MATCH STATISTICS

- Number of positions available: 2708
- 1465 US seniors and 3662 independent applicants ranked at least one FM program
- 94.4% of all positions were filled in the initial Match
- The successful applicants: 48.0% US seniors, 33.8% foreign-trained physicians, and 11.4% osteopathic graduates
- Mean USMLE Step I score: 213
- Unmatched rate for US seniors applying only to family medicine: 2.4%

Data from National Resident Matching Program.

Faculty Development

This fellowship program prepares family physicians for a career in academic medicine, frequently as a medical student or resident educator. As a relatively new specialty, departments of family medicine are constantly forming and training new faculty members. If this sounds like a career for you, this fellowship provides experience in research, teaching, leadership, and management.

Obstetrics and Women's Health

A fellowship in obstetrics allows the family physician to acquire intensive training in performing cesarean sections, amniocentesis, tubal ligation, and other obstetrical procedures. Without this experience, most family physicians that include obstetrical care in their practice only perform normal vaginal deliveries and manage fewer high-risk pregnancies.

Research

Research fellowships provide additional scholarly training for family physicians interested in developing careers as independent researchers. Family physician researchers frequently participate in clinical research, health services research, and public policy research. These fellowships last from 1 to 3 years, depending on the availability of local and grant funding.

Rural Medicine

Typically 1 year in duration, rural medicine fellowships are growing in popularity as family physicians seek to build upon skills specific to practicing family medicine in the rural setting. The core curricula focus on community development, procedural skills, local leadership, and quality improvement.

Sports Medicine

Similar to fellowships in sports medicine offered to emergency medicine and internal medicine residents, this program provides additional experience in the care of sports-related injuries. The approach, of course, is much more primary care and medical, rather than surgical.

Other areas that family physicians have chosen for specialty training (but not necessarily through formal accredited fellowships) include preventive medicine, substance abuse, hospice and palliative care, primary care outcomes research, occupational/environmental medicine, community medicine, health policy, medical informatics, family systems medicine, medical education, public health, minority health policy, osteopathic manipulative medicine, health psychology, family planning and reproductive health, emergency medicine, and family medicine hospitalist.

WHY CONSIDER A CAREER IN FAMILY MEDICINE?

Since its creation as an official specialty in 1969, family medicine has fluctuated in popularity. Driven by technical and financial incentives, most medical students chose to enter medical or surgical specialties (and subspecialties) instead of careers in primary care. But medicine became far too fragmented with the increase in specialization; therefore, in the late 1980s, a movement began that encouraged students to consider entering primary care fields again. It worked. The popularity of family medicine jumped accordingly. More and more graduating physicians became family physicians. Family medicine is again enjoying a resurgence in popularity among medical school graduates. Since 2010, family medicine has seen increases in the number of US graduates entering its ranks.[22] After all, family medicine is the perfect specialty for those who love everything about medicine and want to apply that knowledge to serve as a patient's primary physician.

Family medicine is an essential specialty that meets much of the nation's health care needs. As the only doctors who orient care toward the family and the community, family physicians treat nearly everyone, whether insured or uninsured. Knowing their patients' life and clinical history better than anyone else translates into higher quality, individualized patient care—treating the patient, not the disease. As the initial point of contact, family physicians guide patients through the complex health care system, directing them to appropriate tests and specialist referrals when necessary. At every step, family doctors treat all problems, unless they require additional testing or evaluation by a specialist. You are, essentially, a patient advocate, making an incredible difference in their lives. Because of the universal need for family doctors across the country, they are well represented in both urban and rural areas, which means you have a great deal of career flexibility.

If you have a desire to be a primary care physician, then definitely consider this specialty. You will provide comprehensive care for a huge diversity of patients, have long-term rewarding relationships, and focus on preventive medicine and health maintenance. You will diagnose all types of diseases in kids and adults, deliver babies, and perform minor surgery. You may even become formally involved in health policy or public health. But most important, as a family physician you will apply concepts of medicine and health care to any community you choose to serve.

ABOUT THE CONTRIBUTOR

Drs Michael Mendoza and Lisa Vargish completed residency training in family medicine at UCSF/San Francisco General Hospital. They are now family physicians practicing in Rochester, NY. A native of the Windy City, Dr Mendoza attended both college and medical school at the University of Chicago, where he served as a national officer of the American Medical Student Association. During this time, he also earned an MPH at the University of Illinois at Chicago. After serving an additional year as chief resident at UCSF, Dr Mendoza went into practice as a National Health Service Corps Scholar on the south side of Chicago, and recently relocated to Rochester, NY, where he is medical director at Highland Family Medicine, the primary teaching site for the University of Rochester Department of Family Medicine Residency Program. Dr Vargish is a native of New York and earned her undergraduate and graduate degrees from the University of Rochester. After teaching elementary school, she decided to enter medical school and graduated from the University of Chicago. After completing her residency at UCSF and her geriatrics fellowship at the University of Chicago, she earned board certification in geriatrics, hospice and palliative care, and home care. She now directs the Home Care Program for the Jewish Home of Rochester and serves as a faculty preceptor for residents in family medicine and internal medicine at the University of Rochester Medical Center. They can be reached by e-mail at Michael_Mendoza@urmc.rochester.edu or lvargish@jewishseniorlife.org.

REFERENCES

1. AAFP Policies on Health Issues. American Academy of Family physicians Web site. Accessed July 20, 2006, from www.aafp.org/online/en/home/policy/policies/f/familymedicine.html; Accessed January 6, 2012, from http://www.aafp.org/online/en/home/policy/policies/f/fammeddef.html; Accessed January 24, 2012, from www.cdc.gov/nchs/data/ahcd/namcs_summary/namcssum2008.pdf.

2. Visits to Primary Care Delivery Sites: United States, 2008 Esther Hing, M.P.H., and Sayeedha Uddin, M.D., M.P.H. Accessed January 24, 2012, from www.cdc.gov./nchc/data/databriefs/db47.htm.

3. Ambulatory Health Care Data, National Center for Health Statistics. Accessed July 19, 2006, from www.cdc.gov/nchs/about/major/ahcd/officevisitcharts.htm; Accessed January 24, 2012, from www.cdc/nchs/data/nhsr/nhsr027.pdf.

4. Rosenblatt, R.A., Cherkin, D.C., et al. The content of ambulatory medical care in the United States. N Engl J Med. 1983;309:892–897.

5. Starfield, B., Lemke, K.W., et al. Comorbidity: Implications for the importance of primary care in "case" management. *Ann Fam Med.* 2003;1:8–14.

6. Fryer, G., Dovey, S., et al. The importance of having a usual source of health care. *Am Fam Phys.* 2000;62:477.

7. Mold, J.W., Fryer, C.E., et al. Family physicians are the main source of primary health care for the medicare population. *Am Fam Physician.* 2002;66:2032.

8. Stange, K.C., Zyzanski, S.J., et al. Illuminating the block box: a description of 4454 patient visits to 138 family physicians. *J Fam Pract.* 1998;46:377–389.

9. American Academy of Family Physicians, Facts About Family Medicine. Accessed July 19, 2006, from www.aafp.org/online/en/home/aboutus/specialty/facts.html.

10. Ferrante, J.M., Gonzalez, E.C., et al. Effects of physician supply on early detection of breast cancer. *J Am Board Fam Pract.* 2000;13:408–414.

11. Roetzheim, R.G. Gonzalez, E.C., et al. Primary care physician supply and colorectal cancer. *J Fam Pract.* 2001;50:1027–1031.

12. Starfield, B. Primary care and health: A cross-national comparison. *JAMA.* 1991; 266:2268–2271.

13. Shi, L., Starfield, B., et al. Income inequality, primary care, and health indicators. *J Fam Pract.* 1999;48:275–284.

14. Health Professional Shortage Area (HPSA) Mapper. http://www.graham-center.org/online/graham/home/tools-resources/hpsa-map.html; http://www.aafp.org/afp/2008/0515/p1378.html.

15. Fryer, G.E., Green, L.A., et al. The United States relies on family physicians unlike any other specialty. *Am Fam Phys.* 2001;63:1669.

16. Family Medicine, Scope and Philosophical Statement. Accessed January 6, 2012, from http://www.aafp.org/online/en/home/policy/policies/p/personalmedicalhome.html.

17. Facts about Family Medicine. Kansas: American Academy of Family Physicians; 2000. Accessed January 24, 2012, from www.aafp.org/online/en/home/aboutus/specialty/facts/4.html.

18. Graham, R., Roberts, R.G., et al. Family medicine in the United States: A status report. *JAMA.* 2002;288:1097–1101.

19. Martin, J.C., Avant, R.F., et al. The Future of Family Medicine: A collaborative project of the family medicine community. *Ann Fam Med.* 2004;2(Suppl 1):S3–S32.

20. Rosenblatt, R.A. Specialists or generalists: on whom shall we base the American health care system? *JAMA.* 1992;267:1665–1666.

21. *The Robert Graham Center, Physician/Assistant and Nurse Practitioner Workforce Trends.* Accessed July 20, 2006, from www.graham-center.org/onepager37.xml.

22. Hawkins, J. Encouraging news about family physician recruitment. *Fam Pract Manag.* 2005 Apr;12(4):56–58.

17

GENERAL SURGERY

Ashish Raju

S urgery is the field of medicine that often determines whether people live or die. From the trauma patient involved in a high-speed motor vehicle crash to the patient with newly diagnosed breast cancer, it is the one specialty that has the capacity to heal and salvage the lives of people afflicted with disease. There is the proverbial saying that "nothing heals like cold steel." This mantra of every surgical resident yearning for operating time rings true on all levels of the surgical hierarchy. Since there is so much at stake with surgical procedures and the care of critically ill patients, the residency training is extremely intense. The demands are physical, intellectual, and at times emotional. The decision to pursue a general surgery career or subspecialty is often difficult, but definitely a rewarding one. Whether you are interested in performing open-heart surgery or inguinal hernia repair, you must first go through rigorous training in general surgery—the foundation and entry point for most areas of surgical training.

SURGERY DISSECTED

Surgery, the treatment of disease by operation, is often definitive therapy—many times curative—for a broad range of conditions affecting all organ systems. The general surgeon treats diseases of the entire body, from the skin to the blood vessels, to the liver, and beyond. The surgical subspecialties focus on specific body regions, that is, cardiothoracic surgeons address problems of the heart, lungs, and other organs within the thorax (chest), whereas other specialties focus on certain body systems or patient populations, that is, vascular surgeons operate on arteries and veins and pediatric surgeons operate primarily on infants and children. No matter the subspecialty, surgeons are knowledgeable in critical care, and often care for their own critically ill patients in the ICU.

For most new medical students and nonmedical professionals, surgery remains somewhat of a mythical realm characterized by scalpels, blood, and constant action. This mystery may be partly why surgery-based television shows and movies remain so popular in society today. What most people do not see or understand is that surgery is, indeed, structured, organized, thoughtful, and meticulously planned. Even during times of apparent chaos, surgeons have a definitive plan of action to reestablish control, to treat complications, and to make a difference in the lives of their patients. This art requires a great deal of time and experience. Surgical residency aims to provide the broad foundation necessary for a successful career.

General surgery remains one of the few fields in medicine that brings together many disciplines in order to treat patients. As a surgeon, you will master several aspects of the medical field in order to be successful. You need to work up and evaluate a patient with the efficiency of a medical internist. Surgeons must order and analyze radiological investigations with the acuity of a radiologist. After making the final decision for surgery, you will prepare patients with their cardiac and pulmonary status in mind in order to assess the relative risk of the procedure. Finally, after the operation, surgeons care for any severe complications with the intelligence of a critical care specialist. Being a surgeon means much more than just operating as a technician or automaton. In fact, the *peri*operative care often alters the course of life and death in high-risk surgical patients. In this regard, general surgeons are indeed the few remaining renaissance individuals in a new medical landscape where super-specialization is becoming the way of life.

THE ART OF SURGERY

Surgery is as much art as it is science. The surgeon has the privilege of experiencing the delicate beauty of the human body, both internally and externally. Although all physicians have a knowledge of anatomy from their gross anatomy class in medical school, it is only in the surgical disciplines that one can feel these structures pulsating with life. It is exhilarating and awe-inspiring to hold the small bowel in your hand and feel the peristaltic waves, or to touch the breathing, spongy lung of a living being. It is even more exciting to watch these structures tolerate the procedures we perform on them. For example, there is nothing more invigorating than spending an hour concentrating on making an anastomosis (connection) between an artery and vein to form a fistula and then feeling the "thrill" of the blood rushing through it. The surgeon has the manual dexterity and sense of spatial relationships necessary to make the correct incision, perform the appropriate operation, and bring the tissues together for a functional and cosmetically appealing result. All the while, the surgeon is prepared for the unexpected; there is no such thing as routine surgery. Complications can occur at any time, even in the "simplest" of all procedures. In becoming a surgeon, you will develop patience, manual dexterity, and the ability to remain calm and composed under intense pressure.

Surgeons thrive on the immediate gratification of operating. When choosing a specialty, medical students who want to see the results of their treatment on a moment-to-moment basis will gravitate toward the fast-paced surgical specialties. The general surgeon relieves a patient's unbearable abdominal pain by resecting an inflamed appendix or by performing a lysis of adhesions to relieve a small bowel obstruction. The vascular surgeon performs a femoral-popliteal bypass and restores blood flow to a patient's ischemic, painful limb, saving him from amputation. Trauma surgeons repair organs damaged in the path of a bullet, and surgical oncologists perform definitive cancer operations, giving their patients the chance of a cure. As a surgeon, there are never-ending opportunities to use your knowledge, your skill, and your hands to make a difference in the lives of your patients.

Few people are born with the innate technical skills to perform surgery well. For the majority of us, learning how to operate requires repetition, self-awareness, dedication, and intraoperative teaching—all of which take place in the setting of an "apprenticeship" during residency. From the first day of internship, new surgeons are taught the proper technique for performing procedures appropriate to their level. Usually, this begins with closing an incision or placing a "central line" (a catheter inserted into large veins and threaded to the heart in order

---

WHAT MAKES A GOOD SURGEON?

✓ Has excellent hand–eye coordination and manual dexterity. .

✓ Can think quickly, act decisively, and remain flexible.

✓ Enjoys mastering new technology.

✓ Demands the highest level of perfection.

✓ Is an energetic, dedicated, and compassionate physician.

THE INSIDE SCOOP

RESIDENCY TRAINING

Residency in general surgery requires 5 years of postgraduate training. There are currently 254 accredited programs. Some programs offer (or require) an additional 1 to 3 years of basic science or clinical research. There is no argument that surgery is a tough residency. Residents arrive at the hospital very early to round on

(continued)

their patients before heading to the operating room. Because patient care and consultations continue after finishing the scheduled operations, the days are long and physically demanding. To comply with the new 80-hour workweek requirements, surgical residents are seeing the emergence of "night float" systems and shift work. In the first year, interns spend little time in the operating room. They see patients in the hospital requiring consultation and master the essentials of postoperative care on the wards and in the ICU. Operating room time increases throughout the year, and cases are usually allocated based upon complexity. Residents spend the first 2 years primarily in general surgery but also rotating through surgical subspecialties such as neurosurgery, urology, and orthopedics. The remaining 3 years are dedicated to rotations in general, vascular, cardiothoracic, pediatric, and transplant surgery. Additional months of training include surgical intensive care and endoscopy. Residency in general surgery provides the gateway to a number of subspecialties that require fellowship training.

THE INSIDE SCOOP

to obtain central venous access for administering fluids and drugs). For all procedures, residents can learn certain aspects from textbooks: landmarks, patient positioning, indications, and risks. But the art of the procedure must be learned as an apprentice. To ensure the development of good technique with minimal risks to the patient, senior residents and attendings teach junior residents how to hold instruments properly, take a stitch, tie knots, and use the "bovie" (electrocautery device). They teach them how to avoid the common technical errors that can result in a bad outcome. There are some "tricks of the trade" that no textbook can illustrate. These subtleties are taught by observation and experience over 5 years of clinical training. Over time, every resident cultivates his or her own style, within the limits of being a safe and skilled surgeon.

THE SURGICAL FIELD IN TRANSITION

With the advent of resident hour restrictions in medicine limiting hours within the hospital to an average of 80 hours a week, the surgical landscape and specialty as a whole are undergoing dramatic changes. Resident duty hour requirements were started in July 2003 by the Accreditation Council for Graduate Medical Education (ACGME).[1] Gone are the days of relatively living within the hospital and 120-hour weeks. This change may be partly responsible for the rising interest and increased applications for general surgery positions around the country.

Individuals who would give up surgery due to the previous time dedication are reconsidering their options and pursuing surgical careers.

A recent survey of residents in surgical programs in New England revealed that their "practice desires" and "lifestyle choices" varied significantly from surgeons already in practice. The majority of them wished to work 60 hours a week or less as attendings.[1] Whether the change in the residency hours is responsible for this outlook is not yet clear.

The shift work associated with the new restrictions and possible lack of continuity in care may reveal new problems to be addressed. For example, serial abdominal examinations on a patient with a questionable abdominal process and pain in prior years could be performed by one surgical resident. Any changes would be apparent because one resident knew the examinations based upon his own assessment earlier in the day. Now, however, within a 24-hour shift, there may be as many as three different residents assessing the patient at successive intervals without exact knowledge of the previous examination's impression. Therefore, "sign-out" rounds in surgical residencies are becoming critical in establishing continuity of care and patient safety. The true long-term effect of the duty-hour restrictions on surgical care remains to be seen.

As technology in the medical field continues to grow, so do surgical techniques and options. What was previously done through large incisions is now being performed through small holes and with cameras. Laparoscopic surgery has revolutionized the surgical field. Old "bread and butter" appendectomies and cholecystectomies, which were done with open incisions followed by a couple of days in the hospital, are now being done laparoscopically. The future of minimally invasive surgery promises "scarless" surgery via natural orifice translumenal endoscopic surgery. Patients recover faster and are discharged earlier. A modern surgeon needs to be apprised of new surgical techniques and discoveries in order to provide his or her patient the best care possible. Therefore, residencies are beginning to incorporate this training with simulator equipment into the curriculum. Surgery is no longer merely scalpels and lap sponges. It is now characterized by trocars, angled cameras, endografts, and robotic machines. As a surgical resident and attending, you will need to stay on the cutting edge of new technology and treatments.

THE "SURGICAL PERSONALITY"

The surgical rotation for many medical students is often viewed as scary and overwhelming. You are expected to arrive early in the morning and often leave late at night. You follow the lifestyle of the residents characterized by hunger and exhaustion. Yet, you share the thrill of being in the operating room, being part of a team, and helping take care of patients. However, attending surgeons are sometimes known to be ruthless during morbidity and mortality rounds by interrogating residents. Some in medical school were told that surgery was a frightening place where you were advised to tread carefully. It is fair to say that much has changed in recent years in the surgical personality.

Most surgeons do not fit the description of being insensitive, overbearing, and arrogant. They are diligent, caring, lively, and driven. They are team players and take personal pride in their work. They are decisive, compulsive, and seek success in all their endeavors. These qualities reflect the level of dedication and personal responsibility surgeons take in the care of their patients. After all, surgeons need the confidence and ability to be assertive when necessary. They have to control their environment when carrying out plans. Remarkably, these characteristics have been extensively studied and well represented in the surgical literature. A recent study, for instance, examined the traits that are more common in surgeons than in the general population. The authors found that surgeons are less neurotic, more extroverted, more open, and more conscientious.[1] They also concluded that surgeons are more likely to be aggressive, to prefer competition, and to express their anger when necessary. It is easy to see how these traits are adaptive in this field.

No matter the stereotype, surgeons are team players. It is ironic that the "typical surgeon" perceived by young doctors-in-training is a lone wolf, self-directed, and independent, where, in reality, the success of the individual surgeon depends on working well as a member of the team. The surgeon is called upon to consult on surgical issues and perform basic procedures for other services. (The placement of chest tubes and difficult central lines are two of the most common such procedures.) This highlights the constant interaction between surgeons and other physicians and the need for a collegial relationship. The surgeon must communicate effectively with referring physicians, whether they are in internal medicine, gastroenterology, pulmonology, or other services. The efficient and accurate transfer of information is essential for the care of the surgical patient, and this requires excellent skills of communication.

Most attendings are no longer unapproachable and feared. The old mentality is being replaced by a supportive and understanding one. Surgeons are demanding and meticulous because they want the best care for their patients. This often requires them to be unyielding and uncompromising in the management of their patients. That is why they are often viewed in such light by peers and outsiders. Make no mistake—surgeons are indeed dedicated, compassionate, and unwavering in their responsibilities to their patients.

SURGICAL PROWESS

Details—it's all about the details! This is what makes a great surgeon. Attending physicians and senior residents remind you of this quintessential point every day of your surgical residency. The correct way sutures are placed, the extra attention paid to a critically ill patient, and knowing when to operate are a few of key qualities that distinguishes an awesome surgeon from an average one.

As a surgeon, you must think on your feet and keep your composure in stressful situations. You cannot always predict what you will encounter during an operation, and therefore you must remain levelheaded and ready for anything. This requires a mastery of anatomy and common anatomic abnormalities, physiology and pathophysiology of disease, as well as of proper surgical technique and options for treatment. For example, to safely perform a laparoscopic cholecystectomy, surgeons must know the common anatomic variations of cystic arteries, hepatic arteries, and the ductal system. They have to understand unusual disorders of the biliary tract such as Mirizzi syndrome and parasitic diseases such as *Clonorchis sinensis* infection to accurately interpret the clinical, radiographic, and intraoperative findings. Surgeons must know when it is appropriate to perform cholecystectomy rather than simply placing a cholecystostomy tube. This question often arises with the elderly and debilitated or those who refuse surgical intervention.

As a surgical resident, you will be tired, sleepy, and hungry. You will stand on your feet for consecutive hours and be asked to stand for many more. You need to know that the road is not easy and is quite long compared with other specialties. However, the impact that surgery can have in the face of illness is great. This is what makes surgery worthwhile for so many residents and students. Moreover, education as a surgery resident occurs constantly. Unlike other medical specialties, surgery demands that you learn in many different ways. In the operating room, your mentors will teach you how to cut, bovie, suture, and tie. Outside the operating room, surgical trainees learn how to manage their patients postoperatively. There will be a great deal of responsibility placed upon you as a resident to identify your strengths, weakness, and areas of improvement.

Like all physicians, surgeons begin with a focused history and physical examination before making the diagnosis and the decision to operate. In a typical day, surgeons may receive a page from the emergency department regarding an elderly patient with abdominal pain, emesis, and increased white blood cell count, and simultaneously receive a request for consultation on an incarcerated inguinal hernia from the medicine clinic. The surgeon must ask focused questions to determine the acuity of the consult and prioritize the order in which patients will be seen. Proper clinical judgment determines what tests must be ordered, if further radiographic studies are appropriate, or if the patient should proceed directly to the operating room. What differentiates surgical disciplines from other fields is the limited time available to integrate reams of information from the history, physical examination, lab results, and radiographic studies to come to the correct diagnosis and pursue the proper course of action. This requires a sense of urgency and self-motivation on the part of the surgeon.

THE DOCTOR–PATIENT RELATIONSHIP

As a surgeon, you meet patients along various points in their medical course. You may be called in consult regarding a gastrointestinal bleed in a patient who is in the ICU setting. Another patient may be on an operating room table, and during a routine hysterectomy, an inadvertent enterotomy (hole in bowel) was created requiring your attention. Outside the hospital in your office, a family physician may refer a patient to you because of a breast lump noted on routine physical examination. The most important aspect of being a surgeon is not knowing just how to operate but also when to operate. Therefore, it is paramount that you educate the patient about his or her illness, assess the risks and benefits, and provide information regarding complications so that they can make an informed decision.

The amount of trust that patients place in doctors, especially surgeons, remains unparalleled in all other professions. Patients who are sick and in pain meet doctors for the first time and immediately reveal the most personal information regarding their lives, habits, activities, and desires. Therefore, it is required that surgeons be understanding and open regarding the wishes of patients and their families. After all, patients have to give up control of their medical care and entrust their welfare to your skill and judgment. They may be frightened about undergoing even relatively simple operations such as hernia repair or setting of a fracture. The surgeon must provide comfort during this time of stress and anxiety. A good surgeon–patient relationship requires sensitivity, compassion, and a gentle hand. Despite all the technology involved in an operation, some of the greatest tools of the surgeon are the physical examination and the history. In the time spent taking a history and performing a physical examination, the physician builds a rapport and trust. During the history, the surgeon learns about the patient's belief system and his or her wishes. Many procedures, such as mastectomy (the removal of a breast), have long-term emotional impact, and so you must be prepared to address these concerns. The surgeon–patient relationship does not end at the close of the case. Patients return to the office with questions regarding postoperative pain and changes in their physiology or physical appearance.

After establishing the relationship between surgeon and patient, it is the duty of the surgeon to follow that patient until surgical issues have been addressed and resolved. Surgeons do not operate and then send patients back to their primary physician. Instead, they typically have close, often long-term relationships with their patients. For example, in the case of a patient who comes into the emergency room with right lower quadrant pain and undergoes an appendectomy, this means following the patient in the hospital until discharge, instructing the patient in wound care, answering all questions, setting them up for follow-up visit, seeing them in the office postoperatively, and addressing any other concerns. In this instance, it may be a relationship that lasts a few weeks. In other situations, such as treating patients with Crohn's disease or colon cancer, it requires patience, compassion, and dedication. These illnesses may require several operations, dealing with complications, and supporting the patients and family members through very difficult times. The end point is hopefully resolution of their illness, but sometimes it requires compassion until the last breath.

LIFESTYLE CONSIDERATIONS AND PRACTICE OPTIONS

It is true that surgery requires intense dedication and residency is a minimum of 5 years in length, but what happens after that? Although there is little control over work hours during residency, afterward surgeons can choose from a multitude of practice settings and decide how much or how little they want to work. Needless to say, if you enjoy what you do, the hours will be less of an issue. While it is ideal to have control over your time and where you spend it, if you are tethered to something you love, it is hardly a punishment. Most medical students are exposed only to the highly specialized practice of academic surgery, but the field of general surgery is practiced in a multitude of ways. As an academic surgeon, you can divide your time between research, clinical duties, and teaching. Academic surgeons are often experts in a certain field, for example, parathyroid surgery or inflammatory bowel disease, and give lectures at other institutions in their chosen subspecialty. You will have residents to buffer you from the minutiae, but you ultimately are in control of the care of the patients. Moreover, teaching in the operating room and in formal lectures is an enjoyable and fulfilling experience.

MEDIAN COMPENSATION

Cardiothoracic surgery	$507,143
Colon and rectal surgery	$366,895
General surgery	$340,000
Oncology	$337,475
Pediatric surgery	$400,591
Transplant surgery (kidney)	$348,000
Transplant surgery (liver)	$433,333
Trauma surgery	$399,558
Vascular surgery	$403,041

Data from American Medical Group Association.

Alternatively, you could become one of many surgeons in a group practice. Surgical attendings usually divide up their hospital week with operating days and office days. They have some days where they operate in the morning and see patients in the afternoon. The size of the practice and volume will dictate how often they operate. In this private arrangement, there is a set on-call schedule and a wealth of patients from established referral patterns. Although private practice surgeons may have less control over when they work, the hours are usually predictable and predetermined. Some of these surgeons also serve as clinical attendings and have resident coverage. Some go into solo private practice where there is maximal control over the work hours, but you are responsible for practice management, reimbursement, and referral patterns, which administrators take care of in the academic and mega-medical-group settings. A rare few leave the clinical arena and dedicate their time to industry or research. Whatever practice you choose, your lifestyle will no longer be that of a surgical resident.

Attending surgeons who are a part of a university hospital may share call responsibilities and rounding on surgical inpatients. The advantages of being part of a university practice includes the ability to teach residents and medical students, engage in research studies, and avoid some of the financial issues and overhead costs associated with private practice. The disadvantages usually include less income or personal freedom with regard to managing the practice. Many surgeons love teaching and shaping the education of residents and students over the years. For them, they desire an academic position over private practice benefits.

FELLOWSHIPS AND SUBSPECIALTY TRAINING

After the completion of general surgery training, there are several options available for subspecialization. Some individuals decide to forgo further training and dive right into practice as general surgery attendings. For others, the difficulty is often

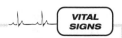

**GENERAL SURGERY
2011 MATCH STATISTICS**

- Number of positions available: 1108
- 1273 US seniors and 1003 independent applicants ranked at least one surgery program
- 99.8% of all positions were filled in the initial Match
- The successful applicants: 81.1% US seniors, 9.7% foreign-trained physicians, and 2.5% osteopathic graduates
- Mean USMLE Step I score: 227
- Unmatched rate for US seniors applying only to general surgery: 14.9%

Data from National Resident Matching Program.

choosing one specific area. Most of the application process takes place during the fourth year of clinical training. By then, the surgical resident has been exposed to a wide range of the available specialties.

Cardiothoracic Surgery

As the name implies, surgery is on the heart and in the chest cavity. It also includes operations on the lungs, esophagus, and major blood vessels in the chest. Heart surgery includes coronary artery bypass grafting, valve replacements, heart transplants, thoracic aneurysm repairs, septal defect repairs, and trauma to the heart. Thoracic surgery includes lung resections, esophageal resections/reconstructions, video-assisted thoracic surgery (VATS), pleurodesis, and similar procedures. The fellowship may be 2 or 3 years depending on the program. There are also fellowships that emphasize cardiac operations. Others focus more on thoracic and lung surgery. It is therefore important to know which interests you more and apply to programs accordingly. If you enjoy cardiac and pulmonary physiology, love meticulous procedures, and become excited with the idea of operating within the chest, CT surgery may be your calling.

Colorectal Surgery

Colon and rectal surgery is growing with the increased screening for colon cancer and other disorders of the lower gastrointestinal tract. Patients will come to you with a variety of pathology, including colorectal cancer, motility disorders, inflammatory bowel disease, diverticulitis, anal fissures and fistulas, constipation, and fecal incontinence. These subspecialists perform colon resections, low anterior resections, abdominal perineal resections, hemorrhoidectomies, operations for Crohn's disease, anal fissures, and colonoscopies. Fellowship training is 1 year in length. Many of these surgeons have working relationships with gastroenterologists so that they have a strong referral base for their practice. Colorectal surgeons take care of patients within a wide range of ages, from a young male with ulcerative colitis to an elderly woman with a colonic mass.

Pediatric Surgery

Pediatric surgeons work in all aspects of the care of children from prematurity to adolescence, such as the repair of congenital defects and treating traumatic injuries and burns. Like true general surgeons, they perform operations on the entire body: abdomen, chest, extremities, and more. Common pathologies encountered include disorders of development such as pyloric stenosis, congenital anomalies such as Hirschsprung disease, and childhood cancers. Known for its delicate precision, pediatric surgery is challenging. These surgeons work with pediatricians, pediatric intensivists, and other surgical subspecialties such as otolaryngology to provide the best comprehensive care for their young patients. As one of the most competitive subspecialties, pediatric surgery is usually 2 years in length following general surgery training. Since there are so few spots throughout the country, many applicants supplant their resume with additional time of surgical research and experience prior to applying for this specialty.

Surgical Oncology

For some patients with cancer, surgery offers the possibility of a cure, while for others, operation means palliation, allowing them to live comfortably with an incurable cancer. Surgical oncology offers additional training in the most complex operations. Like their colleagues in medical and radiation oncology, surgical oncologists deal with strong emotions, particularly when their patients' cancer is unresectable, recurs, or has metastasized. Many surgical oncologists work in academic medical centers and conduct cancer research. Fellowships in this subspecialty require 2 years of additional training.

Transplantation Surgery

With a particular emphasis on complex medical management, this subspecialty encompasses kidney, liver, pancreas, and small bowel transplantation. Transplant surgery is a very exciting field that relies on many medical disciplines for its success. With immunology as one of its scientific bases, it calls upon knowledge of anatomy, physiology, infectious disease, and basic sciences. Fellows usually train in 2-year programs that focus on performing organ transplants for patients with end-stage organ failure, caring for them perioperatively, and treating any complications that may arise following transplantation. The transplant surgeon works as a part of an integrated team of professionals, including nurses, social workers, and medical subspecialists (nephrologists, endocrinologists, and hepatologists).

Trauma Surgery and Critical Care

These subspecialists care for victims of traumatic injuries, such as gunshot and stab wounds, crush injuries, motor vehicle accidents, electrical injuries, and many more. Scenarios requiring operative intervention will call upon you to operate efficiently and quickly in order to save lives. Trauma surgeons are general surgeons who operate throughout the entire body in order to resuscitate their injured patients. In the emergency department, they usually lead the "trauma team" to stabilize and resuscitate critically ill patients before taking them to the operating room. Trauma surgeons also coordinate care with various consultants including neurosurgery, orthopedics, vascular surgery, plastic surgery, and oral–maxillofacial surgery. Trauma fellowships are usually 1 year in length. In addition to acute management of emergency situations, you will receive extensive training in the intensive care management of critically ill patients.

Vascular Surgery

Vascular surgery involves the arteries and veins of the entire body, from the neck to the distal extremities. Surgical procedures include carotid endarterectomies, arteriovenous fistulas, abdominal aortic aneurysm (AAA) repairs, bypass procedures to revascularize threatened extremities, angiographic procedures, amputations for ischemia, repair of pseudoaneurysms, and repair of any type of disruption of blood vessels. Vascular surgery is now characterized by procedures including endovascular AAA repairs, carotid stent grafting, peripheral endovascular therapies, and advances in vascular technology and research. There is an increasing demand for vascular surgeons given the aging population with vascular diseases. Due to the fact that the vascular disease process is not limited to specific parts of the body, patients often have heart, pulmonary, and comorbid conditions such as diabetes, hypertension, and increased cholesterol. Therefore, these patients are very sick and high-risk operative candidates. Vascular surgeons are skilled operators who operate despite dangerous conditions in hopes of improving the lives of their debilitated patients. The fellowship is 2 years in length. If you are confident in pursuing a vascular surgery career, you may want to consider applying to several integrated vascular surgery residencies that now exist. They are 5 years in length and the first 2 years cover core general surgery rotations. The last 3 years are dedicated to vascular surgery training.

WHY CONSIDER A CAREER IN GENERAL SURGERY?

As a field of medicine, surgery is never stagnant. Since it is constantly evolving, surgeons must learn to change and adapt as well. From day 1 as a lowly intern, there will always be perpetual training, teaching, and learning. It continues into your subspecialty, practice, and eventual livelihood as a surgeon. Those who choose general surgery understand that this is a lifestyle decision. You cannot change the lives of patients without giving some of your own in the process. Surgeons come to terms with this sacrifice and find great satisfaction in positively and immediately impacting the lives of their patients.

Surgery is an intellectually, physically, and emotionally challenging specialty that surgeons love to be a part of. Nothing is greater than the unbelievable surge of adrenaline that occurs while scrubbing in, stepping into the operating room, and gowning up. Within the hospital or private practice, being a surgeon means being the master conductor in the care of surgical patients. It calls upon an individual who enjoys working with and at times directing various other specialties toward the common goal of curing illness. Surgeons combine the knowledge of a scientist, precision of a technician, passion of an artist, and empathy of a physician. They demand nothing but the best for the patients, and they give nothing but the best in all of their efforts. Although challenging and demanding, surgery will amply reward all the effort you put into it.

ABOUT THE CONTRIBUTOR

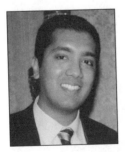

Dr Ashish Raju is a fellow in vascular and endovascular surgery at Montefiore Medical Center, New York. He completed his general surgery residency at the University of Medicine and Dentistry of New Jersey/Robert Wood Johnson Medical School. After growing up in Queens, New York, Dr Raju completed a 6-year accelerated BA/MD program through Lehigh University and Drexel University College of Medicine. He enjoys following sports, writing, traveling, and spending time with family. He can be reached by e-mail at ashish.raju@gmail.com.

REFERENCE

1. McGreevy, J., Wiebe, D. A preliminary measurement of the surgical personality. *Am J Surg.* 2002;184:121–125.

SOURCES

1. Breen, E., Irani, J.L., et al. The future of surgery: Today's residents speak. *Curr Surg.* 2005;62(5):543–546.

2. Johansen, K.H., David, M. *So, You Want To Be a Surgeon.* American College of Surgeons. 2001–2003.

18

INTERNAL MEDICINE

Jennifer Tong and Ian Tong

Even well-seasoned medical students are impressed by internal medicine for both its broad scope and immense depth. If you are unsure what the discipline of internal medicine really includes, you are not alone! Many medical students, patients, public policy makers, and even physicians in other fields of medicine find internal medicine difficult to define. Terms such as internist and internal medicine often elude patients. In fact, nearly half of all patients confuse these physicians with family practice doctors, general practitioners, or even interns (first-year residents).[1] Despite this superficial level of confusion, if you ever closed your eyes and dreamed of 1 day being a caring doctor who builds meaningful relationships with his or her patients . . . then the doctor you envisioned was likely an internal medicine doctor.

Internists take care of the general medical problems of adults. In a single day, they can act as a diagnostician, an educator, a director, an advocate, a motivator, a healer, and a comforter. In the clinic, they treat their patients' aches, pains, and sniffles. They also come to their bedsides in the hospital and manage their inpatient care. Some internists spend their time providing acute and chronic primary care, while others become subspecialists in cardiology, gastroenterology, endocrinology, and more. Whether focusing on one organ system or taking care of the whole patient, internists approach everything with great intellectual curiosity. Sick patients with complex medical problems turn to internists for high-quality care.

INTERNAL MEDICINE IS REALLY "ADULT MEDICINE"

In 1999, the American College of Physicians (ACP) initiated a public relations campaign called "Doctors for Adults" to help patients understand the true role of the internist within the medical community.[2] This catchphrase captures the underlying common denominator within internal medicine—physicians who are experts in the nonsurgical health care needs of anyone older than 18 years. In many ways, internists are similar in practice style to pediatricians—but the kids have grown up. There is less asthma and more emphysema; the neonatal intensive care unit has been replaced by the coronary care unit; and instead of worried parents, there are concerned adult children.

Internists provide comprehensive medical care over a long period of time. Their primary responsibility is to diagnose and treat acute and chronic medical conditions. A number of illnesses invariably comprise the core of most internal medicine practices. These diseases can range from acute problems such as upper respiratory tract infections, influenza, viral gastroenteritis, and urinary tract infections to more chronic problems such as diabetes mellitus, chronic obstructive pulmonary disease, hypercholesterolemia, and hypertension. In fact, a large proportion of medical patients are elderly with complex, chronic comorbidities. Common illnesses treated in the young-adult and middle-aged populations include gastroesophageal reflux disease, peptic ulcer disease, hyper- or hypothyroidism, depression, musculoskeletal injuries, sexually transmitted diseases, and the acute infections listed earlier. Despite the usual plethora of common complaints and illnesses, internists also have many opportunities to diagnose and treat rare diseases such as babesiosis or Still's disease. This is why a general internist's daily practice spans a number of medical disciplines. You receive the challenges (as well as the rewards) of treating a broader range of illnesses than in almost any other specialty.

As you can tell, internists are more than just doctors for adults. This specialty is all about diversity: a varied group of patients spanning late adolescence to the end of life, a number of practice settings from the clinic to the hospital, a broad range of illnesses from acute to chronic, and 21 board certified subspecialties in which one can specialize. For example, a physician trained in general internal medicine will evaluate a 24-year-old woman presenting with weight loss and night sweats, while a colleague who specialized in cardiology treats a 70-year-old heart-attack victim in the cardiac catheterization lab. On a given day, a general internist with a special interest in sports medicine will treat a 40-year-old male with a torn rotator cuff, while another colleague gives preventive influenza vaccinations to the residents of a nursing home.

No matter the subspecialty, all internists have a similar set of clinical responsibilities. Most important, they provide complex medical care while diagnosing and treating acute and chronic problems, whether in the office or hospital. Internists were traditionally responsible for taking care of their own patients when they were admitted to the hospital (for problems such as congestive heart failure, pancreatitis, asthma, bacteremia, unstable angina, and pneumonia). Some office-based internists still care for their patients in the hospital, but others rely on general internists who specialize in hospital medicine (hospitalists). Most internists practice preventive medicine, which involves health maintenance and disease screening. Although some internists may have a subset of patients who fall within that physician's area of expertise, most rely on colleagues in other subspecialties for consultations on advanced problems. General internists must be aware of their own limitations and know when to seek specialized help on a given organ system disease. But do not think that these internists just spend their time consulting others. In fact, they are often asked by surgeons and obstetricians to see patients who have difficult general medical conditions.

Internists and family practitioners both take care of adult patients. So what makes a career in internal medicine unique? Internists have highly detailed knowledge about how to manage the most complicated of medical problems found in the adult population. Family practitioners, on the other hand, care for people of all ages throughout their entire lives. Because they have broader training across other disciplines (obstetrics–gynecology, surgery, psychiatry), family practice doctors have less depth of training in internal medicine. Internists, of course, do not treat young children or deliver babies. Another distinguishing feature of internal medicine is the option to subspecialize in a vast array of fields after residency. Although many internal medicine residents choose to enter a subspecialty fellowship, others remain in the broad field of general internal medicine and become known as general internists.

READY TO EXERCISE YOUR BRAIN?

Internal medicine is perhaps the most cerebral of all specialties. It requires a high level of critical thinking. Many students are drawn to internal medicine for the intellectual stimulation. There are always interesting cases that require a lot of problem solving and interpretation of signs, symptoms, and other pieces of data.

WHAT MAKES A GOOD INTERNIST?

✓ Likes physical diagnosis, pharmacology, and physiology.
✓ Is a thorough, cautious problem solver.
✓ Can interact well with people and maintain long-term relationships.
✓ Likes working with his or her mind.
✓ Is a good, patient listener.

THE INSIDE SCOOP

Internists are very intellectually curious doctors. They always like to ask questions of themselves and others during the differential diagnosis process. Fascinated by the science of medicine, internists love exploring details—such as the mechanisms of drug therapy or the pathophysiology of disease. To make the best diagnosis, internists tend to read quite a bit. Keeping abreast of the latest advances in general medicine requires a career-long commitment to reading journals such as *JAMA* or *The New England Journal of Medicine*.

Critical thinking is necessary because internists take a scientific approach to being master diagnosticians. They thrive on making a great diagnosis, analyzing a fascinating big case, and solving complex medical problems. Internists love to sit around and discuss disease. They get excited by putting together a patient's signs, symptoms, and laboratory findings and trying to come up with a long list of possible differential diagnoses. Students who love to solve problems and mental puzzles find internal medicine a fascinating specialty.

Internists are experts at taking patient histories and performing physical examinations. It is with the information derived from the history and physical (H&P) that they make most diagnoses. After talking to the patient, the internist constructs a list of differential diagnoses for each of the patient's problems. This process allows them to clearly organize in their minds what is going on with the patient and how to address each issue; many patients have multiple medical problems or complaints. To finalize a diagnosis from a list of many, the internist relies on a great deal of critical thinking and deductive reasoning from the data at hand. They take pieces of evidence from the history, physical examination, laboratory data, and imaging studies to rule in or rule out various disease states. It very much resembles detective work. An academic internist colleague commented that "figuring out how all the pieces to a patients' clinical puzzle fit together is extremely rewarding."

With a confident diagnosis in hand, the internist then moves on to treating the patient. Across the subspecialties of internal medicine, therapeutic interventions take the form of either pharmacologic agents or procedures. General internists, for instance, keep up with the advances in treating high blood pressure with the newest medications and are experts at figuring out the proper antibiotic for a patient with bacterial meningitis. Although this specialty requires thorough, organized thought, internists are more than just thinkers; they are also proficient in many technical skills essential for the diagnosis and treatment of illness. These skills include a number of inpatient procedures, such as thoracentesis, paracentesis, lumbar puncture, and central line placement, and outpatient procedures, such as flexible sigmoidoscopy, endometrial biopsy, and intra-articular injections. Subspecialists such as cardiologists open blocked arteries through percutaneous transluminal coronary angioplasty, and gastroenterologists excise cancerous colon polyps through colonoscopy or stop upper gastrointestinal bleeding through esophagogastroduodenoscopy (EGD), try saying that three times fast!

THE DOCTOR–PATIENT RELATIONSHIP

The ability to listen, understand, explain, advise, and educate are central to the role of an internist. Without strong interpersonal skills, it would be difficult to diagnose an underlying substance abuse problem, help a patient start an exercise program or quit smoking, encourage healthier eating habits, or guide a patient's decision to sign a do-not-resuscitate order and abandon aggressive treatment. Through comprehensive history taking and physicals, internists spend a great deal of time with their patients—talking with them and gaining insight into their lives, their values, and their concerns. Internists often use techniques such as motivational interviewing to provide an environment in which patients can effect lasting behavior change. This approach, which repositions the internist as a guide or coach for the patient, has come to be known as *patient-centered or relationship-centered care*.[3] Physicians using these approaches enjoy life-long, trusting relationships with their patients.

Having close relationships with patients and their families is one of the best things about a career in general internal medicine. Unlike the patient of an emergency medicine physician or anesthesiologist, your patient has the potential to stay with you until old age and death. You can imagine the immense amount of trust that builds in healthy doctor–patient relationships. Patients will share with you their secrets, their fears, and their insecurities. In moments of crisis, you will guide your patient through illness amidst what can sometimes be paralyzing fears. Internists must respect the privilege of this trust and the enormous responsibility that comes with it.

Much in the same way an expert climber will guide the novice rock climber in where to place their feet, what type of grip to use, when to use safety measures, an experienced internist helps patients find traction through the health care system and the myriad of subspecialty care and treatment options. This concept of providing an interface between patients and the health care system has recently been given the term "systems-based practice." Internists with strong systems knowledge are very skilled at helping patients avoid unnecessary or redundant tests. Their patients rarely feel lost or isolated, because they trust their doctor knows where to find help and what to expect next.

Although the action of internal medicine practice is not always as tangible as performing a liver transplant, delivering a baby, or intubating a patient before surgery, it is still complex and challenging. Within this specialty, the goal of intervention may not necessarily be to cure disease but to help the patient understand the disease and cope with its psychosocial ramifications. Beyond thinking and communicating, internal medicine requires exploring patients' cultural beliefs, recognizing the impact of socioeconomic status, educating patients about diseases and treatments, motivating lifestyle changes, and organizing multidisciplinary care.

As an internist, you will pride yourself on your ability to solve difficult problems under intense pressure and sensitive circumstances. Take the following example. An internist in private practice was evaluating a new patient in the hospital—a Taiwanese man visiting his family in the United States who became acutely and gravely ill but did not have health insurance. The patient's family members were divided on the decision of whether to continue hospital treatment versus caring for the patient at home due to financial concerns. Although the family was concerned about the patient's lack of insurance and the cost of continued care, they were also guided by cultural values to pursue every option to preserve the patient's life. As demonstrated by this case, the internist's role not only requires challenging medical management but also skills such as cultural competence, family mediation, health care economics, and a holistic view of care.

BEING ON THE FRONT LINE OF MEDICINE

An internist is often the first physician a patient turns to when an illness or symptom arises. By being on the first line of defense, the internist's initial interaction can influence the likelihood the patient will follow up after this visit. An internist with limited patience, poor communication skills, and skepticism toward the validity of the patient's complaint may discourage the patient from seeking further medical care. In contrast, the internist who expresses an appropriate level of concern validates the patient's complaint and offers an understandable follow-up plan that may improve the likelihood that the patient will return for needed medical care. If you enjoy helping others solve problems while providing encouragement, patience, and guidance, then definitely consider a career in internal medicine.

Being on the front line of medicine also offers the intellectual stimulation and challenge of diagnosis. As the first physician to hear and understand the patient's complaint, your skill as a diagnostician directs the treatment plan. Being an effective diagnostician requires skill as an historian and examiner as well as the ability to synthesize history, physical examination findings, laboratory data, and study results. For example, internists are commonly presented with chief complaints of cough and heartburn. Although many of these cases can be attributed to upper respiratory infections or gastroesophageal reflux, the detail-oriented internist recognizes the necessity of a thorough history and physical examination to determine whether further workup is needed. But in today's health care environment of conservative resource utilization, only good clinical judgment can guide the appropriate decision to explore a patient's complaint further with laboratory tests and technological studies.

Preventive medicine is another extremely important part of being on the front line of medicine. Some patients may say "Stop smoking—are you joking?!" or "Colonoscopy? You must be crazy!" But among the global goals of medical care, the prevention of disease has recently achieved a status equal to that of diagnosis and treatment. The difficulty of addressing chronic, multisystem illnesses in the limited time allotted for patient visits makes preventive health care one of the most challenging (and sometimes frustrating) areas of internal medicine. Suggesting a patient replace a weekly meal of fried chicken with grilled fish or convincing a patient it is worthwhile to have a 2-ft scope inserted through the rectum can make you feel more like a salesperson than a physician! The lack of short-term, recognizable results also tends to make prevention a lower priority for patients as well as physicians. If you can envision yourself educating and motivating patients to change their lifestyle, internal medicine certainly provides abundant opportunities to do so. The future of this specialty undoubtedly involves an increase in the number and complexity of screening tests, as well as the opportunity for research on motivating and achieving changes in lifestyle.

THE INTERNIST AS "HEAD COACH"

Because many patients have multisystem diseases requiring specialized care, the team of physicians and other health care providers can easily become fragmented and disorganized, which in turn may seem confusing and frustrating for patients. An organized internist with leadership skills can prevent or at least minimize this frustration and confusion. By tracking medications prescribed by other physicians, monitoring potential drug interactions, following up on studies or procedures performed by subspecialists, and responding to their recommendations, the internist orchestrates multidisciplinary care and helps the patient navigate a complex system of health care delivery. In addition, the internist acts as the patient's advocate within the complex health care environment of resource utilization and restricted access to care.

Internists not only serve as leaders of a multidisciplinary team but also determine which physicians are on the playing field, coordinating care similar to the way National Football League (NFL) coaches used to send in plays with wide receivers (prior to the use of in-helmet radios). As an internist you must provide an appropriate level of specialized care, then recognize your limitations and refer the patient to a subspecialist for optimal care. This can become a fine line for any internist—requiring an impressive breadth of knowledge but a willingness to admit limitations as well. You can imagine a dermatologist being dismayed when an internist could not treat a patient with simple eczema or an infectious disease specialist frustrated by an internist's insistence on treating HIV even though the internist was not up to date on the standard of HIV care. To provide the best care, internists must learn to turn to subspecialty care when it is appropriate and establish professional, mutually respectful relationships with subspecialists.

THOUGHTS ON INTERNIST CAREER SATISFACTION

A recent commentary suggests that general internal medicine is truly at the "cross-roads of prosperity and despair."[4] Prosperity is evidenced by the growth of academic general internal medicine, increasing research opportunities and funding, and the success of the "hospitalist" movement. Despair, however, might be an overly dramatic descriptor for the state of general internal medicine. In recent years, studies have found that career satisfaction among general internists has declined.[5] The reasons are variable, but the most common are reduced autonomy over treatment decisions, less time allotted for patient visits, and more time required for administrative paperwork. None of these challenges is specific to internal medicine. Because today's economic environment places less value on cognitive services than on procedural or diagnostic services, the decrease in the duration of individual clinic visits has compromised the management of psychological aspects of disease. At the same time, the growing elderly population presents more complex comorbidities, and the traditionally valued continuity of care has been disrupted, as changes in patients' insurance now often require a change of physician as well.

There are indications, however, that advances within general internal medicine could improve job satisfaction. The option to divide inpatient and outpatient practice between hospitalists and primary care physicians has the potential to decrease both on-call responsibilities and total work hours. This separation of roles could also allow the outpatient-based internist more time to spend with each patient during clinic visits.[6] Additional role changes are now being seen in the wider use of team-based care models. In these models, the internist is more like a consultant advising and supervising an interdisciplinary team of providers (registered nurse practitioners, RNs, pharmacists, social workers, etc). Many physicians practicing within these medical home models are beginning to report improved job satisfaction.[7] As training in psychosocial and preventive medicine becomes a central component of residency, internists will be better prepared to address these issues as aspects of multiple complex medical problems. Finally, the job satisfaction of all physicians depends on their ability to regain control over medical management decisions. This would allow an internist's time to be devoted to practicing medicine rather than constantly negotiating insurance coverage and financial reimbursement.

LIFESTYLE CONSIDERATIONS AND PRACTICE OPTIONS

The day-to-day life of a practicing internist is quite varied. It really depends on whether the physician is a cardiologist, rheumatologist, critical care specialist, general internist, and so on. Nearly all work long hours. Cardiologists and gastroenterologists are frequently called into the hospital in the middle of the night to perform cardiac catheterizations for heart attack victims and endoscopies for patients with gastrointestinal bleeding. The general internist in private practice is, in a way, on call all the time. When one of their patients is admitted to the hospital, they receive a phone call letting them know.

Because of the broad nature of internal medicine, residents often have a tough time responding to the question "Where do you intend to practice?" After all, the answer may change during your training and even over the course of your career. Your initial career plans may be your choice during residency to pursue a subspecialty fellowship or to remain in general internal medicine. For physicians who choose to remain in general medicine, other fellowship opportunities are available in fields such as end-of-life care, medical education, and medical informatics.

Once a general internist is prepared to enter the workforce, the decision between academic medicine and private medicine must be made. Both have many practice opportunities to explore. Some academicians are mainly educators, spending most of their time in the outpatient or inpatient setting seeing their own patients and supervising residents in clinic or on the wards. Others are researchers with few inpatient or outpatient responsibilities who spend most of their

RESIDENCY TRAINING

Residency in internal medicine requires 3 years of postgraduate training. There are currently 386 accredited programs in the United States (excluding combined programs with other specialties). Residency programs are offered by both academic medical centers and community hospitals. The training includes experience in both general internal medicine and subspecialty areas. It is a rigorous program, requiring in-house overnight call every fourth to fifth night while on an inpatient rotation. The first year is the most intense. Rotations in general patient medicine, subspecialties (consults and clinic), intensive care, geriatrics, and emergency medicine are required. Residents must demonstrate technical proficiency in a number of procedures, including abdominal paracentesis, thoracentesis, central venous line placement, and lumbar puncture. Because of the current emphasis on primary care, one-third of the residency must take place in an ambulatory setting. All categorical residents spend one-half day per week in a continuity clinic where they manage their own panel of patients over the course of 3 years. The decision to subspecialize and apply for fellowship typically occurs during the second postgraduate year.

THE INSIDE SCOOP

time conducting research in areas that are not generally addressed by subspecialty research but broadly applicable to medicine: evidence-based medicine, psychosocial aspects of care, doctor–patient communication, medical ethics, management of medical errors, cost-effectiveness, and the impact of socioeconomic status or race on medical care.

General internists who choose private practice also have several options. In the current health care economic environment, solo private practice is becoming much less common. Instead, most internists belong to a group practice such as multispecialty groups or health maintenance organizations. Some private internists have contracts with hospitalists to provide all inpatient care for their patients, and other private internists continue to see patients both in the clinic and in the hospital. Others hold a salaried position at a health maintenance organization.

In both private and academic practice, the generalist initiative of the last decade gave rise to the rapid growth of a new type of internist: the hospitalist. These internists practice only inpatient (hospital-based) medicine. Similar to consultants, they are called on to provide expert management for the care of sick patients admitted to the hospital. Instead of following a clinic schedule, hospitalists have a shift-work lifestyle similar to emergency medicine physicians. Patients can benefit from having a hospitalist take care of them instead of their own private doctor, since hospitalists work in the hospital on a daily basis and develop an expertise in this area of medicine. With good communication between hospitalists and primary care physicians, hospitalist care has been associated with lower costs, improved patient outcomes, and lower short-term mortality.[8] In academic institutions, hospitalists often oversee utilization management and quality improvement initiatives. They also supervise resident training in patient care, systems-based practice, and procedures. While fellowships in hospital medicine are available, the completion of a fellowship is not required to practice hospital medicine. The American Board of Internal Medicine offers a unique board certification for physicians who have a focused practice in hospital medicine. Hospitalists can apply for this focused practice certification after 3 years of experience in hospital medicine and must maintain an average of 1000 encounters with hospitalized patients per year for ongoing certification.

FELLOWSHIPS AND SUBSPECIALTY TRAINING

Internal medicine is composed of many subspecialties. In 2000, roughly half of all graduates from internal medicine residency programs sought fellowship training within one of ten subspecialties.[9] Currently, there are 18 possible areas of subspecialization. Before jumping into one of these disciplines, take a moment for some honest self-evaluation. It is essential that you give some thought to your field of interest and the type of personality most suited to it. You would also do well to consider who you think you might be in 20 to 30 years. Medical students rarely factor in their own evolving interests as they select their specialty or subspecialty. Many believe that their interests as well as skills are "fixed" rather than dynamic. Carol Dweck, a Stanford University psychologist and author of *Mindset*, would caution us that happier and healthier outcomes

VITAL SIGNS

INTERNAL MEDICINE 2011 MATCH STATISTICS

- Number of positions available: 5121
- 3870 US seniors and 6284 independent applicants ranked at least one internal medicine program
- 98.9% of all positions were filled in the initial Match
- The successful applicants: 58.1% US seniors, 34.2% foreign-trained physicians, and 561% osteopathic graduates
- Mean USMLE Step I score: 226
- Unmatched rate for US seniors applying only to internal medicine: 2.7%

Data from National Resident Matching Program.

may exist within what she refers to as the "growth mindset."[10] Whether subspecializing or remaining a general internist, the belief that a doctor's mind will grow and change is well aligned with the medical school mantra of "life-long learning."

General Internal Medicine

No subspecialty embraces the tradition of "life-long learning" more readily than the general internist or just "internist." When medical students encounter a "complete" internist, their consistent feedback sounds something like "She (or he) knows everything!" It is with good reason that internists develop a broad and deep knowledge base. They are constantly confronted by patients who defy what is "known" about a given illness. In response, these curious and humble professionals accept their new knowledge and consider themselves better prepared for the next interesting patient.

Internists enjoy the advantage of flexibility over their subspecialized colleagues. Traditionally, they function as primary care providers, following patients over many years as their health coach, friend, and advisor. However, many residents upon completion of training programs find themselves opting for careers as hospitalists (discussed above). In addition, an internist can choose to specialize (without formal fellowship training or board certification) in an area of medicine just because it interests her (or him). For instance, many internists specialize in obesity, hypertension, diabetes, heart failure, occupational medicine, and the list really goes on. Others will elect to join hospital administration and focus on medical delivery systems. The choices are endless and it is not uncommon to meet an internist who has enjoyed two or three major phases of his or her career.

Adolescent Medicine

Whatever generation gap you might be experiencing, it should be comforting to know that the medical profession has physicians specialized in addressing the issues of your adolescent children. Physicians from pediatrics, internal medicine, psychiatry, and obstetrics and gynecology all share this domain in an acknowledgment of the complex issues that confront young adults. Their patients usually are caught between puberty and living independent adult lives. Medical issues often are related to behaviors such as eating disorders, drug use, pregnancy, and sexually transmitted diseases to name a few. Ethical issues may also arise in cases where teenagers wish to make independent decisions about their medical care before they achieve legal adulthood. In these cases, adolescent medicine doctors must act in the interest of the patient, with respect and compassion for the parents.

Adolescent medicine providers share a strong interest in advocacy for their patient population.[11] Training programs typically are 2 years in duration.

Allergy and Immunology

Millions of people suffer from allergies, which ultimately affect their workplace productivity and results in billions of dollars lost each year. These reactions include respiratory diseases (asthma, sinusitis, rhinitis), adverse drug effects, and unusual skin rashes. Because allergies have an underlying immunologic component, these specialists are also experts on antibodies, antigens, and other complex aspects of the immune system. They perform skin tests and drug desensitization protocols.

A career in allergy and immunology offers immense intellectual satisfaction, as well as good working hours. Here, there is a strong bond between basic laboratory research and its clinical application. When treating patients (both kids and adults), these specialists witness dramatic improvements in physical functioning. Results are usually fast, positive, and much appreciated. Today, more and more people suffer from asthma and other allergic disorders. As such, there is an extremely high demand for internists with formal training in this discipline. Career options are broad and include private practice, academics, and clinical or basic science research. Some allergist–immunologists also practice general internal medicine in addition to their subspecialty. A fellowship in allergy and immunology lasts 2 years.

VITAL SIGNS

MEDIAN COMPENSATION

Allergy and immunology	$241,138
Cardiology	$398,034
Endocrinolgy	$212,281
Gastroenterology	$389,385
General internal medicine	$205,441
Geriatrics	$211,425
Hematology/ oncology	$315,133
Hospitalist	$211,835
Infectious disease	$222,094
Nephrology	$246,049
Pulmonary medicine/ critical care	$268,250
Rheumatology	$219,411

Data from American Medical Group Association.

Cardiovascular Disease

Like fighter pilots, cardiologists take calculated risks while exercising skill and precision. As experts in the diagnosis and management of cardiovascular diseases, they take care of life-threatening medical conditions that affect a large majority of the population. These disorders include congenital heart defects, arrhythmias, valvular problems, hypertension, and coronary artery disease. Many of the treatment options, whether pharmacologic or interventional, have immediate life-saving benefits. A procedure-oriented specialty, cardiology requires a great deal of manual dexterity. It is a perfect field for those who love gadgets. You will perform cardiac catheterization, electrocardiograms, nuclear stress tests, and echocardiography. You will place stents within the coronary vasculature, open clogged arteries with balloon angioplasty, and even electrically convert patients into normal sinus rhythms through defibrillation.

Life as a heroic cardiologist, however, can be physically draining. They work extremely long, arduous hours taking care of very sick patients. Due to the large numbers of patients admitted to the hospital with heart attacks, cardiologists frequently come to the hospital in the middle of the night. In the intensive care unit, they help critically ill patients maintain their blood pressure through the administration of vasopressors and other powerful drugs. Despite the rigors of the profession, cardiologists maintain long, intimate relationships with their patients. They also practice preventive medicine by identifying risk factors for early diagnosis of heart disease. If you enjoy studying the anatomy and physiology of the heart and love mastering technical procedures, then cardiology is the subspecialty for you. Fellowships in cardiology last 3 years and are extremely competitive. Additional 1-year fellowships are offered in interventional, clinical electrophysiology and advanced heart failure/transplant cardiology.

Endocrine, Diabetes, and Metabolism

This subspecialty involves the study of hormones, endocrine glands, and their effects on whole-body homeostasis. You will find an intimate connection between the latest basic science research and its application in bedside clinical practice. Endocrinologists are experts in treating disease states in which glands (pituitary, thyroid, adrenal, pancreas, gonadal) are either overproducing or undersecreting hormones. These problems include diabetes, thyroid dysfunction, gonadal disorders, pituitary tumors, adrenal gland dysfunction, and disorders of bone metabolism. Patients often live with chronic endocrine diseases that may not declare themselves for weeks or even years (other than a few subtle symptoms). Many of these diseases are treatable, often even curable.

Like great detectives, endocrinologists make use of an extensive array of diagnostic testing. They study adrenocorticotropic hormone (ACTH) stimulation tests, dexamethasone suppression tests, bone densitometry, and thyroid function panels. Aside from cases of diabetic ketoacidosis, adrenal crisis, and thyroid storm, there are few endocrine emergencies. This allows the clinician ample time to think about and prepare appropriate treatment regimens. Endocrinologists enjoy long-term relationships with their patients, who are typically on the younger side. As part of their patients' therapy, they often have to address the behavioral and psychosocial aspects of endocrine disease. For instance, patients with poorly controlled diabetes need to be taught (and encouraged) to modify their lifestyle, comply with their medication schedule, and use home glucose monitoring. Although much of their time is spent in the clinic setting, endocrinologists also serve as inpatient consultants for endocrine emergencies and diagnostic or treatment challenges. If you are interested in this highly scientific subspecialty with many positive outcomes, there are 2-year fellowships in endocrinology.

Gastroenterology

Specialists in gastroenterology treat diseases of the entire digestive system—from the esophagus to the anus, as well as the liver, gallbladder, and pancreas. Depending on the disease process, their relationships with patients may range from a single consultation (eg, a patient presenting with pancreatitis or upper gastrointestinal bleeding) to long-term close relationships (eg, patients with ulcerative colitis, hemochromatosis, or chronic liver failure due to alcoholic cirrhosis). They often see patients on the surgical wards following liver transplants and in the intensive care unit with massive gastrointestinal bleeding or fulminant hepatic failure. Because of the delicate nature of the subject matter, gastroenterologists often have to pay close attention to psychosocial aspects, particularly when discussing the implications of bowel disease for the patient's lifestyle.

As in cardiology, exciting technical procedures are an integral part of the management of gastrointestinal disorders. You will become quite adept at inserting tubes into your patients' mouths and rectums and seeing their diseases right before your very eyes. Colonoscopy, flexible sigmoidoscopy, and EGD allow the clinician to directly visualize disease, take tissue biopsies for diagnosis, and even provide immediate treatment by excising polyps or cauterizing bleeding vessels. Patients rely on their gastroenterologist to screen for precancerous lesions and to remove them before they become malignant. Whether draining fluid from an abdomen filled with ascites or recording intraesophageal pressures, there are many other diagnostic procedures. With new technology on the horizon, gastroenterologists will soon be able to perform endoluminal surgery with lasers and use built-in ultrasound probes to provide new views of our digestive organs. Gastroenterology is a perfect specialty for students who love this combination of technical interventions and cerebral challenges. Fellowships in gastroenterology require 3 years of training. Additional 1 year training is available in hepatology (liver disease) and advanced endoscopy.

Geriatrics

Rather than treating a particular disease or organ system, geriatricians care for a specific population—the elderly, the largest growing proportion of the US population. Patients within this age group typically have many complex medical problems, ranging from degenerative neurologic disease such as dementia to systemic diseases such as high blood pressure and diabetes. Because older patients take a fair number of medications, geriatricians must be experts on drug interactions, adverse effects, and how drugs are metabolized in an older person. At times, they must be selective about which diagnostic procedures and therapeutic undertakings their patients can tolerate. Using a multidisciplinary approach, they address the physical and psychosocial needs of their patients amidst an extensive constellation of medical issues. After all, the elderly have their own special set of problems, such as delirium, dementia, incontinence, and decline in functional status. Geriatricians are intimately familiar with nursing home settings and dealing with Medicare. The practice options for these highly sought-after specialists include traditional outpatient care, consultations at nursing facilities, and academics. Fellowships in geriatric medicine require 1 additional year of training.

Hematology

The faint of heart need not apply for hematology fellowship. This subspecialty treats some of the deadliest and potentially curable cancers known to medicine. When a blood cell cancer strikes, the sickest patients can get deathly ill quickly. However, if you are lucky enough to get a variant that is amenable to treatment you could enjoy an excellent prognosis, thanks to the many basic science research discoveries by the doctors of hematology.

Patients with diseases of the blood, bone marrow, and lymphatic systems require the expertise of a hematologist. Hematologists are comfortable reading blood smears, interpreting cytogenetic testing, and performing bone marrow biopsies. They stay current with the latest chemotherapy regimens and can provide hope when patients need it most. The disorders they treat include anemias, clotting abnormalities, leukemias, lymphomas, and bleeding disorders such as hemophilia. Fellowship is 2 years.

Hospice and Palliative Care

Palliative care specialists focus on providing the highest quality of life as long as possible. Rather than assume all patients fear death and wish to avoid discussing it, palliative care specialists will invite these discussions. They place a strong emphasis on the alignment of the care plan with the patient's goals of care. Common issues addressed are pain control, emotional support, and dignity to dying patients while also addressing the needs of their family members. Practice settings most commonly include inpatient hospice facilities and home hospice care. However, palliative care specialists can also impact chronically ill patients such as those suffering from congestive heart failure and cancer in outpatient clinic visits. These clinics offer patients a comanagement model where the palliative care specialist is embedded within the cardiology or oncology clinic. Patients are not always comfortable discussing death and dying with physicians. As a skilled palliative care specialist, you can help the dying patient accept the passing of his or her life rather than fear and suffer it.

Hospital Medicine

Probably, the fastest growing subspecialty of internal medicine is hospital medicine. Further information about this subspeciality is provided earlier in this chapter.

Infectious Disease

If you love studying bacteria, viruses, parasites, and fungi, then the subspecialty of infectious disease is for you. These physicians take the basic science of microbiology and apply it to clinical situations. In their diagnostic workup, they approach the patient's disease process by taking into consideration recent travel, geographic region, country of origin, and cultural practice. They are experts in the proper collection and analysis of culture specimens, plus a variety of laboratory tests, such as antibiotic sensitivity tests, CD4 counts, and infectious serologies. Their treatment regimens are largely pharmacologic and draw on the latest developments in antibiotic therapy. Through the use of vaccines, they practice a great deal of preventive medicine.

Most patients who require the expertise of these clinicians have diseases that are short term in nature. Thus, infectious disease specialists typically serve as consultants for other physicians. In the summer of 2002, they were on the front lines of the new West Nile virus outbreak in the United States. They consult on patients in the hospital for diagnostic challenges (eg, fever of unknown origin) and for treatment regimens of specific infectious diseases (eg, bacterial endocarditis, meningitis, cellulitis, sepsis). Many infectious disease physicians maintain longer relationships with patients suffering from chronic diseases, such as HIV/AIDS and tuberculosis, who require extensive follow-up. Some practice travel medicine, serving as consultants to patients preparing for international travel and to those who acquired illnesses while overseas. Other areas of expertise include infection control within health care settings, international public health, and the prevention of antibiotic resistance through education and research. They are also involved in the tracking and epidemiology of certain communicable diseases. As the threat of biological attack becomes a growing concern, the prevention, recognition, and treatment of bioterrorism are now focal points of infectious disease. Fellowships require 2 years of training after residency.

Nephrology

Fascinated by urine, the kidney, and complex renal physiology? Nephrologists are masters of fluid, electrolytes, and acid–base homeostasis. After all, the kidneys are responsible for filtering out impurities from the blood. As part of their diagnostic workup, they analyze acid–base studies, electrolyte panels, and urine collections. In this highly intellectual specialty, they treat all types of diseases of the renal system, such as infection, kidney stones, alkalosis/acidosis, autoimmune disorders, and renal artery stenosis. The nephrologist must understand how systemic diseases such as hypertension and diabetes affect the kidneys, as well as be able to identify renal toxic effects of any medication. Long-term relationships are formed with patients who require chronic dialysis, and life-saving interventions such as acute hemodialysis are often provided within the intensive care setting. Nephrologists also treat postrenal transplant patients and manage the complications of chronic immune suppression secondary to posttransplant medical therapy.

There are several procedural skills to master, particularly the placement of hemodialysis and peritoneal catheters and the ability to biopsy tissue from the kidney. Some nephrologists gain additional interventional training and perform thrombectomies and even angioplasty of renal arteries. Although it requires technical skill, nephrology is also one of the most cognitive subspecialties within internal medicine. You can practice as a consultant, direct a dialysis center, work as an intensivist, or practice both nephrology and general medicine. Although dialysis patients can be demanding at times, solving their complex medical problems is highly gratifying. Nephrology fellowships require 2 years of training.

Oncology

Medical oncology involves the evaluation and treatment of neoplasms, both benign and malignant, of every organ system, from the brain to the kidneys. Some oncologists develop specific expertise in a particular type of cancer, such as malignant mesothelioma. They are experts on the latest forms of chemotherapy available, particularly those currently used in experimental clinical trials. Regardless of the area of oncology, you will no doubt acquire both a philosophical and practical approach to life and death.

Oncologists recognize that the therapy they prescribe is often harmful to the patient. They have to reconcile the benefit of every treatment option with the harm involved, which means exercising courage and faith in their patients' ability to cope with the burden of disease and its treatment. This specialty, therefore, requires the highest level of sensitivity, compassion, and empathy. While helping patients through a difficult time, oncologists must tell them the truth about their disease in an easily understandable and compassionate manner. They must guide patients and their families through the dying process, easing the process by providing good pain control and maintaining the patient's dignity. Oncology is especially rewarding for those who can handle the challenge that despite your best efforts and medical care, many of your patients will not survive. Your efforts will never be in vain, for there are patients whom you will indeed cure or whose lives you will prolong. Despite being specialized, oncologists provide a broad base of general internal medicine. Fellowships in oncology are 2 years in length.

Pulmonary and Critical Care

Despite taking care of the most critically ill patients, these technically superb specialists never lose their cool under pressure. Although considered two separate subspecialties, most clinicians undergo training in both fields. Pulmonology entails the diagnosis and treatment of diseases of the lungs and upper airways, whether infectious, inflammatory, or cancerous in origin. Every day, they interpret arterial blood gas studies and pulmonary function tests. These specialists often serve as consultants to patients requiring expert management of emergent problems such as pulmonary hypertension, hemoptysis, and pulmonary embolism. Continuity of care is also important in pulmonary medicine, particularly for patients with chronic problems such as asthma, emphysema, and occupational lung damage. In the multidisciplinary world of critical care, these physicians deal with more than just disorders of the lung. They take care of very sick patients who have life-threatening multi-organ system problems, from septic shock to heart failure to metabolic abnormalities.

If using high-tech monitors and interventional skills to solve complex clinical problems sounds appealing, then consider a career in pulmonary and critical care. In both areas, you become quite adept at performing many procedures. These specialists are experts at bronchoscopy, thoracentesis, ventilator management, and the placement of central lines and Swan–Ganz catheters. You will witness life-saving interventions as well as prolonged and agonizing death, and you will learn to meet both outcomes with the same level of professionalism. You will also become seasoned in end-of-life decision making. As they try to cope with the imminent death of their loved one, the families of your patients will be grateful for your care and guidance when addressing issues regarding goals of care and resuscitation limitations. Be warned, however, that working with critically ill patients—with its demanding pace and intense emotion—can lead to rapid burnout. Fellowships require an additional 3 years of training. You can also earn certification in only one of the two disciplines through 2 years of fellowship.

Rheumatology

Rheumatologists treat diseases of the musculoskeletal system such as osteoarthritis and gout in addition to complex systemic diseases such as lupus and rheumatoid arthritis. They deal mainly with people with chronic diseases that are not curable. Diagnostic challenges are common in rheumatology, as evidenced by the treatment of rare diseases such as scleroderma, amyloidosis, vasculitides, and polymyositis. They interpret complicated rheumatologic blood tests and perform joint aspirations and steroid injections. What are complex presentations of disease for your colleagues, will, in your eyes, appear as routine manifestations of common rheumatologic disorders. Depending on your orientation to laboratory research, you may find yourself working within an overlapping world of rheumatology, immunology, and genetics. The treatment of rheumatologic disease most often consists of immunosuppression as well as adequate pain control. Future advances in gene therapy could potentially revolutionize therapeutic options within the field of rheumatology. Fellowships in rheumatology require 2 years of additional training.

Sleep Medicine

No laying down on the job in this specialty. After Reggie White, former All-Pro defensive end for the Green Bay Packers, lost his life to sleep apnea, sleep disorders have been an increasingly popular diagnosis. Typical disorders include restless leg syndrome, narcolepsy, insomnia, snoring, and sleep apnea. Historical underdiagnosis of these disorders has resulted in a large growth in the sleep study industry. Sleep specialists can emerge from the specialties of psychology, internal medicine, pulmonary, and neurology. The critical role sleep plays in hormonal regulation is bringing to light a host of chronic diseases that may improve with better sleep hygiene. The sleep specialist will enjoy a practice niche, but will likely have to remain rooted in his or her specialty as well. This is a 1-year fellowship.

Sports Medicine

Sports medicine is the practice of preventing and treating sports-related injuries, as well as promoting exercise as preventive medicine for the general population. Those internists practicing sports medicine often provide acute care of injuries during athletic events. Most work closely with orthopedic surgeons, although most athletic injuries, as many studies have shown, do not require surgery. The treatment of basic medical problems is considered to be sports medicine if the patient is an athlete or the problem is related to exercise. This is a 1-year fellowship.

"HORIZONTAL" SUBSPECIALTY AREAS

In recent years, new fellowship opportunities within internal medicine have multiplied. Unlike the organ-based orientation of traditional subspecialties (such as cardiology or pulmonary medicine), the focus of these fellowships is specific patient populations and aspects of health care delivery that are applicable across many areas of general medicine. Training opportunities are becoming more abundant and diverse each year. Because the American Board of Medical Specialties does not officially recognize these subspecialties, board certification examinations are not available. Instead, graduates of these fellowships earn a certificate of added qualifications. Programs typically last 1 to 2 years.

Addiction Medicine

Internists with specific expertise in addiction medicine provide treatment for those addicted to alcohol, tobacco, and illicit drugs on an inpatient and outpatient basis. Because medical professionals have a high rate of substance abuse, some addiction specialists focus on the prevention and treatment of addiction among health care providers.

Clinical Decision Making

Internists specializing in clinical decision making attempt to optimize health care delivery through analysis of cost-effectiveness, health care policy, the development of clinical guidelines, and evaluation of clinical outcomes. Practice settings include academic departments, government policy-making agencies, health insurance companies, and managed care organizations.

Clinical Nutrition

Clinical nutrition focuses on the prevention and treatment of nutritional deficiencies, food allergies, eating disorders, and malnutrition of chronic disease. Some practitioners approach the subspecialty from a public health standpoint, whereas others develop expertise in nutritional aspects of specific diseases such as diabetes mellitus, inflammatory bowel disease, or chronic renal failure.

Medical Informatics

Internists with a specific expertise in medical informatics attempt to improve the storage and communication of medical data and imaging modalities. They integrate this data to yield biostatistical and epidemiologic outcomes. Most subspecialists in medical informatics have a background in computer science or biomedical engineering.

WHY CONSIDER A CAREER IN INTERNAL MEDICINE?

There are many misconceptions about internal medicine, probably because it is such a broad field. A study by the American College of Physicians and American Society of Internal Medicine (ACP–ASIM) found that only 18% of patients surveyed thought that general internists could provide primary care, and 56% believed that general internists were subspecialists.[12] Some internists, in fact, have a patient base composed of older children and adolescents, whereas others primarily see elderly patients in their practices. As a result, internists have the flexibility to work in many different settings: the ambulatory clinic, the inpatient ward, the intensive care unit, nursing homes, and hospices. Internal medicine, therefore, is much more than a specialty devoted to chronic illness without possible cures. Instead, this very personally satisfying field of medicine allows a physician to help patients achieve the best quality of life possible.

Internists are knowledgeable in many aspects of medical care. They treat acute and chronic conditions, not to mention common and rare disease entities. Even if you choose another specialty, no physician can avoid the basics of internal medicine. For instance, orthopedic surgeons have to treat hypokalemia, obstetricians–gynecologists need to be well versed in the management of hypertension, and psychiatrists must be able to recognize the signs and symptoms of hypothyroidism. Internal medicine is, in a way, the foundation for all fields of medicine. If you are excited by the prospect of providing care for adults as a diagnostician, healer, motivator, and patient advocate, you would certainly find a career in internal medicine rewarding.

Medical students who are undecided on a specialty should take into account that training in general internal medicine provides the foundation for a long list of career options. Within one career, you could practice general medicine, provide primary preventive care, specialize in one organ system through formal fellowship, or even independently develop a specific expertise. By deciding to enter internal medicine, medical students ensure themselves a career filled with intellectual stimulation, diagnostically challenging patient interactions, and rewarding relationships. The focus on the patient makes practicing the art of internal medicine an extraordinary privilege.

ABOUT THE CONTRIBUTORS

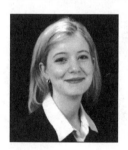
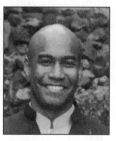

A native of southern Illinois, Dr Jennifer Tong received her BS from the University of Illinois—Urbana-Champaign before entering medical school at the University of Chicago. She completed residency training in internal medicine at Stanford University Hospital. As a nocturnal hospitalist at Santa Clara Valley Medical Center, she provides inpatient care for an underserved population by night. By day, Dr Tong is a happy mother of three children. After earning a BA in English from the University of California, Berkeley, Dr Ian Tong also received his medical education from the University of Chicago. After completing residency and chief residency in internal medicine at Stanford University, he became medical director of veterans outreach for the Veterans Affairs Palo Alto Health Care System. Ian Tong is clinical assistant professor and Educator-4-CARE faculty mentor at Stanford. Jennifer and Ian live in the Santa Cruz Mountains with their three children. They may be reached by e-mail at jrlambmed@hotmail.com or itong@stanford.edu.

REFERENCES

1. Salerno, S.M., Landry, F.J., et al. Patient perceptions of the capabilities of internists: A multi-center survey. *Am J Med.* 2001;110(2):111–117.

2. If you think an internist is an intern, would you choose one as your primary care physician? American College of Physicians, 1999, Pamphlet.

3. Beach, M.C., Inui, T., et al. Relationship-centered care: A constructive reframing. *J Gen Intern Med.* 2006;21(S1):S3–S8.

4. Larson, E.B. General internal medicine at the crossroads of prosperity and despair: Caring for patients with chronic diseases in an aging society. *Ann Intern Med.* 2001;134(10):997–1000.

5. Wetterneck, T.B., Linzer, M., et al. Worklife and satisfaction of general internists. *Arch Intern Med.* 2002;162(6):649–656.

6. Goldman, L. Key challenges confronting internal medicine in the early twenty-first century. *Am J Med.* 2001;110(6):463–470.

7. Marsteller, J.A., Hsu, Y.J., et al. Physician satisfaction with chronic care processes: A cluster-randomized trial of guided care. *Ann Fam Med.* 2010;8:308–315.

8. Meltzer, D., Manning, W.G., et al. Effects of physician experience on costs and outcomes on an academic general medicine service: Results of a trial of hospitalists. *Ann Intern Med.* 2002;137(11):866–874.

9. Sox, H.C. Supply, demand, and workforce of internal medicine. *Am J Med.* 2001;110(9):745–749.

10. Dweck, C. Mindset: *The New Psychology of Success.* New York: Random House; 2006, pp. 6–7.

11. Consensus Statement. A position statement of the society of adolescent medicine. *J Adolesc Med.* 1995;16–413.

12. Arenson, J., McDonald, W.J. Can we educate the public about internal medicine? *Am J Med.* 1998;105:1–5.

19

NEUROLOGY

Tomasz Zabiega

Neurology is the practice of medicine that concentrates on the human brain and nervous system. From higher cognitive disorders (such as Alzheimer dementia) to diseases of nerve and muscle (neuropathies and myopathies), neurologists serve as nervous system specialists at every level. With compassion and dedication, neurologists take care of patients presenting with a wide variety of complaints: headaches, numbness, weakness, tremors, seizures, speech difficulty, and changes in consciousness. Although they deal with some of the most distressing and debilitating diseases in medicine, neurologists tend to have an upbeat, calm, and casual attitude. They typically combine a sophisticated level of intellectual curiosity with down-to-earth friendliness and optimism.

Many medical students, after completing their rotation in neurology, are familiar with the stereotype of neurologists as excellent diagnosticians who cannot treat the underlying neurologic disorders. This observation may have been somewhat true 30 years ago. Today, therapeutics is equally as exciting as diagnostics. In the past several decades, new developments in neuropharmacology, as well as invasive and noninvasive technology, have revolutionized the modern practice of neurology. As our understanding of neurologic disease continues to expand, neurology stands as one of the most stimulating fields in medicine.

NOT JUST FOR "BRAINIACS"

The variety of diseases that fall under the expertise of neurologists is staggering. Because the nervous system controls other organ systems, this specialty overlaps with an entire range of other medical disciplines. For instance, neurologists must be comfortable with psychology when treating dementia and hysteria, with genetics when diagnosing muscular dystrophy and cerebral palsy, and with urology when evaluating a neurogenic bladder. They draw upon their knowledge of immunology to treat patients suffering from multiple sclerosis and myasthenia gravis. They use important concepts from otolaryngology to diagnose dizziness and dysphagia, from ophthalmology to evaluate visual problems, and from dermatology to manage neurofibromatosis. For patients with strokes, intracranial hemorrhage, or spinal cord transection, neurologists often serve as consultants to their surgical colleagues. They interact with oncologists to treat brain tumors. They also must be up on the latest methods of antibiotic therapy to treat patients with meningitis or the neurologic manifestations of AIDS. As you can see, this list goes on and on.

To deal with such a diversity of disorders, neurologists must become experts in an equally varied array of skills. They have to maintain a solid understanding of the basic sciences, particularly neuroanatomy, neuroscience, and physiology. These clinicians are superb history takers and examiners. After all, the neurologic physical examination is by far the most elaborate and important. In addition, the neurologist is called upon to interpret complex diagnostic studies, such as magnetic resonance imaging (MRI), computed tomography (CT), electroencephalography (EEG), sleep studies, and blood tests. Manual dexterity is required when neurologists perform spinal taps and electromyography (EMG) on their patients. On top of all these skills, the neurologist must treat these disorders with many types of medications and therapies, such as intravenous immunoglobulins, plasmapheresis, or infusion of powerful thrombolytic agents for acute stroke management.

The seemingly insurmountable amount of knowledge to master often discourages medical students from choosing a career in neurology. But they should be aware that neurology does not call for genius. Instead, it simply requires the physician to analyze intricate clinical findings in a systematic manner. A neurologist must integrate results from the history, physical examination, and diagnostics—all obtained from a single, logically structured organ system.

Mastering the intricacies of the nervous system is similar to learning the rules of a particular sport. Once you understand the set of laws within neurology, you find that diagnosing disorders and analyzing complications become a relatively simple and enjoyable task. Neurologists do not simply memorize terms, but are thinkers at heart.

NUTS AND BOLTS: THINKING AS A NEUROLOGIST

To diagnose and treat neurologic disorders, neurologists draw upon their solid understanding of the basic neurosciences. This scientific discipline includes the

anatomy, physiology, embryology, biochemistry, pathology, and pharmacology
of the human nervous system. Does this
mean that you have to learn the name and
position of every small structure found
in the brain and spinal cord? Absolutely
not. Neurologists who have failed to grasp
the simplicity of their specialty often
propagate this misconception. By understanding the different components of the
nervous system, the most competent neurologists can more easily manage complications that may result from disease processes occurring in those structures.

Neurology is a perfect specialty for
aspiring physicians who like to delve into
analysis and figure out rational solutions.

WHAT MAKES A GOOD NEUROLOGIST?

✓ Likes to figure out problems logically.
✓ Can deal with diseases that may have minimally effective treatment.
✓ Is intellectual and inquisitive.
✓ Likes serving as a consultant or seeing patients by referral.
✓ Enjoys long-term care of patients.

THE INSIDE SCOOP

The art of practicing clinical neurology is perhaps the most logical and structured of all fields of medicine. When a patient presents with a complaint related to the nervous system, the first step is to distinguish whether damage has occurred in the brain, spinal cord, peripheral nerves, neuromuscular junction, or muscles. Then, the differential diagnoses and thought process ascend cerebrally. Was the damage central (brain and spinal cord) or peripheral (nerve and muscle)? If the lesion is in the spinal cord, could it be localized within the cervical spine (upper extremity symptoms) or the lumbar region (lower extremity symptoms)? If suspected problems involve the brain, neurologists localize the lesion further to subsections of the brainstem or cortex. When a neurologist understands clearly the function of larger brain structures, he or she can more easily pinpoint defects within more intricate components.

This methodical approach to diagnosis is an integral part of the profession. It makes the job of the neurologist both relatively easy and extremely rewarding. A neurologist evaluates patients whose seemingly complex presentation often baf- fles other medical professionals. By systematically analyzing pieces of the clinical picture, these specialists often make rapid diagnoses (or at least greatly narrow the differential list) to the amazement of other doctors. They do so by showing how the pieces of the patient's puzzle correlate with each other through neuroanatomic relationships. But neurologists do not dabble in anatomy out of a masochistic thrill in learning every minute structure by heart. Instead, they engage in a life-long study of nervous system structure to provide the best patient care and most accurate diagnoses.

THE COMPLETE NEUROLOGIC EXAMINATION

If you like using your hands to solve clinical puzzles, if you enjoy playing with reflex hammers and tuning forks, this specialty may be the perfect choice. In addition to the necessity of a thorough knowledge of neuroanatomy and accurate history taking, neurology is famous for its savvy methods of physical diagnosis. After conducting a complete physical examination, good neurologists pride themselves on knowing the exact localization of the problem prior to any laboratory or imaging studies.

Although modern medicine draws heavily on information derived from computers, advanced technology, and highly sophisticated diagnostic procedures, a neurologist armed with just a reflex hammer, safety pin, vibratory fork, and penlight often makes a more accurate diagnosis. Many neurologists have had the experience of findings from a physical examination revealing a specific lesion when every other test pointed to somewhere else. They integrate these findings with a precise patient history, which is usually as important and crucial as the examination. Neurologists who stick to their original diagnoses are often eventually proven right.

Combined with a careful history, the physical examination becomes truly meaningful. At this point, findings such as abnormal deep tendon reflexes and impaired cranial nerves begin to make sense. A thorough neurologic examination involves many complex parts, but a skilled neurologist can quickly conduct it without losing accuracy. The neurologic examination has remained relatively unchanged over the past 100 years, since the days of Charcot and Babinski, the fathers of neurology. This examination provides great insight into a patient's problems. It is an irreplaceable weapon in the diagnostic arsenal of an experienced neurologist.

NEUROLOGIC DIAGNOSIS: TECHNOLOGY AT ITS BEST

Neurology is a wonderful specialty for students interested in combining a slick physical examination with the latest advances in medical diagnostics. Neuroimaging and neurophysiologic studies are essential to the practice of contemporary neurology. A skilled neurologist can evaluate sophisticated radiological tests, such as MRI, magnetic resonance angiography (MRA), CT, and cerebral angiograms.

The ability to do so rapidly and precisely is crucial for patient outcome. For instance, neurologists must distinguish intracranial bleeds from benign calcifications, strokes from cancers, and swelling caused by head trauma from infectious or autoimmune processes. These clinicians often consult with their colleagues in radiology to narrow their list of differential diagnoses further.

Unlike other fields of medicine, neurology has immense potential for amazing advances in diagnostic technology. Every day, there are new breakthroughs in neuroimaging modalities. Neurologists are now using tools that allow them to specify further the nature of a lesion. As a result, fewer invasive biopsies are performed. These advances include positron emission tomography (PET), single photon emission computed tomography (SPECT), and MRI spectroscopy. In the research labs, neuroscientists and neurologists are joining forces to perfect the use of functional MRI, which may be used in the future to determine which parts of the brain light up when stimulated by certain movements, thoughts, experiences, or substances.

For a neurologist, making use of the latest advances in medical technology involves more than just a trip to the radiology department. Their diagnostic repertoire also consists of many tools unique to the practice of neurology, all of which fall under the domain of electrophysiology. The most common is EEG, a test that evaluates the electrical activity of the brain by placing electrodes on the head. The electrical discharges detected by these electrodes determine whether or not a patient has epilepsy and decipher the type and location of seizure activity. This test can also quantify cognitive function, determine brain death, and aid in the detection of difficult-to-diagnose disorders such as Creutzfeldt-Jakob disease (mad cow disease). Neurologists specializing in epilepsy often send their patients for long-term EEG monitoring in the hospital or at home. Here, they record seizure activity to determine the patient's candidacy for neurosurgery or implantation of a vagal nerve stimulator (a pacemaker-like device designed to activate the vagal nerve and stop seizures from occurring).

Although the EEG evaluates neural discharges within the brain, EMG analyzes the electrical activity of the peripheral nerves and muscles. In the first part of this test, known as the nerve conduction study, neurologists apply small shocks via electrodes to determine the strength of stimulus conduction by sensory nerves. During the actual EMG, the physician inserts small needles into different muscles of the patient's neck, back, arms, and legs. By introducing electrical stimuli, it becomes possible to detect abnormalities in neuromuscular conduction. This test enables neurologists to evaluate a patient for peripheral nerve and muscle disorders as well as radiculopathies (pinched nerves due to a slipped disk within the spine). Debilitating diseases such as myasthenia gravis are picked up by special EMG studies that make use of repetitive stimuli and single-fiber stimulation. By guiding the physician specifically to the affected muscle, the EMG allows for more effective treatment of patients with dystonia and severe muscle spasms.

SPECIAL PROCEDURES IN NEUROLOGY

Similar to most subspecialties of internal medicine, neurology is particularly rewarding for aspiring doctors who prefer using their minds more often than their hands. Regardless, there are several important procedures that all neurologists perform on a daily basis. The most common is the famous spinal tap (lumbar puncture). During this procedure, the physician carefully inserts a needle into the thecal sac below the termination of the spinal cord to withdraw cerebrospinal fluid. Unchanged for the past 100 years, this technique can diagnose patients with certain acute infections, particularly meningitis, as well as multiple sclerosis, intracranial bleeding, and neuropathies. Furthermore, the spinal tap can also serve as a therapeutic measure by removing fluid to relieve conditions such as hydrocephalus (water on the brain) or increased intracranial pressure. It also provides a means by which the physician directly injects chemotherapeutic agents or antibiotics to treat infections and cancers of the central nervous system directly (by bypassing the blood–brain barrier).

If sticking long needles into the backs of your patients is not enough, neurology also offers other types of procedures for medical students with great manual dexterity. In addition to EMG testing, neurologists perform injections of Botulinum toxin, a neuromuscular relaxant, to treat patients with severe muscle spasms or headaches. Within the emerging specialty of neurologic intensive care, these clinicians make use of even fancier procedures: placement of intracranial probes and shunts, evaluation of transcranial Doppler studies, and even performing cerebral angiograms and directly treating intracranial blood clots.

THERAPEUTICS: "CAN YOU CURE ME, DOC?"

In the 1950s, physicians often jokingly defined a neurologist as "a specialist in the differential diagnosis of incurable disease."[1] When asked about their reasons for not choosing a career in neurology, many medical students still cite this perceived lack of treatment for patients afflicted with neurologic disease. Perhaps, they completed their rotations with attending physicians who concentrated too much on finding the exact anatomic position of the predicament rather than determining treatment choices. Contrary to this misinformed belief, neurologists can do much to treat their patients' wide variety of disorders. Over the past several years, the wealth of therapeutic options has risen dramatically.

Neurologists often consult with neurosurgeons and vascular surgeons to discuss treatment alternatives related to excision and repair of neurologic deficits. However, they also have an extensive array of neuropharmacologic choices in their therapeutic regimen. Whether the presenting disease is a complex pain syndrome, debilitating multiple sclerosis, or Parkinson disease, neurologists use powerful new medications to alleviate symptoms. In addition, they can also counter these diseases with more aggressive therapies, such as high-dose steroids, strong acute blood thinners, intravenous immune therapies, plasmapheresis (for cleaning out the blood), vagal nerve stimulators, and many others.

Unfortunately, there still remains no effective treatment for many extremely debilitating, and usually fatal, neurologic diseases. These include amyotrophic lateral sclerosis (Lou Gehrig disease), muscular dystrophy, certain brain tumors, Alzheimer dementia, and Creutzfeldt-Jakob disease. Yet this is part of the reason why neurology is an exciting field for future physician–scientists. Because clinical research in these areas is extremely active, therapies for these diseases may exist by the time current medical students begin their residency training in neurology.

THE DOCTOR–PATIENT RELATIONSHIP

In many fields of medicine, such as oncology, patients sometimes present with severe disease and die within months to years. In neurology, most of the disorders are not outright terminal. Instead, they generate significant disability over time. If they are mortal, death may take many excruciating years to occur. Sometimes, the neurologic disability presents with an acute, shocking nature; other times, it is slowly progressive. More than any other specialty, neurologists are confronted with a wide spectrum of progressive and disabling diseases. The paralyzed, wheelchair-bound young person is a neurologist's patient. The stiff, trembling elderly man with Parkinson disease is a neurologist's patient. The severely demented grandmother is a neurologist's patient.

What does all of this mean for the clinician? Good neurologists always approach their patients with empathy, compassion, and patience, which are just as important in this profession as having a scientific, cerebral bent. When there is little hope for significant improvement, they engage in honest discussions with patients and their families about the patient's medical care and future ability to function. After all, the most common reasons for a neurologic consultation are the sudden development of confusion, a gradual slip into a comatose state, or the determination of brain death. Patients, therefore, seek neurologists who are good, patient listeners, especially when the afflicted person (or family member) expresses frustration.

In neurology, patience is the golden rule. Hasty decisions often have detrimental consequences. Many physicians in other specialties are often surprised when their neurologist consultant advises a wait-and-see approach to their patients. When treating certain disorders, such as an acute stroke, neurologists often hold off on aggressive treatment while waiting for improvement. At other times, it is the neurologist who initiates aggressive therapy. For example, if presented with a patient who has just suffered a stroke, an overanxious physician who intervenes by decreasing the blood pressure or giving powerful blood thinners may actually worsen the stroke or cause bleeding into the brain, while the neurologist may do little and simply watch for improvement or actually implement intravenous therapy to increase the patient's blood pressure to supply the damaged brain with more blood. It is the neurologist who needs to make a sound decision based on the specific clinical picture of the patient.

Neurologists practice by virtue of not giving up on their patients, no matter how little improvement has been achieved. Health professionals with little background in neurology often dash the hopes of patients and their families in cases of acute confusion, disability following a stroke, or progressive multiple sclerosis. Instead, the neurologist knows that even the most severely disabled patient may eventually recover substantially. But these physicians do not necessarily practice on the basis of common sense alone. Rather, all neurologists need to strive for a combination of calmness and initiative, compassion and objectivity, the ability to communicate clearly, and the skill to listen quietly.

The intimate physician–patient relationships make neurology an extremely rewarding profession. By treating disease and holding the best interests of your patients in mind, you become their ally. A neurologist in private practice believes that "all neurologists should provide a shoulder to cry on. We are here to serve our patients, to discuss their doubts openly, and to be someone whom they can rely upon and trust."

CURRENT CONTROVERSIES IN NEUROLOGY

Medical students interested in neurology should feel comfortable dealing with end-of-life care and the withdrawal of life support. Neurologists are frequently consulted to evaluate the cognitive and brainstem status of comatose or brain damaged patients. It is neurologists who are asked to make a determination whether the patient has sustained brain death, irreversible brain damage, or whether there is some potential for recovery of neurological functioning. These are not easy decisions and they have to be made carefully, as sometimes even a subtle neurological finding observed over several examinations may reveal that a patient's neurological status may be slowly improving. Meanwhile, the hospital, other physicians, and family may be pressuring the neurologist to make a hasty decision that is not in the best interest of the patient. More and more research is showing that the complexities of brain functioning are often difficult to assess and that someone who on initial evaluation may seem unresponsive may in fact be fully aware of what is occurring around him or her. New pharmacological and interventional techniques (such as deep brain stimulation) are being utilized to awake patients from their comatose state.

Consider the following example. A woman lying in a coma state after suffering a severe brain injury may appear still and unable to communicate. In this case, families often wonder about the meaningfulness of any existing brain activity. What measures should be taken to maintain that patient's life? Do we give her medications for her assumed discomfort? Do we let her die peacefully? Is starvation and withholding medicine, in fact, a peaceful death or actually torture? Are we allowed to make any proactive decisions in this matter whatsoever, especially ones possibly bordering on euthanasia? Neurologists are the doctors who must cope with these difficult questions. As a neurologist, you should apply your own ethical and religious standards, not any norms determined by medical or legal ruling bodies, to provide the most appropriate patient care.

The other current topic of heavy debate in contemporary neurology is the question of research utilizing stem cells.

From these preprogramed cells, nerve and other tissues could be grown to replace damaged organs. A few years ago, the focus was on embryonic stem cells, but more recent techniques have determined that cells obtained from a patient's own tissues, such as skin, can be reprogramed to produce other cells, such as dopamine-producing cells that can be implanted into the brain of a patient suffering with Parkinson's disease. Unlike embryonic or other foreign derived stem cells, there would be less risk of rejection by the patient's immune system if a patient's own cells were used. Because most neurological diseases would require only certain cell lines for treatment, not a need to produce entire organs, successful treatments using stem cells will probably occur sooner in neurology than in many other specialties. As research progresses, neurologists will be at the forefront on the debate regarding the use of stem cells, cloning, and gene therapy.

LIFESTYLE CONSIDERATIONS AND PRACTICE OPTIONS

What can a neurologist expect when entering the job market after residency? Among the possible options, academic neurology draws a significant percentage of specialists. After all, neurology is a field of medicine heavily intertwined with the basic sciences. Because much of the research in this specialty is still based in the laboratory, as opposed to a clinical setting, many neurologists are MD–PhD trained scientists. In academic medicine, most neurologists concentrate on their clinical and basic science laboratory research responsibilities more than their clinical duties. To maintain their clinical competence, they typically hold outpatient clinics a few times a week and supervise residents and medical students as attending physicians on inpatient and consult neurology services.

The role of the neurologist in the private sector is quite different. In the community hospital setting, the neurologist is a consultant; they do not usually admit patients under their own name. Instead, neurologists consult on patients admitted to the hospital by primary care physicians. After rounding on these patients, they spend the bulk of their day in the clinic. They see new and returning patients, review relevant radiologic studies, and perform EEGs and EMGs. Although the workload may, in fact, border on staggering in some hospitals and clinic settings, neurologists are less likely to be woken in the middle of night for patients with neurologic emergencies. Thus, most neurologists maintain an enjoyable lifestyle with plenty of time to pursue outside interests.

Due to the aging population, new developments in brain science, and further subspecialization, the specialty of neurology is expanding rapidly. A recent study predicts that the demand for neurologists will greatly exceed the supply by nearly 20% in the next decade.[2] As a result, more neurologists are greatly needed in most regions of the country. Today, the average waiting period for a clinic appointment can range from a few weeks to several months. There are many job openings with excellent salaries and high earning potential in all types of markets, from urban to suburban to rural.

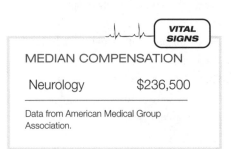

VITAL SIGNS

MEDIAN COMPENSATION

Neurology $236,500

Data from American Medical Group
Association.

FELLOWSHIPS AND SUBSPECIALTY TRAINING

Since the founding of the National Institute of Neurologic Disease and Stroke in 1950, subspecialization within neurology has developed at an accelerating rate. According to the American Academy of Neurology (AAN), the most common areas of clinical focus among neurologists were headache, epilepsy, stroke, and neurophysiology. Most fellowships in neurology last 1 to 2 years following completion of residency training. For medical students interested in a career in academic neurology, a research-oriented fellowship in a subspecialty is almost imperative. Only two of the following fellowships (clinical neurophysiology and headache/pain) are Accreditation Council of Graduate Medical Education (ACGME) approved and lead to board certification.

Clinical Neurophysiology

For the procedure-oriented clinician, this extremely popular subspecialty, involving both EEG and EMG, allows the neurologist to incorporate a greater number of procedures into his or her practice. By mastering how to perform and to interpret these tests, you will become a better diagnostician of epilepsy, sleep disorders, and neuromuscular disease. Clinical neurophysiologists often monitor EEG rhythms and interpret evoked potentials prior to and during surgical procedures. They also are sometimes trained in the evaluation of sleep studies. Some neurophysiologists assist neurosurgeons inside the operating room by monitoring EEGs and evoked potentials during surgeries to remove brain tissue that is the source of a patient's seizure activity. These neurologists become well versed in the evaluation and treatment of patients with epilepsy, peripheral neuropathies, muscular dystrophy, myasthenia gravis, and amyotrophic lateral sclerosis. Clinical neurophysiology is a highly sought after fellowship, particularly by those interested in private practice.

Stroke/Neurointensive Care

According to the AAN, the prevalence of stroke in the general population is roughly 250 out of every 100,000 people. Thus, stroke and intracranial hemorrhage comprise the majority of neurologic admissions to the hospital. The advanced study of stroke and mastery of neurointensive care are often combined under a single fellowship. This is because many patients admitted to a neurologic ICU typically have cerebrovascular disease. Neurointensivists serve as a bridge

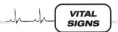

between neurology and neurosurgery. They are intense, hands-on specialists who direct patient care in the ICU by working closely with the neurosurgeons. These physicians can interpret transcranial Doppler studies and insert intracranial catheters and monitors. They are also very capable in the skills typical of any other critical care specialist, particularly those related to ventilator management, intubation, and other interventional procedures. Some academic centers also train their fellows in performing cerebral angiograms and interventional therapeutic procedures associated with this technique. These neurovascular specialists are often at the forefront of care for patients with acute strokes, utilizing techniques that can remove clots from blocked arteries in the brain.

Movement Disorders

Nearly 1% of the population older than 65 years has Parkinson disease. Neurologists interested in specializing in these types of diseases often complete a fellowship in movement disorders. They gain knowledge on the cutting-edge treatment for Parkinson disease, particularly the newest pharmacologic therapy. They also develop expertise in managing other disorders that cause abnormal movements or body distortions, such as progressive supranuclear palsy, dystonias, essential tremor, Huntington chorea, and Wilson disease. Because close observation of the patient is crucial to this subspecialty, movement disorder specialists are particularly fond of their video cameras. They are keen observers of abnormal tremors, jerks, muscle spasms, positions, and other unusual motions. In addition, these physicians also gain skill in performing Botulinum toxin injections to treat dystonias. Recently, movement disorder specialists have became increasingly involved in helping neurosurgeons in the new technology of deep brain stimulation for Parkinson's disease and other neurodegenerative disorders.

Neuroimmunology

Specialists in neuroimmunology concentrate on patients with autoimmune neurologic disease, particularly multiple sclerosis. According to the AAN, roughly 350,000 to 500,000 people suffer from multiple sclerosis in the United States. The neuroimmunologist also evaluates and treats patient with other autoimmune neurologic problems, such as myasthenia gravis, lupus, and Sjogren disease. Due to the complexity of these diseases, neuroimmunologists are also knowledgeable in their complications, including depression, psychosis, spasticity, incontinence, sexual dysfunction, and pain. This field is expanding dramatically, with new, effective treatments being approved nearly every year.

Behavioral Neurology

Specialists in this research-oriented academic specialty are mostly confronted with dementia, including Alzheimer disease, vascular dementia, dementias

RESIDENCY TRAINING

Residency in neurology requires 4 years postgraduate training. There are currently 120 accredited programs. It requires an internship year (PGY-1) plus 3 years of clinical neurology. The PGY-1 year (either internal medicine or transitional) must include a 6- to 8-month internal medicine. Some medical centers offer categorical 4-year tracks that include a preliminary medicine year at the same institution, while others have combined neurology programs with internal medicine, psychiatry, and radiology. During the last 2 years of training, overnight call may be taken from home. The typical monthly rotations include inpatient neurology, consults, outpatient clinic, pediatric neurology, EEG/EMG, neuropathology, neuroradiology, and neurointensive care.

THE INSIDE SCOOP

associated with prion disease (mad cow disease), and reversible metabolic dementias. The AAN reports that more than 4 million people in the United States have Alzheimer dementia. The behavioral neurologist concentrates on evaluation of the patient's mental status, often using complex neuropsychological tests. Many of the skills these specialists have overlap with those of neuropsychologists and neuropsychiatrists. Advanced imaging and biochemical techniques are being utilized to help neurologists understand dementia and determine new avenues for diagnosis and treatment.

Headache/Pain

In the general outpatient clinic, headaches are the main complaint evaluated by neurologists. More than 45 million people suffer from chronic headaches. This fellowship allows the clinician to gain further skill in treating chronic pain syndromes, including headaches. Some programs provide training in interventional pain techniques, similar to those learned by anesthesiologists. These procedures include epidural injections, trigger point injections, denervation procedures, spinal cord stimulation, botox injections, and others. Many hospitals offer special headache clinics staffed by neurologists.

WHY CONSIDER A CAREER IN NEUROLOGY?

The future looks extremely bright for neurology, one of the fastest growing fields within medicine. Because of the rapid expansion of clinical information, neurology will increasingly rely upon its many subspecialties to provide the best patient care. Most neurologists agree that with proper training, primary care physicians should manage certain uncomplicated neurologic problems.[3] However, more and more aging patients are presenting with complicated and chronic neurologic diseases. As a result, neurology may shift its focus from being a consultation specialty to one of long-term primary care by a subspecialist. For instance, many general neurologists, who consult on simple patients for primary care physicians, acknowledge that even their skills in treating severe intractable epilepsy and its complications are not enough. Instead, they refer their patients to specialized epilepsy centers, where research and clinical trials are usually held, for long-term continuity of care.[4] This cost-effective subspecialization is essential to both the progress of neurology and the improvement of patient care.

What entices physicians to become neurologists? For many, it is their fascination with the tremendous depth and complexity of the nervous system. Others enjoy using basic sciences to solve neurologic puzzles. Neurologists are physicians who are never bored. Every day, they encounter some of the most severely ill patients found in medicine. Despite the frequent interactions with pain, dysfunction, and disability, neurology is full of many wonderful rewards and intense satisfaction. Patients with neurologic disease challenge your scientific knowledge, diagnostic ability, and therapeutic skills. They express an immense sense of dependence and appreciation for your guidance that is unrivaled by any other patient population. You will learn to cherish and admire your patients. They teach all neurologists about the importance of appreciating, loving, and enjoying the quality of one's life, even if it is compromised by disability.

If you are a medical student fascinated by the complexities of treating nervous system disorders, then neurology awaits you. By learning the language of neurology, you will join a group of specialists who are true medical detectives. They continue every day to be amazed by the depth and variety of patients and diseases they encounter. In the near future, neurologists will find themselves at the forefront of a revolution in therapeutics. This is an exciting and exhilarating time to be a neurologist!

ABOUT THE CONTRIBUTOR

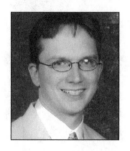 Dr Tomasz Zabiega is a neurologist at the Joliet Headache and Neuro Center in Joliet and Morris, Illinois. He has spent much of his life here (California and Illinois) and in Poland. After earning his undergraduate and medical degrees at Southern Illinois University, he completed his neurology residency at the University of Chicago Hospitals. Dr Zabiega acknowledges his wife Maria Antonia Mariscal de Zabiega; children Stanislaw, Vitaliana, Maria Jozef, and Jose; parents Andrew and Helena (a neurologist and neurological nurse); and sister Margaret (also an MD) as his sources of inspiration and support. He can be reached by e-mail at tzabiega@hotmail.com.

REFERENCES

1. Herndon, R.M. Neurology should not become a consulting specialty. *Arch Neurol.* 1995;52:205–206.

2. Bradley, W.G. Neurology in the next two decades: Report of the workforce task force of the American Academy of Neurology. *Neurology.* 2000;54:787–789.

3. Ringel, S.P., Vickrey, B.G., et al. Training the future neurology workforce. *Neurology.* 2000;54:480–484.

4. Menken, M. Neurology as a consulting specialty. *Arch Neurol.* 1995;52:206–207.

20

NEUROSURGERY

Kiarash Shahlaie

Amazing. There are few experiences in medicine more awe inspiring than gently incising the dura to reveal the delicate and beautiful anatomy of the human brain. This mysterious organ houses our memories, thoughts, and desires and gives us the ability to interact with the world around us. The brain, via the spinal cord and peripheral and cranial nerves, animates us. It is with our brains that we think, hope, and wonder, and it is because of our brains and spinal cord that we are able to walk, talk, run, and play. Neurosurgeons not only operate on the brain, spinal cord, and nerves but they are also experts in diagnosis and management of diseases that affect this delicate system. They are scientists, clinicians, and surgeons who are dedicated to treating diseases of the central and peripheral nervous system—this is the unique challenge and reward of being a neurosurgeon.

WHAT IS NEUROLOGICAL SURGERY?

Unless you seek out experiences in neurosurgery during medical school, you may not have a good understanding of what exactly neurosurgeons do. Are they brain surgeons? What about spine surgeons? There are nerves all over the body—do they operate on those too? Most hospitals have a neurosurgical ICU—are they the physicians who take care of those patients as well? Do neurosurgeons treat all neurological diseases? What is the difference between a neurosurgeon and a neurologist? Briefly, the answers to these questions are yes, yes, often, absolutely, no, and a scalpel (well, not exactly!).

Neurosurgery is not a required clerkship in medical school, but it is a service in the hospital that you will likely encounter on a regular basis. During a rotation in family practice, for instance, medical students may see a patient that recently underwent decompression and fusion of a herniated disk that was pressing on

WHAT MAKES A GOOD NEUROSURGEON?

✓ Likes the immediate gratification of surgical outcomes.
✓ Is creative, detail oriented, and holds him- or herself to high standards.
✓ Can remain relaxed and confident under intense pressure.
✓ Enjoys incorporating highly technical procedures into patient care.
✓ Has good manual dexterity.

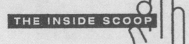

THE INSIDE SCOOP

the nerves in his low back. While learning pediatrics, you will probably care for a child who had a ventriculoperitoneal shunt placed shortly after birth to treat her congenital hydrocephalus (a condition in which cerebrospinal fluid accumulates in the brain). During your surgery clerkship, you may witness the neurosurgery team racing the victim of a bad car accident to the operating room to rapidly evacuate an epidural hematoma that threatens her life. After spending some time in the hospital, you soon realize that neurosurgeons play a critical role in treating a variety of disorders in a very diverse group of patients, and they very frequently interact with physicians from many different specialties.

Since most medical students do not complete clerkships in neurosurgery, their opinion of neurosurgeons is often influenced by what other residents tell them ("neurosurgeons have no lives"), what the nurses say ("those neurosurgeons think they are gods"), or what they have seen on television (the scandalous exploits of "Dr McDreamy" on ABC's *Grey's Anatomy*). As with most stereotypes, however, these notions rarely hold much truth. In fact, neurosurgery residents work under the same hour limitations as all other specialties, they all know too well that they are not gods, and not all of them live the life of those neurosurgeons in television dramas. What is true, though, is that neurosurgery is an intense and high-stakes field of medicine. It is intellectually fascinating, personally rewarding, and requires significant compassion and empathy for patients suffering from serious and potentially disabling conditions. Neurosurgeons are the only physicians in the hospital that interact daily with the most amazing and intriguing anatomy and physiology in the human body: the central and peripheral nervous systems.

NEUROLOGICAL SURGERY: TREATING THE NERVOUS SYSTEM

Neurosurgery is a specialty that is all together challenging, exciting, interesting, stressful, invasive, focused, and, yes, fun. Neurosurgery is brain surgery. But it is also spine surgery and even peripheral nerve surgery. The brain and spinal cord are composed of extremely complex and delicate pathways that may result in devastating consequences when struck with disease. Although psychiatrists and neurologists also help diagnose and treat patients with neurological disorders, it is only neurosurgeons that physically navigate around and through its delicate structures to treat their patients. Neurosurgeons care for traumatic injury to the nervous system, manage some of the most critically ill patients in the hospital, and focus their efforts on preserving or improving their patients' ability to walk, talk, and interact with the world around them.

Since neurosurgery is a specialty focused on a physiological system rather than a specific anatomical region, neurosurgeons treat diseases that affect all types of patients in various parts of their bodies. For example, a typical neurosurgeon not only operates on the brain and spinal cord but may also perform procedures on the skull, face, neck, spine, arms, and legs. Neurosurgeons care for some of the youngest patients in the hospital, such as a premature infant with a congenital malformation, as well as young and elderly adults suffering from trauma, tumors, infections, vascular anomalies, or degenerative disorders. The level of care provided by neurosurgeons is similarly broad—some patients do not require an operation at all (observing a patient after mild head injury), some undergo outpatient surgery (carpal tunnel release or lumbar microdiscectomy), while others may be very unstable and critically ill for days and weeks during their treatment (ruptured intracranial aneurysm, traumatic brain injury). Therefore, neurosurgery is a very diverse field with varying and unique challenges.

Neurosurgeons not only *operate* on the nervous system but must also understand its structure and function better than any other physician in the hospital. Neurosurgeons must thoroughly examine their patients (performing the infamous "neurological exam," an "art" they share with neurologists), interpret many different types of diagnostic studies, and identify the correct diagnosis for their patients' ailments. Neurosurgeons are experts of basic neuroradiology and must carefully review diagnostic studies such as CT, MRI, angiograms, or EMGs. Neurosurgeons provide care to patients in the neurosurgical ICU and must develop a strong understanding of advanced critical care medicine. Therefore, neurosurgery is a specialty focused on improving neurological outcome through caring for a broad range of patients and diseases in varied clinical settings, accomplished with the use of highly advanced and constantly improving technological tools.

CHOOSING NEUROSURGERY

Most neurosurgeons say they chose this specialty because it brought together their interest in neuroscience with their desire to be a surgeon: neurosurgery equals

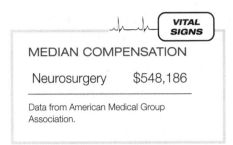

"neuro" plus "surgery." However, this is far from a complete answer. The truth is that neurosurgery is such a unique field of medicine, such a rare thing to do with one's life, that it is difficult for most residents (and attendings) to put into words exactly why they chose this career. Neurosurgery is a specialty rooted in basic and clinical science, surgical technique, and expert clinical skills—due in large part to its history in the modern era.

Although neurosurgical procedures date back to the earliest stages of human history (skull trephinations were successfully performed by many ancient societies), modern day neurosurgery developed in the late nineteenth century following advancements in general surgical techniques. In the early twentieth century, Harvey Cushing became the first surgeon in the United States to specialize in neurological surgery. A highly gifted neuroscientist, neurophysiologist, surgeon, and author, Cushing's insight and innovation propelled neurosurgery into the modern era. He is affectionately referred to as "the founding father" of neurosurgery. Cushing's contributions to medicine are numerous. He first introduced the practice of anesthesia record keeping during surgery (as a medical student!), developed electrocautery techniques to minimize operative bleeding (the infamous "Bovie" instrument essential to all surgeons was developed by Cushing and the physicist William T. Bovie), and significantly advanced our understanding of intracranial physiology and pathology (he characterized diseases of the pituitary gland and classified hundreds of brain tumors based on pathological characteristics).[1] Harvey Cushing decreased mortality following brain tumor surgery from 40% to 7%, and was even recognized with a Pulitzer Prize in Literature for a biography he wrote of his instructor Sir William Osler.[2] Cushing was not only a clinician but also a talented writer, an intelligent scientist, and a gifted surgeon—the culture of modern day neurosurgery in many ways reflects aspects of the great Harvey Cushing.

Although very few modern day neurosurgeons can be compared with Dr. Cushing, his legacy lives on in the way neurosurgeons strive to practice their art. A classic neurosurgeon is part neuroscientist, part surgeon, part clinician, part critical care specialist, and part ethicist. To operate on the nervous system is a huge responsibility, and neurosurgeons must not only master their basic sciences but also develop superb surgical skills, learn to communicate effectively with their patients and families, understand how to carefully manage patients before and after surgery, and recognize when their operative skills should not be used (eg, in the face of devastating or irreversible neurological dysfunction).

What typically drives medical students into neurosurgery is a strong desire to better understand neuroanatomy and neurophysiology. However, this does not mean that all neurosurgeons were those medical students who quickly and easily memorized detailed pathways in neuroanatomy class (most of us still cringe at the thought) — instead they were the ones that found neurophysiology to be fascinating in its complexity. Similarly, neurosurgery residents did not memorize every subtle aspect of cross-sectional neuroanatomy while in medical school (remember the claustrum and extreme capsule?), but they were likely the ones who marveled at the subtlety of these structures. Neurosurgery is a career in neuroscience and neurophysiology, so a desire to continue learning about neural pathways and neural structure rather than an "innate" ability to memorize it all in medical school is an important aspect of choosing a career in neurosurgery.

However, many residents and attendings will tell you that a good neurosurgeon is not necessarily the one who has the pathways of the vestibulospinal tract memorized, but the one who has a good understanding of the aspects of neuroscience that are clinically relevant and can apply them to patient care. Indeed, neurosurgeons are not simply scientists, but they are clinicians, and they must use relevant aspects of neuroscience to provide thoughtful, compassionate care to their patients. Neurosurgery is a field that continues to advance with new scientific discoveries and technological developments. It is important that neurosurgeons not only determine how these advancements should impact patient care but also have the ability and skill to explain these issues to their patients. This common theme in clinical medicine is particularly challenging in neurosurgery, since diseases of the nervous system are often poorly understood by patients (the brain is a "black box" to most) and may result in debilitating symptoms such as confusion, seizures, paralysis, or chronic pain. In the extreme situation, neurosurgeons may care for patients who are deeply comatose (or even brain dead), and must carefully consider many end-of-life issues when helping families make difficult decisions. An effective neurosurgeon, therefore, is far more than someone who loves neuroscience and surgery. Neurosurgery does *not* simply equal "neuro" plus "surgery"!

NEUROSURGERY AND TECHNOLOGY

When first wandering into the operating room during a neurosurgical procedure, some medical students are surprised by the amount of highly advanced technologies that are used by neurosurgeons. In fact, neurosurgery is one of the most technologically oriented surgical specialties, constantly improving as new diagnostic and therapeutic tools are developed. For example, when examining a patient and planning treatment for a brain tumor, neurosurgeons will begin by reviewing conventional studies such as CT, MRI, and angiograms. Some patients, however, will also have spectroscopic studies that measure the chemical composition of various regions in the brain, functional images that indicate which areas of the brain are active during various tasks, or specialized scans that accurately depict the location and direction of white matter fibers that connect brain regions. Some patients may even undergo placement of brain electrodes prior to their primary operation to "map" areas of electrical activity during seizures episodes. Highly advanced technologies also guide neurosurgeons during an operation. For example, to more accurately understand the specific function of various brain regions surrounding an area of interest, neurosurgeons may use neuromonitoring (to ensure that adjacent pathways are not affected during surgery), brain mapping (to identify the function of various regions of the cortex adjacent to the area of interest), or stereotactic techniques such as neuronavigation (to identify the precise location of various intracranial structures during surgery based on CT or MRI technology). Some modern-day operative suites use live MRI or CT scanning or robotic arms that assist during surgery.[3] Surgery on the nervous system's surrounding structures is similarly advanced. Neurosurgeons may correct cranial defects using custom-designed implants (based on 3D CT scan reconstructions obtained prior to surgery), replace intervertebral discs in the spine with artificial articulating joints or stem cells (these are currently in clinical trial!), or fuse an unstable lumbar spine using percutaneous techniques and live CT imaging (passing instruments through the skin rather than making a large incision and painfully dissecting through tissue).

After surgery, technological advancements continue to guide neurosurgical care. For example, blood flow velocities through cerebral vessels can be measured using transcranial ultrasound; electrical signaling in the brain can be monitored using electroencephalograms; or the exact levels of extracellular glucose, tissue temperature, tissue pH, or intracranial pressure can be directly monitored in the brain using tiny microdialysis catheters and probes. Therefore, technological advancements play a large role in neurosurgery and make this a particularly exciting field of medicine. The way neurosurgery is practiced continues to evolve. As newer technologies are introduced, the practice of neurosurgery will continue to evolve, placing neurosurgeons on the forefront of scientific advancement.

NEUROSURGERY AND NEUROSCIENCE RESEARCH

Although most neurosurgeons in practice are not actively involved in neuro-science research, the culture of this specialty is such that most neurosurgeons highly value neuroscience and constantly keep up to date with scientific literature. As a result, most residency programs look favorably upon students who demonstrate an interest in contributing to neuroscience, and most medical students who apply for neurosurgery residencies have some degree of research experience. Although it would be ideal to apply with a handful of first author publications in high-impact journals, most programs understand that it is difficult to achieve this lofty goal during medical school. Instead, a strong interest (and track record of experience) in basic or clinical science research is an important factor in most residency programs' selection criteria, although the research accomplishments of those who successfully match into neurological surgery vary significantly.

NEUROTRAUMA AND NEUROCRITICAL CARE

Neurosurgeons are at the frontline of treatment for traumatic injuries to the brain. Some of these injuries, such as epidural or subdural hematomas, require emergent operations that can save a patient's life. For example, a patient with an epidural hematoma who is brought to the emergency room on the brink of brain death may be awake and back to normal the very next morning if he is urgently taken to the operating room for evacuation of his clot. Other injuries require placement of drains or small probes into the brain to monitor brain swelling, oxygenation, pH, temperature, and changes in metabolites — these monitors are used to guide therapy in hopes of preventing additional insults to the brain during its recovery process. Some patients with milder injuries may not require surgery at all, but instead close observation and consultation with a neurosurgeon.

Just as trauma surgeons provide nonoperative care for patients who have suffered injuries to the chest or abdomen, neurosurgeons similarly care for patients with brain or spinal cord injuries that do not always require an operation. This is an interesting aspect of neurosurgery because it requires a strong foundation in general principles of trauma and critical care and results in significant collaboration with physicians from other specialties. For example, a patient struck by a car while riding his bicycle may present with a moderate head injury, multiple orthopedic fractures, a small splenic laceration, and a pulmonary contusion. In such multitrauma situations, neurosurgeons play an important role in helping to prioritize a patient's injuries (and treatment) so that the chances of neurological recovery are maximized while not compromising other care issues. To be effective in this role, neurosurgeons must understand the pathophysiology of neurotrauma and the many subtle aspects of neurological recovery that can be affected by other systemic issues (fluid status, oxygenation, ventilation, electrolyte balance, etc). Since traumatic brain and spinal cord injury continue to be very prevalent in modern day society, neurosurgeons will continue to play an important role in operative and nonoperative management of these patients.

HIGH STAKES: LIFE AND DEATH

Neurosurgery is an emotionally demanding specialty. There are times that are very rewarding. Seeing a pediatric patient run around the wards 2 days after resecting a tumor from her brainstem is a feeling one cannot put into words. There are also times of frustration, anxiety, and sadness. For instance, it is extremely difficult to tell a young woman that she will never walk again or to tell an elderly man that his wife's head injury is so severe that nothing can be done to prevent her death. Damage to the central nervous system can be severe and devastating, and our abilities to reverse or repair damage to the brain and spinal cord are still quite limited. As a result, neurosurgeons are often involved in providing end-of-life care and neurosurgery residents typically witness more patients die than any other group of physicians-in-training in the hospital. Delivering unfortunate news to families can be an extremely challenging aspect of neurosurgery.

THE NEUROSURGEON–PATIENT RELATIONSHIP

The close relationships neurosurgeons have with their patients are particularly special. For example, imagine meeting a patient with a newly diagnosed brain tumor in your clinic. What follows is a very intimate discussion with them about what you have found and how you can help them. You finally explain their symptoms to them ("that's why you've been getting weak in your arm"), and you share with them your hopes ("I think we can remove it completely") and your concerns ("this may be a malignant tumor"). You talk frankly about the risks of what you will do ("you may get worse after surgery," "you may lose the ability to talk," "you may become paralyzed"), and you discuss all alternative treatments with them in detail. Such an intimate discussion between a physician and patient—between two human beings—is an amazing experience that is unique to being a physician. What amplifies this experience in neurosurgery, however, is that the discussion is so deeply personal ("you may not be able to talk or recognize your wife's face") that the relationship between a neurosurgeon and his or her patient is one of the most intimate of all medical specialties. Patients are generally *very grateful* to the surgeon that repaired a painful hernia in their groin or the one who bypassed the blockage in their coronary artery, but they are somehow *connected* to the surgeon who carefully navigated along their language cortex to delicately remove an abnormal growth that was pushing on part of their brain. It is typical, therefore, for neurosurgeons to remember every detail about the patient they operated on many years ago ("he had horrible nausea for two weeks," "his daughter recently graduated from kindergarten," "they recently went on vacation to Europe"), and patients will often begin their follow-up visit with a big hug or tears.

NEUROSURGERY, NEUROLOGY, AND PSYCHIATRY

The range of diseases that affect the nervous system is large, and not all of them are primarily treated by neurosurgeons. This is where the neurologist's role comes into play. The neurologist is an expert of clinical diagnosis and manages neurological disease in predominantly noninvasive ways. For example, a patient diagnosed with Parkinson's disease will be treated medically by a neurologist for many years. It is only after they have exhausted medical management and are still refractory to medications that the neurosurgeon implants a deep brain stimulator (DBS) into the basal ganglia to relieve the patients of their tremor. When a mysterious disease strikes a patient, neurosurgeons may be asked to biopsy the brain to help find answers. Some patients with certain types of epilepsy may also exhaust medical treatments by neurologists and require surgical treatment to improve or even cure them of their condition. As a result, neurosurgeons have a deep appreciation for neurology and clinical neuroscience, but their efforts on diagnosis and treatment through are more invasive, surgical means.

A similar relationship exists between neurosurgery and psychiatry. Psychosurgery—operating on the brain to treat psychiatric disorders—is a fascinating field in neurosurgery that has a very interesting history. There was much interest in psychosurgery at the turn of the twentieth century, particularly in the late 1930s when Antonio Egas Moniz began to describe the therapeutic effects of lesions in the frontal lobes to treat various psychiatric disorders (he was later awarded the Nobel Prize in Physiology and Medicine in 1949 for "the discovery of the therapeutic value of prefrontal leucotomy in certain psychoses"). Adverse side effects from the widespread use of these therapies, coupled with the development of better antipsychotic medications, resulted in a shift away from surgical therapies for psychiatric disorders. However, the benefits of surgical intervention for many disorders have been well described, and select patients today undergo surgical intervention for obsessive compulsive disorder, severe depression, or intractable pain.[4] Functional neurosurgery, therefore, has a very promising future as a minimally invasive therapy for a host of mental and behavioral disorders and presents a very interesting and exciting subspecialty of neurosurgery.

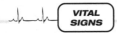
VITAL SIGNS

NEUROSURGERY 2011 MATCH STATISTICS

- Number of positions available: 195
- 208 US seniors and 75 independent applicants ranked at least one neurosurgery program
- 98.5% of all positions were filled in the initial Match
- The successful applicants: 91.1% US seniors, 9.0% foreign-trained physicians, and 0% osteopathic graduates
- Mean USMLE Step I score: 239
- Unmatched rate for US seniors applying only to neurosurgery: 11.8%

Data from National Resident Matching Program.

LIFESTYLE CONSIDERATIONS AND PRACTICE OPTIONS

Although interesting and rewarding, neurosurgery training is also challenging and difficult at times. Most residents take in-house call every third night during the early years of their training, and they are very quickly given significant responsibility for patient care. Since most neurosurgery programs tend to be very busy (and always in need of more residents), the workload can be quite substantial. For example, on a typical night, a neurosurgery resident may be caring for 10 to 20 ICU patients and 20 to 30 floor patients while seeing consults in the emergency room and urgently taking a patient to the operating room for surgery. The ability to prioritize and multitask is therefore critical, and the inherent stress of this responsibility is significant at times. This type of training is critical and invaluable for neurosurgeons, but it can also affect one's mood both at work and at home. Coupled with the responsibility and stress of learning the basic and clinical science of neurosurgery (ICU management, perioperative care, surgical anatomy and techniques, etc), this can result in the resident who "lives in the hospital" or "has no life." This issue, however, is not unique to neurosurgery as many specialties in medicine can be quite demanding.

It is important to note, though, that residency training in general has changed significantly over the past few years, in large part due to an increased emphasis on limiting resident work hours and improving educational experiences and quality of life in general. Although the acuity and spectrum of diseases neurosurgery residents treat are generally the same as before, neurosurgery residents work the same number of hours per shift/week as other residents in busy programs. Changes to resident work hours have resulted in improved quality of life for surgical residents,[5,6] and many feel that the learning experience is enhanced when residents have time to prepare for cases and are less tired when performing them. Although many neurosurgeons continue to debate the effects of work hour limitations on neurosurgical resident training, it is clear that the exhaustive work hours that resulted in many of the old stereotypes ("neurosurgery residents live in the hospital," "they're always tired," "they have no lives") are clearly a thing of the past.

After the completion of residency training, life as a neurosurgeon varies significantly based on where and how the physician chooses to practice. Fortunately, one very positive aspect of neurosurgical career planning is the wide array of job opportunities for graduating neurosurgeons. A study published in the *Journal of Neurosurgery* reported an increase in neurosurgical job opportunities, a decrease in the number of active neurosurgeons, and a constant supply of residents finishing training each year.[7] This means that salaries remain among the highest in all medical specialties and there is some ability to negotiate and establish the type of career one would like (call schedule, work hours, pay, etc). A survey performed by the American Association of Neurological Surgeons (AANS) found that 63% of members worked in private practice, 17% in academic affiliated private practices, and 17% in full-time academic appointments.[8] Most neurosurgeons work in either a small group of two to five practitioners (34%) or have a solo practice (29%), and almost all neurosurgeons have their practice located at a hospital (97%).[8] Therefore, there is considerable flexibility and generally good compensation for neurosurgeons in most regions of the United States. Coupled with decreased resident work hours, this has resulted in a significant improvement in the lifestyle of a neurosurgery resident, and it is not infrequent to meet neurosurgeons who devote much of their time to family, friends, and outside hobbies.

FELLOWSHIPS AND SUBSPECIALTY TRAINING

Spine Surgery

Most medical students may be surprised to learn that the majority of neurosurgical operations performed are on the structure that supports and protects the spinal cord and nerve roots: the spine. Surveys by the AANS have found that spine surgery accounts for approximately 65% to 75% of all cases performed by neurosurgeons, although this clearly differs based on training and clinical interest.[8] Spine surgery is a highly technical subspecialty of neurosurgery, focused on treating congenital, acquired, and degenerative diseases of the cervical, thoracic, and lumbar spine. Spine surgeons treat congenital disorders such as scoliosis, neoplastic disorders such as primary and metastatic tumors of the spine (bony elements) and spinal cord, traumatic injuries to the spine (fractures, dislocations), and neural elements (spinal cord injury), and many degenerative disorders such as herniated discs or osteoarthritis. Basic spine surgery is practiced by most general neurosurgeons, although more advanced techniques may require fellowship training. In fact, spine surgery has experienced some of the most rapid technological advancements in surgical technique over the past 10 years, with less invasive (minimally invasive, percutaneous techniques) and more physiologic (artificial disc replacement) treatment options being developed and studied (clinical trials in stem cell therapy are underway to help regenerate the spine). Spine surgeons are at the forefront of many biomedical engineering developments and are helping to guide the evolution of this exciting field of neurosurgery.

Spine surgery is a unique subspecialty in that both orthopedic surgeons and neurosurgeons operate on the spine. Historically, orthopedic surgeons focused on the bony aspects of spine surgery (exposing and fusing unstable levels), while neurosurgeons would primarily focus on treating neurological symptoms (decompressing the spinal cord and nerve roots and treating lesions within the neural elements themselves). This distinction no longer exists in most hospitals, as neurosurgeons and orthopedic surgeons both perform bony removal, decompression, and fusion techniques (lesions of the neural elements are primarily treated by neurosurgeons). Whether there is much of a difference between an orthopedic or neurological spine surgeon is unclear, but there are some fundamental differences in residency training for spine. For example, orthopedic surgery residents do not participate in as many spine cases during their residency as neurosurgery residents, largely due to the distribution of neurosurgery cases annually.[9] Also, neurosurgery residents gain earlier exposure to spine cases (typical spine cases are far less dangerous than cranial procedures, so junior residents are more often involved) and become very comfortable with most spine operations early in their senior years of training. However, it is unclear if this results in better spine surgeons (orthopedic surgery residents typically do a fellowship after their general training), and the reality is that some of the best spine surgeons today come from both orthopedic and neurosurgical backgrounds. As a result, those who are interested in spine should carefully consider many other fundamental differences between orthopedic and neurological surgery when choosing the best path toward a career in spine surgery.

Neurosurgical Oncology

Most cranial neurosurgical procedures are performed for tumors of the brain and surrounding structures including the meninges and skull (27%).[8] Brain tumor surgery is an exciting subspecialty of neurosurgery that continues to advance, with increased emphasis on developing techniques that allow for safer and more accurate tumor resections. Surgical planning often involves advanced neuroimaging to determine the best way to approach within the brain tissue, and surgery is often performed with the use of intraoperative neuronavigation ("GPS for the brain," which allows surgeons to know exactly where they are at all times based on a three-dimensional map of the brain and tumor). Neurosurgeons who specialize in treating tumors often have a particular interest in treating gliomas—tumors that arise from glial cells that normally support nerve function in the brain. The most common primary brain tumor in adults is glioblastoma multiforme, a high-grade lesion that despite advancements in treatment is associated with a dismal survival time of 6 to 12 months.[10] As a result, neurosurgeons who focus their careers on treating brain tumors work closely with radiation and medical oncologists and are often involved in exciting and promising cancer research or clinical trials.

RESIDENCY TRAINING

Residency in neurological surgery requires 6 to 8 years of postgraduate training. There are currently 97 accredited programs. The first year (internship) is spent in general surgery (usually 6 months) and other surgical subspecialties. Most programs are small and spread the residents across several hospitals. This translates into a fairly rigorous call schedule. In most programs, a q3 schedule (overnight call every third night) for junior residents is very common. Compared with other surgical junior neurosurgery residents, residents are expected to become relatively independent earlier in their training. One resident described the arduous training as "the only residency in which the internship year is the easy year." In most programs, residents gain experience in the various subspecialties: pediatric, oncology, spine, cerebrovascular, and stereotactic neurosurgery. The program typically involves at least 36 months of inpatient neurosurgery, 6 months of electives such as neurology and neuroradiology, 6 to 24 months of research (basic science or clinical), and 12 months as chief resident. Neurosurgery residents spend most of their time performing surgery in the operating room. When not scrubbed in for surgery, they see patients in the outpatient clinic, neurological ICU, emergency room, and hospital floors.

THE INSIDE SCOOP

Cerebrovascular Surgery

Along the ventral surface of the brain lies the Circle of Willis, a network of cerebral vessels derived from the internal carotid and vertebral arteries. It is at the branch points of this circle that most cerebral arterial aneurysms are located, and when these lesions rupture, they result in subarachnoid hemorrhage (patients present with the "worst headache of my life"). Critical lesions that can easily lead to death or severe disability, aneurysms, are treated by surgical clipping or intravascular coiling, a procedure performed by both vascular neurosurgeons and neurointerventional radiologists. Vascular neurosurgeons perform some of the most difficult and risky procedures in neurosurgery: they treat diseases that affect the vessels of the central nervous system.

Vascular neurosurgeons are experts in treating a range of diseases that affect the brain's blood vessels, including cerebral aneurysms, various vascular malformations, and carotid stenosis. A highly technical subspecialty of neurosurgery, cerebrovascular surgery is extremely challenging, carries significant risks, and requires an excellent understanding of vascular anatomy and physiology. Advanced surgical approaches are required to safely treat most vascular lesions, and many modern-day neurosurgeons are seeking fellowship training in both open and endovascular techniques (treating blood vessel abnormalities using catheters that are passed up to the brain via the groin). Most neurosurgery residents interested in vascular neurosurgery will perform fellowship training after residency.

Skull Base Surgery

The most complicated and amazing anatomy in the human body is that of the skull base—the area between the ventral undersurface of the brain and the cranial vault that cradles the brain and its supporting structures. In what resembles a complicated downtown interchange where many freeways overlap and connect with one another, the skull base is home to all of the major arteries that supply the nervous system, most cranial nerves that exit the central nervous system to innervate the face and neck, and structures of the lower brain including the pituitary gland, midbrain, medulla oblongata, and pons. Operating on the skull base is extremely challenging—the approach is often difficult, the anatomical relationship complicated, and the consequences of inadvertent damage to vessels, cranial nerves, or the brainstem can be devastating. Once considered "no man's land," skull base surgeons use advanced techniques (microscopes, endoscopy, approaches through the face or sinuses) to treat various diseases in this area, including aneurysms and tumors. Skull base surgery has witnessed an exciting transition in the past decade, with new minimally invasive endoscopic techniques that allow neurosurgeons to access this complicated region through the nose, eyebrow, or from behind the ear. Many skull base operations are performed by a multidisciplinary surgical team that includes otolaryngologists (head and neck surgeons). Neurosurgeons interested in skull base surgery typically complete 1 year of fellowship training after residency.

Pediatric Neurosurgery

Pediatric neurosurgeons treat an array of neurological diseases that affect children, many of which are similar to those that occur in adults (eg, tumors) while others are unique to children (eg, spina bifida). These patients can be as young as a premature infant born with intraventricular hemorrhage (due to immaturity of the germinal matrix along the lateral ventricles of the brain) or hydrocephalus. Pediatric neurosurgeons have a very strong understanding of embryology and central nervous system development, and enjoy the challenges and rewards of caring for sick children. They tend to develop a unique relationship with their patients and their parents, treating their conditions and closely following them into adulthood. Fellowship training is necessary for residents interested in pediatric neurosurgery.

Functional Neurosurgery

As discussed earlier, functional neurosurgery is an exciting and rapidly advancing field that provides surgical treatment options for diseases that are also treated by neurologists and psychiatrists. Functional neurosurgeons perform surgery for severe cases of epilepsy and implant DBS electrodes into the brain that act as "pacemakers" of brain activity. DBS is currently performed for various movement disorders (eg, Parkinson disease) and severe cases of obsessive-compulsive disorder; it is also in clinical trials for treatment of Alzheimer's disease, coma, severe depression, and epilepsy. Many specialists feel that functional procedures represent the future of neurosurgery, due to both scientific research and technological advancements in this subspecialty. It is a rapidly growing field, and one that often requires fellowship training after residency.

Peripheral Nerve Surgery

Peripheral nerve surgery is a highly subspecialized field of neurosurgery, accounting for approximately less than 5% of all procedures performed by neurosurgeons.[8]

As a result, there are very few neurosurgeons who exclusively perform peripheral nerve surgery, but there are many neurosurgeons who occasionally treat patients with peripheral nerve syndromes. Some of the more commonly performed procedures include carpal tunnel release (removing pressure on the median nerve at the wrist) and ulnar nerve transposition (moving the ulnar nerve out of its anatomic position over the extensor surface of the elbow). Peripheral nerve surgeons may also decompress or anastomose cranial nerves in the face or neck and resect tumors of the brachial plexus or peripheral nerves.

WHY CONSIDER A CAREER IN NEUROSURGERY?

So how do you decide if neurosurgery is right for you? Unfortunately, there is no simple answer. Just as most of us did not *really* know what it would be like to be a medical student, most medical students do not *really* know what a particular residency is going to be like. The fact remains that many of these decisions are made by "gut instinct." Although certain personality types tend to be more or less prevalent in various specialties, these trends are not as important as evaluating your personal career goals.

Neurosurgeons share qualities with trauma surgeons (head injury and neurocritical care), orthopedic surgeons (spine surgery), otolaryngologists (skull base operations), and surgical oncologists (brain tumors). They hold themselves to very high standards in order to develop a very strong understanding of operative neuroanatomy. After all, neurosurgeons must understand brain and spinal cord anatomy in situ—not simply what their gross anatomy cadaver's brain looked like on a tray! Their expertise must also include elements of neuroradiology, neurology, and pathology, because good neurosurgeons need to read their own films, perform thorough neurological assessments, and interpret basic brain and spinal cord specimens.

So what makes a neurosurgeon happy with his or her career choice? These surgeons treat the most challenging, enigmatic, and humbling system of the human body: the nervous system. They enjoy having a strong background in neuroanatomy and neurophysiology, understanding how the brain works, why it does not work in certain disease processes, and what they can (and cannot) do to the brain and spinal cord to help it recover from disease. Neurosurgeons assume responsibility for some of the sickest and most critically ill patients in the hospital and they enjoy the responsibility that comes along with that. As a result, they experience the most rewarding outcomes (saving a young person's life that is minutes away from death due to an intracranial bleed) and are witness to patients succumbing to the severity of their illness (brain cancer, severe head injury). Neurosurgeons are, therefore, the last line of care for diseases of the central and peripheral nervous system. They thrive in their specialty because it is highly technical, constantly advancing, and full of high stakes. Remember that these specialists provide care with the goal of optimizing neurological outcome. Neurosurgical patients suffer from debilitating diseases—they have the most to gain or lose—and neurosurgeons, therefore, enjoy the challenge and reward of caring for such patients.

ABOUT THE CONTRIBUTOR

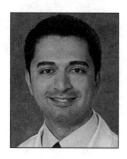

Dr Kiarash Shahlaie recently completed medical school and residency in neurological surgery at the University of California, Davis Medical Center in Sacramento. He then completed fellowship training in functional neurosurgery at UCSF, followed by a fellowship in minimally invasive skull base surgery at the John Wayne Cancer Institute. Dr Shahlaie joined the faculty at UC Davis last year, where he directs functional and skull base neurosurgery and is actively involved in premedical student advising, medical student education, and resident training. In his free time, Dr Shahlaie enjoys traveling, playing golf, and spending time with his friends and family. He can be reached by e-mail at kiarash.shahlaie@ucdmc.ucdavis.edu.

REFERENCES

1. Fulton, J.F. *Harvey Cushing: A biography.* Springfield: Charles C. Thomas; 1946.

2. Black, P.M. Harvey Cushing at the Peter Bent Brigham Hospital. *Neurosurgery.* 1999;45:990–1001.

3. Nathoo, N., Cavusoglu, M.C., et al. In touch with robotics: Neurosurgery for the future. *Neurosurgery.* 2005;56:421–433.

4. Mashour, G.A., Walker, E.E., et al. Psychosurgery: Past, present, and future. *Brain Res Brain Res Rev.* 2005;48:409–419.

5. Irani, J.L., Mello, M.M., et al. Surgical residents' perceptions of the effects of the ACGME duty hour requirements 1 year after implementation. *Surgery.* 2005;138:246–253.

6. Breen, E., Irani, J.L., et al. The future of surgery: Today's residents speak. *Curr Surg.* 2005;62:543–546.

7. Gottfried, O.N., Rovit, R.L., et al. Neurosurgical workforce trends in the United States. *J Neurosurg.* 2005;102:202–208.

8. American Association of Neurological Surgeons. *National Neurosurgical Statistics: 1999 Procedural Statistics*. 2000.

9. Dvorak, M.F., Collins, J.B., et al. Confidence in spine training among senior neurosurgical and orthopedic residents. *Spine*. 2006;31:831–837.

10. Deorah, S., Lynch, C.F., et al. Trends in brain cancer incidence and survival in the United States: Surveillance, Epidemiology, and End Results Program, 1973 to 2001. *Neurosurg Focus*. 2006;20(E1):1–7.

21
OBSTETRICS AND GYNECOLOGY
Kelly Oberia Elmore

Every woman needs a great obstetrician–gynecologist. These multidisciplinary specialists practice preventive medicine, deliver new lives into the world, and perform life-altering surgery. Half of their patients are healthy young women who come for prenatal care or annual physical examinations. However, with the longevity and desire for a healthier life, the rest of the practice consists of physically active mature women who are concerned about "life surrounding and after menopause." More than just experts on the pelvic region and reproductive tract, obstetrician–gynecologists must handle problems that require highly technical medical and surgical skills, and at the other end of the spectrum, be sensitive observers who can give psychological support. They are compassionate, highly focused listeners and clinicians who render the highest quality medical and surgical care. Whether in the clinic, operating room, or the labor and delivery ward, their methods of diagnosis and treatment options are rapidly expanding.

ONE WOMAN—TWO SPECIALTIES

Prior to 1930, these two areas of medicine were separate and unequal. Obstetrics was considered a subspecialty of internal medicine and surgery departments claimed authority over gynecology. At that time, however, obstetricians were thriving on new developments in reproductive physiology and endocrinology, and many gynecology patients did not require surgery for their diagnoses (such as sexually transmitted diseases). For this reason, the newly formed joint specialty of obstetrics and gynecology was born.

WHAT MAKES A GOOD OBSTETRICIAN-GYNECOLOGIST?

✓ Likes working with his or her hands.

✓ Can deal with tense situations involving sensitive subject matter.

✓ Likes to see immediate results from his or her efforts.

✓ Has the ability to make fast, confident decisions.

✓ Enjoys taking care of women.

THE INSIDE SCOOP

After completing their clerkship, medical students often comment that participating in their first laparoscopic supracervical hysterectomy then quickly hurrying through the hospital to assist in the miracle of childbirth feels like an exhilarating adrenaline rush. The mind of every obstetrician is organized into three time frames: prenatal, intrapartum, and postpartum. The management of pregnancy, labor, and puerperium (the time period directly following childbirth) all fall within the realm of obstetrics. Obstetricians have the privilege of taking care of not one but two patients—mother and fetus. But the diagnosis of pregnancy is sometimes not as simple as a urine or blood test. Obstetricians must monitor the physiologic changes of the mother and her fetus during each stage of pregnancy. With an understanding of the symbiosis of pregnancy, they can better manage and determine its viability.

Although the outpatient component of obstetrics may seem like excessive watching and waiting, the transition from monitoring to action can occur faster than you might imagine. If the pregnancy is not viable, the physician must provide immediate medical or surgical care. In times of urgent crises, such as a preterm patient with uncontrolled hypertension or multiple gestations, obstetricians must react quickly and decisively. Because there are many ways in which a pregnancy can go wrong, each patient presents a new challenge.

Gynecology focuses on the overall health the female and her reproductive organ systems, and in particular, the diagnosis and treatment of female-specific diseases. Ambulatory gynecology incorporates well woman exams, ultrasound and colposcopy; surgical gynecology involves pelvic surgery by either the vaginal or abdominal route. Gynecologists do more than just conduct pap smears, prescribe oral contraceptives, perform hysterectomies, and dilatation and curettages (D&C). They also treat sexually transmitted diseases, manage pain disorders, sexual and urinary dysfunction, menopausal symptoms, and discuss psychosocial issues, such as domestic violence. Remember—women look to their gynecologists for assurance, guidance, and understanding of how to care for their bodies. These physicians assume great responsibility in helping women of all ages find pride in themselves and their bodies.

Obstetrics–gynecology is a hands-on specialty full of many surprises. There is never a dull moment. You must be able to keep your cool while dealing with many varied situations and personalities simultaneously. To excel in this specialty, medical students have to tolerate touching many gravid abdomens, performing unlimited vaginal examinations, and getting their hands dirty (after all, any type of bodily fluid is game). During the third stage of labor, obstetricians may find the delivery area covered in blood, vomit, urine, and even fecal matter. Like their colleagues in emergency medicine, obstetrician–gynecologists are ready for anything when it comes to women's health. Whether the case involves an infant failing to deliver head first, a placental abruption, or a new patient with imminent delivery of twins, obstetrician–gynecologists have to think fast and react quickly and competently in life-threatening situations.

Many medical students enter obstetrics–gynecology because they are attracted to its integration of both surgery and medicine within the context of women's health. For example, a serious antepartum obstetric complication, such as gestational diabetes or preeclampsia, requires careful thought for its diagnosis and management. In other situations, such as nonreassuring fetal heart tones or complete placenta previa, surgical methods are necessary to bring both the patient and the fetus to a successful outcome. Although obstetrician–gynecologists perform many specialized procedures, such as hysterectomies, pelvic reconstructions, and exploratory laparotomies, the hands-on aspect of the specialty is not necessarily confined to the operating room. In the clinic or hospital ward, you also engage in many pelvic examinations, pap smears, colposcopies, and radiologic evaluations to help diagnose incontinence, infertility and various endocrinologic abnormalities. Several aspects of primary care and emergency medicine are also very important in this specialty. Despite subspecialty development, the vast majority of physicians who train in this field consider themselves generalists, meaning that they assume the role of obstetrician, gynecologist, and primary care doctor for women, or all three. "In this specialty, you can really do a lot for your patients," remarked one gynecologist in private practice. In a single day, you may be delivering a baby, treating a sexually transmitted disease with an antibiotic, evaluating unusual vaginal bleeding in the emergency room, or counseling a woman on the psychological effects of menopause. However, the most difficult situations may be the mental anguish of telling a woman that she has ovarian cancer or a mother that there is no cardiac motion at her 32-week prenatal care visit. Thankfully, more than 90% of the outcomes are success stories. In all cases, the obstetrician–gynecologist listens to the patient and empathizes with health issues that are unique to women.

IS IT PRIMARY OR SPECIALTY CARE?

Obstetrics–gynecology is unique in being highly specialized — in the medical and surgical treatment of female health problems — while still categorized as primary care. The majority of reproductive-age women in this country consider their obstetrician–gynecologist as their primary care provider. In a recent survey of obstetrics–gynecology residents, 87% believed that obstetrics–gynecology was primary care, while 85% intended to establish a balanced practice drawing on all of the skills they learned in residency,[1] with a special focus on health maintenance, screening, and disease prevention.

The first encounter with an obstetrician–gynecologist can mean the difference between a lifetime patient and an unsatisfied client. As a primary care physician, you use compassion, understanding, and patience to forge close interpersonal relationships. You promote a healthy lifestyle and continuously remind the mother of the best ways to care for both herself and her unborn child. They also provide annual screening services related to blood-pressure and cholesterol screening, cervical cancer prevention, breast examination and review of the breast self-awareness, and referral for mammography or other specialized services. They spend time discussing work-related health risks, smoking, seat belt use, safe sex and sexually transmitted disease prevention, and genetic screening for family planning.

Continuity of care is extremely important in obstetrics–gynecology. Following delivery, the obstetrician holds a responsibility to the mother for at least 6 weeks. The physician must continue to evaluate not only her anatomy but also her psychological well-being. Most patients of gynecologists are either initially transferred from their obstetric clinic or referred from nurse practitioners or internists. The patient usually remain with their gynecologist throughout the course of their lives. Thus, patient relationships may be as short as one delivery or continue through the lifetime of several generations.

OBSTETRICS–GYNECOLOGY IN THE OPERATING ROOM

The art and science of surgery forms the core of this specialty. Without it, obstetrics and gynecology would probably remain under the jurisdiction of internal medicine. Because of the thrilling rush of the operating-room experience, some obstetrician–gynecologists like the surgical aspect of their specialty the best. Cesarean delivery has become the most common hospital-based operative procedure in the United States and now accounts for about 32% of all live births, and with the advent of primary cesarean by request, the numbers have increased.[2] Gynecologists also use their surgical skills to carry out many types of operations, such as an exploratory laparotomy or laparoscopy for a ruptured ectopic, diagnosis of infertility, hysterectomy, and pelvic reconstructive surgery. One academic physician stated, "in most cases, my surgical efforts cure problems, usually with good outcomes." She reiterates that many students are attracted to this specialty because of the immediate ability to fix problems using surgery.

Medical students should disregard condescending comments made by other surgical subspecialists. The manual dexterity required for obstetric or gynecologic surgery may not approach that of, for example, neurosurgery or otolaryngology. However, the notion that gynecologists are not true surgeons is a myth. Despite the reduction in operating-room time due to new primary care educational requirements, graduating residents in this specialty are still well-trained, competent surgeons of the abdomen and pelvis whether by laparoscopy or an open technique. And if you desire further training in any subspecialty, obstetrician–gynecologists can take the initiative of completing a 1- to 3-year fellowship.

LIFESTYLE CONSIDERATIONS AND PRACTICE OPTIONS

A medical student who had completed his required clerkship in obstetrics–gynecology commented that the attending physicians "seem like very energetic and outgoing people." Self-confidence and a strong personality are necessary to deal with the stressful events and tense situations you face daily. There is little room for indecisiveness, meekness, or timidity within this specialty. Because gynecologic surgeries start quite early in the morning and deliveries or ruptured ectopic pregnancies can occur during the middle of the night, you must be able to function at all times of day or night. Even when tired or agitated, obstetrics–gynecology physicians have to be sensitive to the emotional and psychosocial needs of their patients. Your common sense and experience are calming and reassuring for an expectant mother about to deliver her first child, a preoperative gynecologic patient, and a woman struggling with the loss of a pregnancy.

The obstetrician–gynecologist's typical day often consists of a mix of surgery, hospital rounds, clinic, and administrative duties. Due to the erratic lifestyle, many medical students strike this specialty from their list of choices. Every

VITAL SIGNS

MEDIAN COMPENSATION

Gynecology	$218,607
Obstetrics	$301,773
Obstetrics–gynecology	$294,190
Reproductive endocrinology and infertility	$317,943
Urogynecology	$301,777
Gynecologic oncology	$406,000

Data from American Medical Group Association.

practicing obstetrician–gynecologist experiences long hours and irregular schedules. Whether at the office or while enjoying the evening at home, your plans may be altered by obstetrical patients in labor or a ruptured ectopic in the emergency room. However, there is some variability depending on your choice of practice. In private practice, the hours of patient care depend on the number of group members, location, and patient load. The number of trips to the hospital by patients in labor correlates with the volume of obstetrics in one's practice. After finishing residency, some doctors choose to practice only gynecology. After all, the delivery of uncomplicated pregnancies also falls under the domain of family practitioners and nurse midwives. In the academic setting, obstetrician–gynecologists who are full-time faculty members spend less time in surgery and clinic. More time is devoted to teaching and mentoring residents, conducting research, and administrative tasks.

Despite the need to balance family and personal time, most obstetricians and gynecologists are extremely fulfilled by their careers. Their high level of career satisfaction and desire to practice is comparable with that of other women physicians, particularly those in surgery.[3] If given the opportunity, the majority would not change their career decision. To honor maternity/paternity leave and family obligations, most hospitals and group practices create contracts with defined schedules including part-time hours, minimal on-call nights, and less operating time. Despite such flexibility, a study found that female obstetrician–gynecologists, compared with other women physicians, worked significantly more clinical hours and call nights; they slept even less when on call.[4] Consequently, domestic responsibilities, such as cooking and housework, and quality time with their children are greatly minimized.[4] According to a recent survey, nearly 76% of both male and female obstetrician–gynecologists were happy with their lives, making them the least satisfied among all specialists surveyed.[5] However, the trend of "work first" is changing, especially with the acceptance of hospitalists (physicians who only take call to allow for 24 hours in hospital coverage) and more physicians are taking time to be with their families.

GENDER ISSUES IN THE WORKPLACE

More and more female physicians are becoming obstetrician–gynecologists. According to the American Medical Association, the percentage of women in this specialty increased from just 7.2% in 1970 to 26.9% in 1994.[6] In current training programs, nearly 70% of the residents are women.[7] By 2014, many predict that the number of female physicians will far exceed that of men practicing obstetrics–gynecology.[8] As they become dominant in this specialty, female physicians, who are perceived as more caring and sensitive, will greatly influence its scope of practice and research.

Gender discrimination in obstetrics–gynecology has undergone a significant role reversal. Not only do male obstetrician–gynecologists feel at times that they are losing ground, but some recruiters from private practice groups have begun discriminating against male physicians. Assuming that women prefer a female obstetrician–gynecologist, these practices aggressively seek female residents. They want to balance their male-dominated staff with female obstetrician–gynecologists, creating a dramatically changed workforce. As a result, many qualified male doctors struggle to secure their preferred career. In fact, one study found that 26% of graduating male residents reported difficulty in finding a job, compared with 17% of female residents.[9]

Should these facts discourage male medical students from considering a career in obstetrics and gynecology? Certainly not—men still have the ability to compete in this field. The idea that female patients feel more comfortable with a female obstetrician–gynecologist is erroneous. In a survey of obstetric patients during their postpartum hospital stay, the majority (58%) had no preference for the gender of their obstetrician; 34% preferred female physicians and 7% indicated a desire for a male doctor.[10] Rather than specifying gender, the attributes most satisfied patients said they wanted in an obstetrician–gynecologist were excellent interpersonal skills, an empathic communication style, the ability to make a connection, and a high level of technical expertise. Men who cultivate traditionally female skills, particularly empathy and good communication, can thrive as obstetrician–gynecologists.

DEALING WITH MALPRACTICE CONCERNS

When asked about any negative aspects of their specialty, most obstetrician–gynecologists were quick to cite the critical and increasingly costly issue of medical malpractice. The current medicolegal climate of our society, with its get-rich quick incentives, makes obstetrics–gynecology a high-risk specialty. In fact, most medical students considering this specialty are especially concerned about the daily potential litigation. Many things can go wrong during the delivery of an infant. Because manifestations of these incidents, such as neonatal brain damage, may not appear until the child is much older, the threat of liability is always present (until the patient reaches 18 years of age). In light of this ever-present malpractice menace, obstetrician–gynecologists must be passionate about their careers and provide outstanding patient care. In many instances, the threat of litigation encourages the development and training of better physicians.

If you look at all the statistics and numbers, obstetrician–gynecologists have the highest incidence of lawsuits throughout their careers. Since the 1950s, the number of malpractice claims filed against obstetrician–gynecologists has increased nearly 15% every year.[11] Approximately two-thirds of these physicians have been sued for alleged medical malpractice; they now have one of the highest (and continuing to skyrocket) malpractice insurance premiums in the nation.[11] Some insurance companies are not only raising premiums but are also refusing to provide liability coverage. In spite of all the negative statistics, there are still glimpses of hope. More than half of all claims were dismissed, settled without payment, or won by the physician.[11]

The rising malpractice claims are severely jeopardizing access to high-quality, affordable health care for women and their newborns. Due to unaffordable liability insurance premiums (or even the inability to obtain insurance), many physicians have curtailed their services. Physicians are forced to reduce the number of deliveries they perform, cut back on high-risk patients, and even stop some surgical services. This loss of access to prenatal and delivery care particularly affects women in rural and inner-city communities, which are typically underserved. As a result, many obstetricians are banning together in various states to pass tort reform bills that cap the restitutions patients can gain. In California, physicians lobbied to enact a series of reforms that curbed soaring liability premiums, stopped physicians from leaving the state, and prevented the decrease in availability of care. The 50-year challenge of malpractice will continue to be an important issue for future obstetrician–gynecologists. However, with tort reform occurring across the country, a change for the better has appeared.

SHARING THE SPOTLIGHT: NURSE MIDWIVES

Due to rising insurance premiums and the overall threat of liability, fewer family physicians are including obstetrical care in their private practices. Many medical students wonder about the role of family practitioners and midwives, however, as providers of pregnancy-related care. A midwife (meaning with a woman) provides prenatal care, attends childbirth, manages her clinic patients during labor and delivery, and supervises the general care of women and children directly after birth. As advanced degree registered nurses, nurse midwives have completed an accredited midwifery program and passed the certification examination. Family practitioners are medical doctors who are trained in comprehensive obstetrics. Although they provide care to women during apparently normal pregnancies and deliveries, they must call on obstetricians if complications develop. All midwives are required by the American College of Obstetrics and Gynecology (ACOG) to have a physician with hospital privileges as part of the maternity team. Nurse midwives, however, attend only about 9% of vaginal births in the United States.[12]

Whether in private practice or affiliated with an independent birthing center, both obstetricians and midwives seek to fulfill the common goal of providing excellent health care for women. As such, their professional relationship should always remain collegial and cooperative. It is one in which the obstetrician—the expert consultant—steps in whenever his or her services are necessary.

FELLOWSHIPS AND SUBSPECIALTY TRAINING

After completing residency in obstetrics–gynecology, one may decide to specialize. Each of the following approved fellowships requires an additional 3 years of training. To earn board certification, graduating fellows must pass the American Board of Obstetrics and Gynecology (ABOG) subspecialty examination.

Maternal–Fetal Medicine

Patients with high-risk pregnancies, who have serious coexisting medical or surgical disease that could prevent delivery of a viable term infant or affect the survival of the mother, fall under the expertise of specialists in maternal–fetal medicine (MFM). These specialists serve as consultants to general obstetricians for referrals involving pregnancies complicated by major disease or for diagnostic or therapeutic procedures.

Although MFM physicians may focus on consultations and sonography, they are specially trained in a variety of intricate procedures. Diagnostically, they perform genetic amniocentesis, fetal blood sampling, obstetrical ultrasound, chorionic villus sampling, and cordocentesis. Therapeutically, they are experts at high-risk deliveries, medically indicated abortions, laparoscopy, fetal gene therapy, and fetal reduction.

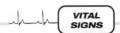

Gynecologic Oncology

Roughly 15% of all cancers found in women involve tumors of the reproductive tract. This area of specialization focuses on the medical and surgical care of women with malignancies arising in the reproductive system: ovarian, uterine, cervical, vulvar, and vaginal cancer. These specialists receive extensive training in the biology and pathology of gynecologic cancer, particularly its diagnosis, treatment, and complications of oncologic care.

Gynecologic oncologists comprise an elite group of surgeons who bring hope to thousands of afflicted women. They are skilled pelvic surgeons who use the latest techniques in radical surgery, chemotherapy, and radiation treatment. They manage the urinary and bowel complications resulting from cancer treatment, as well as pain, palliative care, and psychosocial issues. Gynecologic oncologists are supported by a multidisciplinary team of medical oncologists, radiation oncologists, and gynecologic pathologists who collaborate to provide optimal care. Gynecologic oncologists practice in a variety of clinical settings—academic medical centers, regional hospitals, and specialized cancer centers.

Reproductive Endocrinology and Infertility

The endocrine system, which is responsible for releasing hormones that modulate the development of the ovum, is one of the most intricate and complex regulatory systems. For the specialist in reproductive endocrinology and infertility (REI), establishing a pregnancy for couples suffering from infertility is extremely rewarding. Their practice also extends to the treatment of hormonal and reproductive disorders affecting women, children, men, and mature women. Reproductive endocrinologists gain special competence in advanced microsurgical procedures, such as reversal of tubal ligation, treatment with fertility drugs, and methods of assisted reproduction (in vitro fertilization and insemination). With vast knowledge and expertise on the physiology of reproduction, REI specialists medically and surgically treat a variety of complex hormonal disorders, such as infertility, endometriosis, recurrent pregnancy loss, menopause, and ovulatory dysfunction.

Female Pelvic Medicine and Reconstructive Surgery

As women age, a history of multiple deliveries and other forms of strain may cause the musculature supporting the pelvic contents to slowly weaken. This can lead to disorders such as urinary incontinence or a prolapsed bladder, uterus, or vagina. To correct pelvic floor dysfunction, women should seek out specialists in female pelvic medicine and reconstructive surgery. Also known as urogynecology, this advanced surgical subspecialty remains on the cutting edge of medicine. It integrates the fields of urology and obstetrics–gynecology in the operating room. To diagnose pelvic prolapse and female voiding dysfunction, these physicians have special expertise in clinical evaluation of genitourinary diseases,

RESIDENCY TRAINING

Residency in obstetrics–gynecology requires 4 years of postgraduate training. There are currently 237 accredited programs. Unlike other surgical subspecialties, a PGY-1 internship in general surgery is not required. Instead, residents immediately begin surgical training in obstetrics–gynecology. Upon graduation, residents are required to prove competency in all surgical and obstetric procedures. The typical monthly rotations include routine and high-risk obstetrics clinics and wards, general office and surgical gynecology, reproductive endocrinology and infertility, gynecologic oncology, urogynecology, primary care, and neonatal intensive care unit. Due to the increasing emphasis on primary care within this specialty, most residency programs now require at least 6 months of outpatient rotations. About 10% of residents continue their training in fellowships.

THE INSIDE SCOOP

cystoscopy, and analysis of urodynamic testing. Because this is a surgical fellowship, specialists in pelvic medicine perform many reconstructive operations to correct pelvic floor dysfunction. They help to improve the quality of life for women with these disorders.

WHY CONSIDER A CAREER IN OBSTETRICS–GYNECOLOGY?

Despite its seemingly specialized nature, the field of obstetrics–gynecology provides much diversity and variety. Medical students should disregard the narrow views of colleagues who may dismiss these specialists as "pap smear providers by day and baby delivery service by night." The breadth of issues includes acute and chronic medical conditions, health maintenance, genetics, operative gynecology, pregnancy and delivery, adolescent and postmenopausal gynecology, infertility, endocrinology, urogynecology, and oncology.

Because of the diverse age of patients, your scope of practice can range from broad (primary ambulatory care) to very focused (concentration in an area of specialization). With so many paths available within this one specialty, there is no limit to what you may be able to offer to obstetrics–gynecology. After all, a single obstetrician or gynecologist cannot provide for all of the needs of a woman. The positive interactions between generalists and subspecialists allow for the highest quality of care for women of all ages.

Our society expects great things from modern medicine to improve quality of life, "nowhere are these expectations higher than in the practice of obstetrics and the desire and expectation of having a healthy child."[13] To achieve these goals, obstetricians–gynecologists must demonstrate superior compassion, intelligence, and the ability to pay close attention to detail. Despite the rigorous lifestyle and the pressure of handling the high-risk responsibility, there are lots of rewards. Future obstetricians–gynecologists will be part of a group of caring, competent, and conscientious doctors who strive for the best patient care for women. Although not every day is filled with success stories, most obstetricians and gynecologists go home each day with the satisfaction of having changed someone's life.

ABOUT THE CONTRIBUTOR

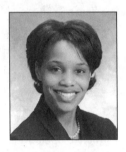

Dr Kelly Oberia Elmore completed her chief residency in obstetrics–gynecology at the Naval Medical Center in San Diego. She grew up in southern California and Chicago, graduated from Xavier University (Louisiana), and attended medical school at the University of Chicago. She actively practices both obstetrics and gynecology. Her focus is obstetrics and women's sexual and reproductive health. Dr Elmore enjoys writing poetry and short stories. She acknowledges her "Trinity" of friends and husband as her main sources of inspiration and support. She can be reached by e-mail at drkellyo@koemedicalconsulting.com

REFERENCES

1. Laube, D.W., Ling, F.W. Primary care in obstetrics and gynecology residency education: A baseline survey of residents' perceptions and experience. *Obstet Gynecol.* 1999;94:632–636.

2. Martin JA, Hamilton BE, Ventura SJ, et al. Births: Final data for 2009. National vital statistics reports; vol 60 no 1. Hyattsville, MD: National Center for Health Statistics. 2011. Available from: http://www.cdc.gov/nchs/data/nvsr60_01.pdf.

3. Frank, E., McMurray, J.E., et al. Career satisfaction of U.S. women physicians: Results from the women physicians' health study. *Arch Intern Med.* 1999;159:1417–1426.

4. Frank, E., Rock, J., et al. Characteristics of female obstetrician-gynecologists in the United States. *Obstet Gynecol.* 1999;94:659–665.

5. Keeton K, Fenner DE, Johnson TR, Hayward RA. Predictors of physician career satisfaction, work-life balance, and burnout. *Obstet Gynecol.* 2004;109(4): 949–55.

6. American Medical Association. *Women Physicians by Specialty.* Accessed April 30, 2003, from www.ama-assn.org/ama/pub/article/171–199.html.

7. Barzansky, B., Etzel, S.I. Educational programs in U.S. medical schools, 2001–2002. *JAMA.* 2002;288(9):1067–1072.

8. Jacoby, I., Meyer, G.S., et al. Modeling the future workforce of obstetrics and gynecology. *Obstet Gynecol.* 1998;92:450–456.

9. Miller, R.S., Dunn, M.R., et al. Employment seeking experiences of resident physicians completing training during 1996. *JAMA.* 1998;280:777–783.

10. Howell, E.A., Gardiner, B., et al. Do women prefer female obstetricians? *Obstet Gynecol.* 2002;99:1031–1035.

11. Finberg, K.S., Peters, J.D., et al. *Obstetrics and Gynecology and the Law.* Ann Arbor, MI: Health Administration Press; 1984.

12. Ventura, S.J., Martin, J.A., et al. Births: Final data for 1999. *Natl Vital Stat Rep.* 2001;49:130.

13. Loring, T.W. My fifty-year odyssey in obstetrics and gynecology. *Am J Obstet Gynecol.* 1997;176:1244–1249.

22

OPHTHALMOLOGY

Andrew P. Schwartz

Imagine the smallest, darkest, hottest room in which you have ever been. The room is so small that you cannot stand up straight and it is so dark that you cannot see your hand in front of your face. The floor has rotted and, with each step, you hope that your weight is not the final insult under which it will give way. You estimate there are hundreds of mosquitoes by the noises near your ear and the bites on your skin. In a way, you are glad for the darkness because it hides depressing details of the scene surrounding you. You turn on your flashlight to reveal a gaunt elderly woman in soiled clothes, lying on a homemade mattress with her knees pressed up to her chest. Her feet are dark, necrotic, and ravaged with ulcerations. Her legs will not fully extend within this confined room. Her blood sugar is markedly elevated and her eyes appear white due to cataracts. A young boy who brings her food explains that she developed "the sugar" 20 years ago and has not left her tiny home since she became blind. A fragile woman, she holds your arms tightly while being brought to the hospital. Without sight, only human touch could assure her that she was not alone.

My encounter with this woman, on a service trip to Belize during medical school, gave me an unforgettable glimpse of the profound impact the loss of vision can have on human existence.

OPHTHALMOLOGY: SEEING THE LIGHT

Ophthalmology is the branch of medicine that provides the complete medical and surgical care of the eye and related structures of the visual system (extraocular muscles, eyelids, orbit, nerves, visual pathways, and more). Yes, they can (and often do) prescribe glasses and contact lenses. But their spectrum of care extends much further. It requires mastery of the anatomy, physiology, microbiology, and

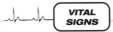

VITAL SIGNS

OPHTHALMOLOGY
2011 MATCH STATISTICS

- Number of positions available: 461
- 99.3% of all positions were filled in the initial Match
- The successful applicants: 88% US seniors, 6% foreign-trained physicians, and 6% US graduates
- Mean USMLE Step I score: 237
- Applicants submitted on an average 52 applications and received 4.4 offers
- Unmatched rate for US seniors applying only to ophthalmology: 12%

Data from San Francisco Matching Program.

pathophysiology of the eye, as well as an understanding of optical physics. To treat ocular and visual disorders, ophthalmologists are really both internists and surgeons.

Most medical students' exposure to the field of ophthalmology is much less dramatic than my experience in Central America. In fact, many students are never introduced to this surgical subspecialty at all. It is unfortunate that every medical school does not actually require the completion of any sort of clerkship in ophthalmology. (And many seniors do not choose to pursue an elective in the specialty either.) Vision is usually only discussed in the context of a broader neuroscience course taught by neurologists and neuroscientists. As a result, most medical school graduates' only exposure to ophthalmologists is through lectures during surgery or outpatient medicine.

In addition, ophthalmology is largely an outpatient subspecialty. Because many hospitals do not have a big inpatient service, a medical center is usually not an ideal learning environment for a medical student who is untrained in eye examination techniques and can therefore have only limited responsibility in the outpatient clinic. Everyone knows how to use a stethoscope to listen to heart, lung, and bowel sounds, but not every physician or medical student can perform a proper eye examination. Despite the limited exposure, ophthalmology is one of the most highly sought after specialties. Why?

Ophthalmology remains highly competitive to match in despite the fact that it is a field that is not easy to get experience in and is not stressed by medical schools. First, it is one of the few specialties in which your practice includes the full spectrum of care, including preventative medicine, medical management, and surgical treatment of patients. For patients at high risk for developing glaucoma, for example, ophthalmologists follow their ocular pressure, visual fields, and cup-to-disk ratios. For patients with diabetes, they monitor for retinal neovascularization. This is what preventive medicine is all about. Once pathology is diagnosed, the physician who made the initial diagnosis now decides if a course of medical treatment is warranted and what that course should be. If medical management fails or is not applicable, the very same physician can now bring his or her patient to the operating room. The ability to provide every single aspect of a patient's care makes ophthalmology an extremely gratifying specialty.

Ophthalmologists' relationships with their patients vary in length, although they tend to be long term. Patients who have deteriorating vision due to diabetes require follow-up with an ophthalmologist several times a year. The young child with severe bacterial conjunctivitis might only be seen a few times over the course of a month and then not for several years.

> **WHAT MAKES A GOOD OPHTHALMOLOGIST?**
>
> ✓ Prefers a highly specialized, detail-oriented discipline.
> ✓ Likes working with his or her hands.
> ✓ Enjoys both medical and surgical approaches.
> ✓ Is a relaxed, patient, and confident person.
> ✓ Has excellent manual dexterity.
>
> **THE INSIDE SCOOP**

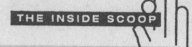

Regardless of the particular patient or disease process, it is important to keep in mind that vision is a sensitive subject. When it comes to problems of the eye of any nature—whether serious or benign—most patients are very frightened of the possibility of going blind. Ophthalmologists must draw on their compassion and sensitivity to alleviate their patients' concerns. Knowing everything about the eye and its diseases is not enough. Patients who are worried or distressed about losing their vision require special attention that medical or surgical treatment alone does not provide.

It should be noted that there are many intangibles that make a specialty desirable to someone. Ophthalmologists are some of the nicest, most relaxed, and generally happiest physicians to be found in the hospital. It is rare to see an ophthalmology resident embarrassed at grand rounds or yelled at in front of his or her peers, in stark contrast to certain other surgical subspecialties. The eye clinic is usually a friendly and collegial environment to work and learn, so if you think you are someone who functions better in that kind of environment, ophthalmology is certainly a field you should consider.

SPECIALIZING IN TWO TINY ORGANS

The eye and its supporting cast make up perhaps the most highly specialized and complicated organ system in existence. Approximately 35% of all the sensory input into the brain is made up by the left and right optic nerve, and roughly

65% of all intracranial disease processes have ophthalmologic manifestations.[1] A plethora of systemic disease processes, therefore, can affect the eye, each in several ways and by different mechanisms.

One of the most important things for medical students to determine when considering ophthalmology as a career is whether or not they would be happy specializing in only one region of the body. This is not to say that there are not vast arrays of disease processes that have ophthalmic manifestations; in fact, quite the opposite is true. Rather, the examination skills, diagnostic tools, and surgical procedures you learn and use as an ophthalmologist involve a small area of the body and one highly specialized organ system.

Unlike in surgical specialties, the ophthalmologists' surgical field is typically measured in millimeters. The lids and skin surrounding the eye and orbit; the eye itself from the cornea back to the optic nerve; orbits with their bone, vascular, sinus, lymphatic, and neural components; and the central nervous system components of vision make up the world of the ophthalmologist. You will become an expert specialist in one particular system and know that structure inside and out. But do not think that it is easy to master the body of knowledge for these two small structures. There is an immense body of knowledge to be learned about the eye.

Ophthalmologists treat a wide range of disorders of the eye. Some of the more common conditions include cataracts (a disorder of lens clarity), glaucoma (a problem of increased intraocular pressure), conjunctivitis (inflammation of the conjunctiva, usually due to infection), and macular degeneration (progressive blindness). For such seemingly small structures, a large number of diseases can affect the eye. Any type of infection—from gonorrhea to herpes—is fair game. Ophthalmologists also deal with all kinds of trauma to the eye, whether it involves the orbit (in which the eye is located) or the eye itself. They operate on detached retinas. They treat intraocular tumors such as choroidal melanoma and retinoblastoma. They treat disorders of the extraocular muscles like strabismus. Even problems of the eyelid, eyelashes, and lacrimal (tear) glands fall under the domain of the ophthalmologist.

To be a good ophthalmologist, you need a solid foundation in general medicine. Many ocular disorders are manifestations of underlying systemic disease, congenital or chromosomal disorders, metabolic defects, connective tissue diseases, diabetes, and hypertension—the list goes on. You will not just find elderly patients with cataracts or glaucoma in an ophthalmologist's office. There will also be patients with inflammatory bowel disease, Graves disease (hyperthyroidism), AIDS, central nervous system tumors, and Bell palsy—all of who have problems involving the eye. Uveitis (inflammation of the iris, ciliary body, and choroid), for instance, is a common ocular presentation of lupus, Crohn disease, and juvenile rheumatoid arthritis. Like dermatologists, who have to know the skin manifestations of underlying diseases, ophthalmologists require a good understanding of the pathophysiology of these primary disorders. Although the eye condition may at times be secondary, these specialists must maintain their general medical and surgical knowledge across a broad range of disorders. This is a recurrent theme within this specialty.

OPHTHALMOLOGY AS A HIGH-TECH FIELD

Ophthalmologists love gadgets and technical breakthroughs. Their offices are filled with a wide range of instruments ranging from simple ophthalmoscopes to complicated operating microscopes. In the last few decades, there has been an explosion of new technology in the visual sciences, which has resulted in several promising new techniques and advances. Diagnostic and surgical breakthroughs in this specialty include laser photocoagulation, micromanipulation, fluorescein angiography, and microsurgery. To be a good ophthalmologist and make the most of this technology, the specialty requires excellent visual and motor skills, depth perception, and color vision.

Pharmacologic treatments are important in ophthalmology. Primary open angle glaucoma, for instance, remains one of the largest causes of blindness in the world, affecting more than 5 million people.[2] Topical beta-blocking medication provides one main form of therapy, and several new medications, including topical carbonic anhydrase inhibitors, alpha-2 agonists, and prostaglandin agonists, have made the medical treatment of glaucoma far more effective. In addition, advances in surgical techniques and the use of antimetabolites, such as 5-fluorouracil and mitomycin C, have greatly improved filtration surgeries and dramatically improved postoperative wound healing. These advances have greatly improved the chances that patients with glaucoma will live into old age with their vision preserved.

The rapidly advancing technology has made surgical visual correction a safe reality for many people. LASIK, or laser-assisted in situ keratomileusis, is a procedure by which an excimer laser emitting ultraviolet beams removes precise amounts of corneal tissue based on a person's refractive error and corneal topography (essentially a road map of the cornea). It is estimated that 148 million people (52% of the population) wear some type of corrective eyewear and approximately 1.8 million refractive surgery procedures were performed in 2002.[3] For those who have near-perfect vision, imagine what it is like for someone to wake up every morning and be unable to see the alarm clock or to differentiate between the shampoo and conditioner bottles while taking a shower. The technology in the practice of ophthalmology—particularly LASIK—is having a dramatic effect on the quality of people's lives. Instead of always relying on glasses and being constantly reminded of their worsening vision, these patients' lives are transformed. They wake up with enormous smiles on their faces and perfect 20/20 vision for the first time in years.

PERFORMING SURGERY ON THE EYE

Like their colleagues in otolaryngology, ophthalmologists practice both medicine and surgery. To be a good surgeon of the eye and its related structures, you must have excellent hand–eye coordination and fine motor skills. Much of the precise, targeted surgery occurs behind the lenses of a microscope. It is a different kind of surgery than in other subspecialties: cleaner, shorter, more controlled, with less worry about bleeding and less of a need to suture fascia or cauterize blood vessels. Like most surgeons, ophthalmologists are action-oriented physicians who like to see fast results. In the operating room, they demand as much or more attention to detail as any other surgeon. In this specialty, all results of surgery are permanent and usually cannot be reversed. Thus, care, precision, and patience are key components to being a good ophthalmologic surgeon.

Many ophthalmologists perform refractive surgery such as LASIK, in which they reshape a patient's cornea to improve visual acuity. Because most of these procedures are elective, ophthalmologists must be aware of the extremely high (or even unrealistic) expectations patients have of refractive surgery. Ophthalmologists need to carefully evaluate their patients and make sure they have realistic expectations and understand the benefits, risk, and alternatives to surgery, because it is irreversible. Most patients, however, are very pleased with the results, especially as the newer techniques continue to improve.

Perhaps the most common surgical procedure ophthalmologists perform is phacoemulsification—the process of modern cataract extraction, in which the opacified lens is removed, usually from the capsule in which it sits. A cataract is considered present when the transparency of the lens of the eye has been reduced to the point that vision is impaired. Opacity of the lens is as much a part of aging as wrinkles in the skin. Reduced transparency is present in 95% of all persons older than 65 years.[4] Usually caused by natural aging, cataracts can also be congenital, secondary to trauma, or caused by systemic disease processes such as diabetes, galactosemia, Wilson disease, and myotonic dystrophy among many others. During phacoemulsification, the hardened lens is broken up using ultrasound and then the remnants are aspirated out of the capsule. Next, a lens implant correctly matched to the person's refractive power is implanted into the evacuated capsular bag. Consider that the entire intraocular procedure is performed through a 3- to 6-mm incision in the cornea in as little as 10 minutes, often using only topical anesthetic drops. Isn't ophthalmic surgery amazing?

Ophthalmologic surgery profoundly changes people's lives. The visual loss for someone with bilateral cataracts could be so profound that the patient may no longer see even the face of her granddaughter. Before phacoemulsification, her cataracts might be so dense that she could only see hand movement in front of her face but not count fingers. For these patients, ophthalmologists return to them the gift of vision. Through modern technology and the miracles of eye surgery, patients like this can now once again see the smile on her granddaughter's face. This is the type of impact ophthalmologists have on their patients on a daily basis.

LIFESTYLE CONSIDERATIONS AND PRACTICE OPTIONS

Although ophthalmology is a legitimate surgical specialty comparable with orthopedics, urology, otolaryngology, and the like, it offers a significantly better lifestyle than virtually any other subspecialty in medicine. It has the advantages of a surgical field, such as procedures, time in the operating room, medicine mixed with surgery, and good financial compensation, but it is generally felt to do so while still allowing free time for endeavors outside of medicine. Equally important, it gives time to remain actively engaged in learning and to stay current on new advances in your field. Relatively few emergencies arise in ophthalmology, and as discussed earlier, only a small minority of patients is admitted to the hospital. A good lifestyle should never be your only consideration in choosing a particular specialty, but it certainly is a nice added benefit of ophthalmology.

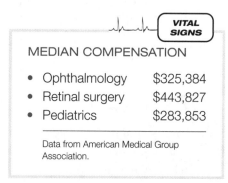

VITAL SIGNS

MEDIAN COMPENSATION

- Ophthalmology $325,384
- Retinal surgery $443,827
- Pediatrics $283,853

Data from American Medical Group Association.

Although jobs abound in many different areas, most ophthalmologists work in private practice. They typically divide their time between seeing patients during regularly scheduled appointments and performing procedures in the operating room. In the office, as internists of the visual system, ophthalmologists take patient histories, examine eyes with slit lamps and other advanced equipment, consider differential diagnoses, and prescribe new lenses and medication (both topical and oral). In the operating room, ophthalmologists take on the role of surgeon as they perform fine, delicate procedures to improve patient's vision. Most ophthalmologists operate 1 or 2 days per week and spend the remaining 3 or 4 days in the office. Because a significant proportion of ocular disorders are the result of underlying systemic medical disease, ophthalmologists also play a role in managing these conditions in close consultation with the patient's internist, pediatrician, or other relevant specialist.

A relatively small field, ophthalmology continues to have excellent job opportunities for its graduating residents. As the American population ages, the demand for ophthalmologists to operate on the exponential number of cataracts and glaucoma continues to increase. Moreover, as new procedures, scientific breakthroughs, and techniques come into practice, more and more people are seeking elective refractive surgery and other procedures involving the eye, like plastic surgery. Historically, ophthalmology has done well to ensure that the number of residents trained every year corresponds to the health care needs of the population. The small number of available training positions is advantageous for graduating residents because it increases the likelihood of entering a good job market. It also helps to explain the highly competitive nature of matching in ophthalmology despite students' limited exposure to the specialty in medical school.

THE OPHTHALMOLOGY–OPTOMETRY DISTINCTION

Many medical students interested in a possible career in ophthalmology are confused by the role of optometrists, who are often mistakenly referred to as eye doctors by the general public. Where exactly do these health professionals fit into the spectrum of vision care? Optometrists, after all, are not licensed to practice medicine—only optometry. Although some states permit optometrists to prescribe limited topical medications, optometrists are generally not given privileges or training in performing ophthalmologic surgery. Their expertise lies in understanding and treating problems with the optics of the eye. They prescribe the majority of corrective lenses in this country and also diagnose diseases of the eye that may or may not require referral to an ophthalmologist.

Instead of competing with each other, most ophthalmologists and optometrists have mutually beneficial relationships. As the medical doctor with extensive clinical and surgical training, ophthalmologists are specialists in every single aspect of the eye and all its diseases. The optometrist, who specializes in optics and the correction of refractive errors, is adequately trained as a generalist to provide primary eye care, leaving the sicker patients and complicated cases (which generally require surgical interventions) for the ophthalmologist. This is an excellent way to run a cost-effective private eye care practice. The ophthalmologist is present as a backup for the optometrist, taking over diagnostic and treatment challenges that involve complex diseases. If they work closely together, they can form an effective health care team.

FELLOWSHIPS AND SUBSPECIALTY TRAINING

It might be surprising that a field as seemingly specialized as ophthalmology could have several fellowship opportunities to specialize even further, but this is the reality. This extra training allows physicians to treat and operate on very different disease processes using equally diverse procedures. Ophthalmology fellowships are generally 1- to 2-year endeavors. Unlike many fields within medicine, completing fellowship training often does not mean limiting yourself only to that subspecialty area of practice. Many ophthalmologists who have completed fellowships choose to integrate that area of expertise into their practice of general ophthalmology.

Cornea and External Disease

This subspecialty involves the care of the cornea, sclera, conjunctiva, and eyelids. Various different types of pathologic problems, both congenital and acquired, can affect these structures of the eye. These include, but are not limited to, corneal dystrophies, corneal tumors, infections, inflammation, and manifestations of systemic disease processes as they affect the anterior segments of the eye. Cornea surgeons are experts in corneal transplant—one of the most precise and delicate procedures one will ever see in an operating room. In this procedure, roughly 30 stitches are placed around an area 10 mm in diameter to anchor a donor cornea into place. Indications for such a surgery include severe bacterial and fungal

RESIDENCY TRAINING

Residency in ophthalmology requires 4 years of postgraduate training. There are currently 117 accredited programs, most of which are very small. It requires 1 internship year (internal medicine, surgery, or transitional) plus 3 years of ophthalmology training. The structure of individual programs varies greatly but must meet the basic requirements set by the American Academy of Ophthalmology. Some programs use full-time faculty for teaching, while others provide instruction through community-based ophthalmologists as part-time or volunteer faculty. Usually the first year of residency is spent in the clinic evaluating a wide variety of patients, mastering examination skills, and seeing consults within the medical center. The resident may also perform minor surgical procedures during this year. The second and third years involve rotations through subspecialties such as pediatrics and oculoplastics, as well as much more time spent in the operating room, assisting with surgery and then later functioning as primary surgeon.

THE INSIDE SCOOP

infections, scars secondary to trauma, corneal dystrophy, and corneal protrusion disorders. Cornea surgeons are also experts in refractive surgery, among many other procedures.

Glaucoma

Fellowships in this subspecialty provide additional training in the medical and surgical management of glaucoma, plus other disorders that may threaten the optic nerve with increased intraocular pressure. Glaucoma is an area of ophthalmology in which a great deal of research is underway. Like other subspecialties, glaucoma specialists have the unique opportunity to work with children and adults, as well as the privilege to care for their patients both medically and surgically.

Neuro-ophthalmology

For students who cannot make up their minds between neurology and ophthalmology, it is possible to have the best of both worlds. Neuro-ophthalmology involves both central nervous system disease and its effect on the visual pathways, as well as disease processes inherent to the nerves and pathways of the eye. Because about 65% of all intracranial processes have ophthalmic manifestations, the importance of this subspecialty is obvious. Although some neuro-ophthalmologists operate on a limited basis and are more involved with the recognition and diagnosis of disease, others perform complicated surgeries on the eye and orbit, such as orbital wall decompressions for Grave eye disease. This procedure involves the precise removal of areas of orbital bone to alleviate the exophthalmos (forward protrusion) of the eye that results from the swelling of orbital tissues—as can occur in thyroid disease.

Ophthalmic Plastic Surgery

Do you have an "eye" for beauty? Those trained in oculoplastics blend ophthalmology and plastic surgery in the treatment of the orbit, lid, nasolacrimal system, brow, and upper face. Oculoplastic surgeons remove the eye in cases of extensive trauma, intractable and severe eye pain, and destruction secondary to neoplastic or inflammatory processes. They reconstruct the orbit, lids, and upper face in cases of tumor, trauma, or other local processes and perform cosmetic surgeries such as orbital wall decompression. They are also trained in the use of radiation and chemotherapy. Optic nerve fenestration, one of the more interesting procedures, helps young patients suffering from pseudotumor cerebri, a condition in which elevated intracranial pressure (for unclear reasons) causes vision loss. In this fascinating procedure, the oculoplastic surgeon dissects back to the optic nerve, rotates the eye laterally and rapidly enough so as to avoid damage due to the lack of blood flow caused by extreme rotation of the eye, and cuts a window on the sheath of the optic nerve to alleviate pressure.

Ophthalmic Pathology

The existence of ophthalmic pathology as a specialty is a testament to the complexity of the eye and visual system. The anatomy and pathophysiology is so complicated that at most major medical centers, a trained ophthalmic pathologist (who has completed an ophthalmology residency followed by a pathology fellowship) examines tissue removed from the eye and surrounding structures.

Pediatric Ophthalmology

This specialty involves the eye care of the pediatric population, as well as the treatment of certain conditions such as strabismus (deviation of the eye from its normal visual axis) that can occur in both children and adults. Pediatric ophthalmologists perform surgery on congenital cataracts, repair ptosis (droopy lids), fix strabismus, diagnose childhood eye tumors such as retinoblastoma, and treat amblyopia. One of the most common problems of amblyopia is defective vision uncorrectable by glasses in an eye that is otherwise normal; it is essentially the result of anything that causes vision in one eye to be better than the other while visual pathways are still developing in early childhood. Because several syndromes have a major impact on vision, this specialty also affords the opportunity to work with special needs children. Last, pediatric ophthalmologists work with premature infants: they monitor and treat the ocular sequelae of prematurity along with retinal surgeons.

Vitreoretinal Disease

Several disease processes affect these two important areas of the eye—the retina and the vitreous humor—including local, systemic, and genetic conditions. Trauma obviously has a profound impact on the retina, resulting in tears and detachments, and systemic diseases such as diabetes and HIV can also cause a variety of problems for this part of the eye. Diagnostic modalities are highly advanced and include fluorescein angiography and electrophysiology. Treatment modalities are equally impressive: cryotherapy, lasers, retinal detachment surgery, and vitrectomy, among many others.

WHY CONSIDER A CAREER IN OPHTHALMOLOGY?

There are many reasons why talented medical students should consider a career in ophthalmology. In a survey of residents,[5] they listed the following factors as the most influential in their decisions to pursue a career in ophthalmology, ordered from most to least influential: surgery, patient contact, lifestyle, junior/senior year electives, previous contact with ophthalmologists, potential income, and status among peers. Extrapolating from this study, the most important factors in choosing a career in ophthalmology are historically those inherent to the practice of ophthalmology and to patient care. Despite the fact that many medical students do not complete electives in this field, the desirability of ophthalmology remains high because of what it has to offer a future physician.

Ophthalmology is an exciting and challenging field that involves the complete care of the patient. It offers physicians the opportunity to practice preventive medicine, medical management, and surgical treatment of a wide variety of disease processes. It is an amazing field in which physicians have a significant influence on their patients' quality of life; as a result, their patients are some of the most satisfied in all of medicine. It also allows the physician to become an expert on one of the most complicated organ systems in existence—one in which miraculous new advances are constantly being achieved. By preserving the health of your patients' vision, you will gain unparallel skills that impact their lives tremendously.

ABOUT THE CONTRIBUTOR

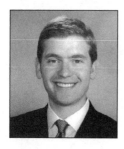

Dr Andrew Schwartz recently completed his ophthalmology training at The Mount Sinai Medical Center in New York City. He is now a comprehensive ophthalmologist and refractive surgeon in private practice in Manhattan as well as a faculty member at The Mount Sinai Medical Center. After receiving his undergraduate degree from Tufts University, he attended medical school at Loyola University Chicago — Stritch School of Medicine. Dr Schwartz is particularly interested in cataract, anterior segment, and refractive surgery. Dr Schwartz would like to thank his father and grandfather (both pediatricians) for inspiring him to pursue medicine and is very grateful for the continued support of his wife, Rebecca, and his children Mikayla, Leo, and Tyler. He can be reached by e-mail at andysmd@aol.com.

REFERENCES

1. Berson, F.G. *Ophthalmology Study Guide for Students and Practitioners of Medicine*, 5th ed. San Francisco: American Academy of Ophthalmology; 1987.

2. Alistair, F.R., Bentley, C., et al. Recent advances: Ophthalmology. *BMJ*. 1999;318:717–720.

3. *Refractive Errors and Refractive Surgery*. American Academy of Ophthalmology website. Accessed April 30, 2003, from www.aao.org/aao/newsroom/facts/errors.cfm.

4. Lang, G.K. *Ophthalmology: A Pocket Textbook Atlas*. New York: Thieme; 2000.

5. Pankratz, M.J., Helveston, E.M. Ophthalmology: The residents perspective. *Arch Ophthalmol*. 1992;110:37–43.

23

ORTHOPEDIC SURGERY

John C. Langland

At some point in their lives, many people require the care of an orthopedic surgeon: little children who fall down on elementary school playgrounds with broken wrists and elbows, high-school basketball players who twist and tear up their knees, and elderly men and women with chronic joint pain. Each of these patients will seek the expertise of a specialist in orthopedic surgery—highly trained physicians who treat the diseases and injuries of the entire musculoskeletal system, from the neck down to the toes. Although considered specialists, orthopedic surgeons actually have a rather broad knowledge base and take care of a wide spectrum of disease.

Although orthopedic surgery implies that most problems seen within this specialty are treated surgically, this notion is far from the truth. In fact, despite the long years of surgical training, most patient care is nonoperative. Cutting and curing is indeed an important part of orthopedic surgery, but medical students should keep in mind that it is not the sole focus of this wonderful specialty.

BONES, MUSCLES, AND JOINTS: THE HEART OF ORTHOPEDIC SURGERY

The specialty of orthopedics basically involves the care of the musculoskeletal system, which includes care of most disorders and injuries in the upper and lower extremities as well as the spine and pelvis. As such, future orthopedic surgeons need a thorough knowledge of the anatomy, mechanics, and physiology of this body system. You master everything there is to know about each muscle, nerve, and blood vessel within all parts of the musculoskeletal system. In addition, proper diagnosis and management of orthopedic injuries requires a solid grasp of forensics and physics to understand the mechanisms of injury. With an understanding of the underlying mechanisms, injury patterns can be predicted and will assist in appropriate diagnoses.

Orthopedic surgery involves more than just broken bones, dislocations, and sprains. It covers a wide array of problems, including conditions that may be congenital, acquired, or simply idiopathic (meaning of unknown origin). The list of orthopedic pathology is quite long and diverse, but a sampling of the diagnoses includes musculoskeletal infections, bone dysplasias, arthritis, neuromuscular disorders, scoliosis, pediatric deformities, meniscus and tendon tears, ligament sprains, compartment syndrome, tendonitis, joint instability, osteonecrosis, bunions, hammertoes, gout, diabetic foot wounds, carpal tunnel syndrome, trigger fingers, rheumatoid arthritis, Dupuytren disease, nerve injuries, musculoskeletal neoplasms, spinal stenosis, herniated disks, spondylolysis, spondylolisthesis, gait disturbance, and osteoporosis.

Because orthopedics covers such a broad array of disorders and injuries, which requires an extensive knowledge base, it has been divided into many subspecialties. Many orthopedists practice general orthopedics and take care of a variety of common injuries and disorders. Other surgeons choose to subspecialize in areas such as sports medicine, back and neck, shoulder and elbow, foot and ankle, upper extremity, adult reconstruction, musculoskeletal oncology, and pediatric orthopedics.

The real joy of orthopedics is the ability to help people with painful disorders and injuries, usually in a very short time period. Injuries cause mechanical problems in the body, and it is the job of the orthopedist to figure out the underlying problem and then correct the abnormality. Some problems can be fixed with simple medications or physical therapy, whereas others require a trip to the operating room. In general, orthopedic surgery includes the repair, reconstruction, and replacement of injured tendons, ligaments, bones, joints, and other anatomic parts.

Many health professionals make the analogy that orthopedic surgeons are like carpenters. If you have always loved working with your hands and building things, then perhaps this specialty is the perfect choice. The orthopedic surgeon is essentially the repairman and construction worker for the limbs and spine. They even have similar tools at their disposal in the operating room—saws, drills, tamps, hammers, chisels, screwdrivers, pliers, vice grips, and so on. With these tools, the orthopedic surgeon can do wonderful and amazing things to make people better. It is the ability to really make a significant change in a person's quality of life that makes orthopedics so enjoyable.

An easy example of the difference orthopedic surgery can make is looking at the result of a simple knee replacement. Knee arthritis can cause very disabling pain that limits a patient's ability to walk, climb stairs, and even get up from a chair. An orthopedic surgeon can perform a total knee replacement on that worn out joint and within 3 months that patient in most cases is pain free. With the alleviation of pain, their quality of life dramatically improves. There are countless other operations in orthopedics that help restore function and improve patient's lives.

EMERGENCY ORTHOPEDICS: BEING PART OF THE TRAUMA TEAM

Most orthopedic surgeons spend the majority of their time in the clinic seeing new and returning patients and, of course, in the operating room performing elective, nonemergent surgeries. However, most still have to live by the pager. After all, emergency care plays a role in the practice of many orthopedic surgeons. Many people—especially those involved in major motor vehicle accidents—come to the emergency room with severe traumatic injuries to their bones and joints, such as fractures and dislocations.

To a medical student, it may seem like the orthopedic residents are always down in the emergency department evaluating patients for possible emergency surgery. Keep in mind, however, that this perspective is a little skewed because most trauma centers are located in academic medical centers—a hospital with which a minority of practicing orthopedic surgeons is affiliated. In many teaching institutions, orthopedic residents handle even basic orthopedic problems such as finger dislocations for educational purposes. The residents and their attendings also work together as members of the trauma team to care for the severe injuries that show up at the medical center. Consequently, orthopedic surgeons who are on staff at a teaching hospital provide much more emergency care than those in private practice.

In the world of private practice and community hospitals, the amount of emergency orthopedic care is dictated by call schedule, hospital size and type, and practice focus. In fact, the emergency medicine physicians in the emergency department handle most minor orthopedic injuries. Many of those problems are simple sprains and lacerations and never need the care of an orthopedic surgeon. Follow-up care is instead arranged with the primary care physicians. Nonurgent problems requiring orthopedic attention are referred to outpatient clinic for follow-up. Urgent or emergent problems are called immediately to the orthopedic surgeon on call. There are only a few orthopedic emergencies: infections, dislocations, open fractures, unstable fractures, compartment syndrome, and progressive nerve compression (spinal cord injuries, myelopathy, cauda equina) are the most common. So in some practice settings with a quiet local emergency room, the orthopedic surgeon may make only rare trips to the emergency room. This is in contrast to what most medical students see in the academic centers.

GOOD OPERATIVE SKILLS ARE ESSENTIAL

Orthopedic surgery obviously requires the ability to perform operative tasks. The surgical responsibilities can range from the very delicate (operating on the hand or spine) to the less intricate (using long rods and heavy hammers to stabilize a fractured femur). The vast array of different operations keeps this specialty interesting and entertaining, and it is continually growing. Every year, new and less-invasive techniques are developed for classic operations. Nonetheless, excellent hand–eye coordination is essential to being a good surgeon.

Currently, the increasing use of minimally invasive techniques has been the focus of many areas of orthopedics, especially in the areas of trauma and arthroscopy. This type of surgery requires the ability to use your hands and your brains. As more and more operations are performed using a scope and smaller incisions, even more precise hand–eye coordination is required. Although many of these motor skills can be acquired, the basic spatial coordination and perception are most often natural in those who seek out orthopedics. These skills—in combination with a thorough knowledge of anatomy—are essential to becoming a good orthopedic surgeon. Computer-assisted surgery is also making some waves in orthopedics. The ability to make more precise cuts in joint replacement may allow better placement of a prosthesis and hopefully a longer lasting joint.

Orthopedic surgeons use their hands in other ways as well. The care of fractured bones makes up a proportion of a typical orthopedist's practice. Reducing broken bones and dislocations and holding them in place can sometimes be just as challenging as surgery. Placing casts and splints is definitely an art form. During

---

WHAT MAKES A GOOD ORTHOPEDIC SURGEON?

✓ Prefers action-based medicine.
✓ Likes working with his or her hands.
✓ Is a confident, decisive individual who can make fast decisions.
✓ Likes seeing the immediate results of treatment.
✓ Has excellent hand–eye coordination.

THE INSIDE SCOOP

residency training, many of these techniques are handed down from the senior resident to the more junior resident year after year. After all, there are many fine subtleties in casting that take dedication and practice. One simple mistake can mean the loss of the reduction or a painful cast sore. The feeling of warm wet plaster often brings a smile of satisfaction to the faces of most orthopedic surgeons. The cast is their creation and their work of art.

THE DOCTOR–PATIENT RELATIONSHIP

As an orthopedist, you have a variety of professional relationships with your patients. Some patients are treated only once, such as a man with a trigger finger who requires a simple injection. Others—such as elderly patients with severe osteoarthritis—may be evaluated repeatedly. Other short-term appointments include preoperative evaluations and postoperative checks. Many patients are seen for painful disorders that are interfering with their life and work, such as an injury obtained on the job. The goal of the orthopedist is to help them get through these troubling times and return them to full function. It is a rewarding and immensely satisfying privilege to do so.

It is interesting that many patients pick their orthopedic surgeon by word of mouth from family members. For instance, a grandmother may come in to see an orthopedic surgeon for her hip replacement because he did such an excellent job taking care of her grandson's broken forearm. When his older brother tears his anterior cruciate ligament while playing football, the family will frequently see the same orthopedic surgeon. Patients also tend to return for other problems as well. These word of mouth referrals are important to help each orthopedic surgeon establish a successful practice. Without a good bedside manner and surgical skills, this would not be possible.

SPORTS MEDICINE: BEING A TEAM PHYSICIAN

The practice of sports medicine is a part of nearly every orthopedic subspecialty. In fact, many athletic medical students choose careers in orthopedic surgery because of their attraction to the glamour of sports medicine. Although internists, pediatricians, and emergency medicine physicians can also pursue fellowships in this subspecialty, only orthopedists manage all types of sports-related injuries from both a surgical and medical (nonoperative) approach.

Within the community, the orthopedic surgeon can assume the role of team physician. Providing care to a local high-school team, for instance, is usually done on a voluntary basis and allows the orthopedist an opportunity to give back to the community. Divided up among different orthopedic practice groups, this service serves as an excellent public relations tool. Despite the lack of direct financial rewards, the time spent with the athletes, parents, and coaches can lead to significant referrals in the future.

Many orthopedic surgeons also take care of college teams and local semiprofessional teams. Depending on the situation, this service can involve a salary or remain strictly voluntary. Medical students should be aware that the amount of time required to be a team physician at this level is not for everyone. Usually, the time scheduled for seeing these athletes is outside of normal office hours and includes patient evaluations at night or early in the morning in the training room. If the medical care also includes sideline coverage, this can add up to extensive time spent with the team and away from family. Despite the commitment, most surgeons find that getting the athletes back into their game at this level is extremely gratifying.

Many aspiring orthopedic surgeons are excited by the prospect of caring for professional athletes. To achieve this dream, you must successfully make it through orthopedic residency training, followed by a sports medicine fellowship that includes care of a professional team, such as one of the members of the National Football League (NFL). Although the job of a professional team physician looks fairly glamorous from the outside, it is usually hard and stressful work. Dealing with owners, agents, players, and the media and balancing the needs of everyone involved can be very difficult. In today's litigious environment, malpractice premiums have skyrocketed for professional team physicians. Because they deal with players making millions of dollars, the potential monetary reward for a malpractice claim often exceeds the maximum limits of an orthopedic surgeon's insurance policy. There is also a trend among professional athletes of traveling to outside sports medicine centers for their operative care. The local team physician, who takes care of the player on the field and in the training room, makes the diagnosis, but if the player requires surgery, it is often the agent who chooses a surgical specialist, undermining the physician–player relationship. Although not every orthopedic surgeon serves as a team physician, most take care of sports injuries in some capacity. Sports injuries span all age groups from young kids playing football, to middle-aged joggers, to elderly tennis players. There is also the fitness boom that is going on. Many people are trying to get healthier and are pursuing training for marathons and triathlons. There are also many current workout regimens that cause a fair amount of injuries in the middle-aged crowd. By treating these problems, you derive immense satisfaction from returning your patients to their sports and livelihood as soon as medically possible. So whether or not you enjoy sports, sports medicine care will make up some part of the everyday practice of orthopedics.

A SPECIALTY JUST FOR DUMB JOCKS?

Despite the very intense competition for residency positions in this specialty, orthopedic surgery has long been labeled as the field for "dumb jocks." Why is this misleading image perpetuated among medical students? Perhaps it is because orthopedic surgery—with its emphasis on sports medicine—also always attracts athletic students. For some, the classic stereotype of an orthopedic surgeon is a large athletic man who is in the bottom of his medical class.

Yet, today this perception is very far from the truth. Orthopedics is one of the most selective and competitive residency programs. Mostly top medical students from across the nation find themselves with a position in this specialty. If you are considering a career in orthopedic surgery, you should worry more about your grades and board scores and less about your physical size, maximum bench press, or other athletic capabilities. More importantly, not everyone in this field of medicine is a white male. In fact, according to the most recent demographic data, residency programs were composed of women (13.6%), Asians (12.3%), African Americans (4.6%), and Hispanics (4.7%).[1] Yet, there are still not enough orthopedic surgeons from underrepresented minority groups, and it continues to remain a challenging problem.

LIFESTYLE CONSIDERATIONS AND PRACTICE OPTIONS

Some medical students are scared away from surgical subspecialties due to their tough residency and busy lifestyles. (However, the residency work hour rules may have dampened this effect.) Many do not realize that the long hours, heavy work, and rigorous call schedule do lighten up after the completion of residency training. Out in practice, the lifestyle of an orthopedic surgeon is quite variable and hard to pin down exactly. It is basically whatever you make of it. It depends on a number of factors, such as subspecialty training, group size, referral area size, reimbursement, competition, and call schedule. According to the American Academy of Orthopaedic Surgeons (AAOS), most physicians practice general orthopedics as part of a group and spend about half of their clinical time in the operating room. They generally work much longer hours in regions of the country where reimbursement is lower and competition is higher.

If you truly love orthopedic surgery, do not be frightened of its rigorous lifestyle, which is typical of most surgical specialties. After long days in the office and in the operating room, taking overnight call is an obligation of nearly every orthopedic surgeon in the country. However, the type and quantity of call can be quite different. In a large group practice, you may only take call once or twice a month. If the group covers a busy hospital, however, you may be up all night operating on patients. Joining a more intimate group practice at a smaller hospital may entail a more frequent call schedule but less of a chance of actually being called in to evaluate a patient. Because there are other combinations within this spectrum, the lifestyle of an orthopedic surgeon depends on the specific practice setting. First determine your life priorities and acceptable work schedule and then seek out the practice of your dreams through careful job selection. It will be out there somewhere, but keep in mind it may not be the first practice you choose in your career.

VITAL SIGNS

MEDIAN COMPENSATION

Orthopedic surgery (general)	$476,083
Orthopedic surgery (pediatrics)	$424,367
Hand	$465,006
Foot and ankle	$399,445
Joint replacement	$580,711
Spine	$641,728

Data from American Medical Group Association.

As the specialist shortage continues to worsen, orthopedic surgeons are still needed now more than ever. This is especially a problem in midwestern rural settings. With the rising numbers of senior citizens in this country, there is plenty of work available for a newly trained orthopedic surgeon, scalpel and hammer in hand. Among the aging population, there are thousands of worn out joints requiring replacement and just as many hip fractures needing repair. Also, with the nation becoming healthier and pursuing recreational sports later in life, orthopedic surgeons have a steady supply of sports medicine injuries to treat. All across the country, rural towns and small cities are clamoring for more orthopedic surgeons. Some hospitals, in desperate need for orthopedic surgeons on staff, are now even willing to pay off student loans and guarantee large salaries.

What about the stability of this specialty and its overlap with other areas of medicine? Aspiring surgeons should keep in mind that orthopedics is really primary care for the musculoskeletal system. As such, it will never get squeezed too hard from other specialties; no other physician has expertise in the entire musculoskeletal system. Over the last 20 years, there has been a limited degree of slow encroachment into orthopedics from other specialists and health professionals. Podiatrists, who have traditionally limited themselves to foot disorders, are now doing ankle work as well. Some neurosurgeons are pursuing advanced training in spine treatment to perform fracture care, discectomies, and laminectomies from the neck down. Some will also perform carpal tunnel releases. In the area of hand care, there is some overlap between orthopedic surgeons and their colleagues in plastic surgery, who are also trained in the management of soft tissue and bony injuries of the hand. Yet, there is still plenty of work to go around for everyone.

FELLOWSHIPS AND SUBSPECIALTY TRAINING

Because of its many areas of subspecialization, there are a variety of orthopedic fellowships. Most residents decide whether or not to pursue a fellowship by the end of their third year in residency training. According to the AAOS, the most popular fellowships are hand surgery, sports medicine, and spine surgery. Each accredited fellowship—no matter the subspecialty—generally lasts for 1 additional year. Some highly academic programs include an additional year of research. The orthopedic subspecialty areas do not have their own board certification examinations. Only a fellowship in hand surgery or sports medicine leads to any sort of recognition (a certificate of added qualification). The others simply provide additional specialized training.

Adult Reconstruction

If you seek additional experience in joint reconstruction of adults, this fellowship is for you. There is a strong focus on complex total joint replacements and revision arthroplasty for failed joint replacements. You will become an expert on the operative treatment of arthritis and deformity. Some programs focus only on knee and hip, while others include other joints such as ankle, shoulder, and elbow.

Foot and Ankle

This fellowship provides advanced training in the care of foot and ankle disorders from simple bunions and fractures to complex deformities and wounds. Subspecialists in foot and ankle surgery are among the most needed orthopedic surgeons across the country.

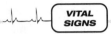

Hand and Upper Extremity

If you have delicate fine motor skills and like to work with microscopes or loupes, then hand surgery may be for you. This subspecialty concentrates on hand and wrist surgery for trauma (fractures, tendon injuries, nerve injuries, replants, flaps), deformity, arthritis, cancer, infection, congenital disease, and occupational injury. Some fellowships are strictly related to hand and wrist, while others include other upper-extremity work involving the shoulder and elbow. These subspecialists do some fine microsurgical work, such as replantation of fingers — which requires delicate nerve and vessel repair or reconstruction.

Pediatric Orthopedics

Pediatric orthopedic surgery provides training in the care of all musculoskeletal disorders and injuries found in children. This includes the care of scoliosis, cerebral palsy, meningomyelocele, osteogenesis imperfecta, and other advanced disorders that can require multiple surgeries. A large portion of the training is focused on pediatric fracture care and treating other disorders such as in-toeing, clubfoot, and developmental dysplasia of the hip.

Musculoskeletal Oncology

This fellowship provides training in the nonoperative and operative treatment of bone and soft tissue neoplasms, such as sarcomas, and tumors that have metastasized to the bone. Many who seek out this fellowship have an interest in cancer research and treatment and enjoy being part of a multidisciplinary cancer treatment team. Your patients will range in all ages from children to the elderly. Most musculoskeletal oncologists practice at academic medical centers.

Spine Surgery

Subspecialists in surgery of the spine have received advanced training in treating disorders of the spine—from the cervical portion down to the lumbosacral area. They repair and reconstruct spinal deformities that have resulted from trauma, infection, cancer, and degenerative disease. There is currently a shortage of specialists in this area of orthopedics.

Sports Medicine and Arthroscopy

Orthopedic surgeons with additional training in sports medicine and arthroscopy focus their practice on the care of athletes of all ages and how to take care of sports-related injuries. The vast majority of their operative experience is related to knee and shoulder injuries, with less work on the ankle, elbow, and hip. Most sports medicine fellowships provide extensive training in arthroscopy and advanced arthroscopic techniques. Many fellowships include time caring for a team, which may be a local high school, college, or even a professional team.

Trauma

This fellowship provides additional training in the management of complex traumatic injuries to the extremities and pelvis. This includes blunt and penetrating trauma as well as industrial accidents. Typical problems seen in the trauma bay are long bone fractures and complex

RESIDENCY TRAINING

Residency in orthopedic surgery requires 5 years of postgraduate training. Some programs mandate an extra year of clinical research. There are currently 153 accredited programs. Although it varies per program, the internship year (PGY-1) usually consists of 3 months of orthopedics mixed with rotations in general surgery, other surgical subspecialties, internal medicine, and radiology. As with most surgical training, residents work long weeks in excess of 60 hours and take in-house call routinely during residency. In the last year or two, senior residents can take most night calls from home. Divided among the different subspecialties of orthopedics, the monthly rotations consist of trauma, adult reconstruction, pediatric orthopedics, musculoskeletal oncology, foot and ankle, hand surgery, sports medicine, and spine surgery. Programs that cannot provide adequate training in each subspecialty may send residents to other hospitals for subspecialty experience to meet accreditation requirements.

THE INSIDE SCOOP

articular fractures, including those of the pelvis and acetabulum. Those who seek out this fellowship should have good hand–eye coordination and excellent spatial orientation. As a member of the trauma team, you will learn how to prioritize multiple orthopedic and other surgical problems.

WHY CONSIDER A CAREER IN ORTHOPEDIC SURGERY?

If you want to get involved in a medical field that is leading the way when it comes to innovations in technology, orthopedic surgery is it. These specialists are now delving into the world of robotic surgery, computer-assisted surgery, gene manipulation, and medical therapeutics. The ability to alter the rate of bone healing or to correct a chromosomal error that causes a collagen disorder is fascinating. New techniques are evolving with which to grow new tissues such as menisci, cartilage, and bone. Because of the tremendous growth in research, many of the basic surgeries learned 10 to 15 years ago are being replaced by new techniques. This requires the orthopedic surgeon to constantly learn and participate in continuing medical education, particularly on topics related to biomechanics and the pathophysiology of the musculoskeletal system.

If you are considering a residency in orthopedic surgery, it is extremely important to know that this is one of the most competitive residencies to obtain. It ranks up there with most other surgical subspecialties. A decision to pursue orthopedics is best made very early in medical school. By making a decision early, you can provide yourself with the tools to match successfully in most cases. Although orthopedic surgery residency is arduous, long, and busy, the lifestyle and satisfaction you obtain is worth the effort. Most important, the ability to restore normal musculoskeletal function in your patients and to improve their lives is definitely worth it all.

ABOUT THE CONTRIBUTOR

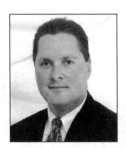

Dr John Langland is an orthopedic surgeon and specialist in sports medicine and arthroscopy at the Steindler Orthopedic Clinic in Iowa City, Iowa. Born and raised in Ottumwa, Iowa, Dr Langland earned his undergraduate and medical degrees at the University of Iowa—Iowa City. He completed his residency in orthopedic surgery at the University of Wisconsin—Madison. During his sports medicine/arthroscopy fellowship at the University of Cincinnati/ Christ Hospital, Dr Langland took care of athletes from the

University of Cincinnati Bearcats, the Cincinnati Bengals (NFL), and the Cincinnati Mighty Ducks (AHL). He currently assists medical students interested in orthopedics by managing the Orthopedic Surgery Residency Ring (www.osrr.org), which provides a gateway to information on orthopedic training. He also moderates the Orthopedic Residency Education Forums at Orthogate.com. Dr Langland is motivated daily by his wonderful wife, Traci, and his three children, Brittani, Christopher, and Brooke. In his free time, he enjoys fishing, water skiing, wake-boarding, and downhill skiing. He can be reached by e-mail at OSRR@orthosurg.net.

REFERENCE

1. Brotherton, S.E., Etzel, S.I. Graduate medical education, 2010–2011. JAMA. 2011;306(9):1015–1030.

24

OTOLARYNGOLOGY

Arjun Joshi and Neil Tanna

W hen medical students begin to consider a career in otolaryngology, they are often met with blank stares from their family, friends, and significant others. It is a specialty that is often difficult to pronounce, much less to understand its scope and subject matter. These physicians are not just "ENT" (ear, nose, and throat) doctors. Technically, the official name of this field of medicine is "otorhinolaryngology" or "otolaryngology— head and neck surgery." This specialty involves both the medical and surgical care of all structures related to the head and neck (basically, above the clavicles and excluding the brain and the eye). It is, quite simply, the best surgical subspecialty within medicine.

If you like treating patients with complex diseases of the oral cavity, larynx, sinus, ears, throat, and other parts of the head and neck, then take a closer look at this specialty. Otolaryngology is perfect for those students who prefer working with their hands and dealing with a lot of "action" in their medical career. Do you see yourself as a specialist? Are you a perfectionist? Do you like to solve a piece of a medical puzzle? Then perhaps the intricate anatomy, physiology, and pathology of otolaryngology are all for you.

A BRIEF OVERVIEW OF OTOLARYNGOLOGY

Formally established in 1924, the American Board of Otolaryngology is one of the oldest medical specialty boards in the country. Prior to its founding, specialists of the head and neck were responsible for treating both otolaryngologic and ophthalmologic diseases. In 1978, to better reflect the increase in breadth of this complex field, the board was renamed "otolaryngology—head and neck surgery." This change came about because skull base surgery, oncology, cosmetic and reconstructive facial plastic surgery, and other forms of head and neck surgery became part of the otolaryngologist's realm of expertise. Although most physicians and patients still refer to these surgeons simply as "ENTs," this specialty is, in reality, so much more than ears, noses, and throats. Otolaryngologists are also experts in the management of head and neck tumors (eg, thyroid and salivary gland), chronic pediatric infections (tonsillectomies, adenoidectomies, and tympanostomy tube placement), facial trauma and cosmetic deformities, and diseases of the airway and phonation (laryngoscopy, bronchoscopy, palate surgery for snoring and sleep apnea).

Otolaryngologists are unique among surgical specialists because they are trained in both surgery and medicine. As a branch of surgery, otolaryngology essentially has no equivalent counterpart in medicine. This is in contrast to their fellow surgeons such as urologists (nephrology), neurosurgeons (neurology), cardiac surgeons (cardiologists), and thoracic surgeons (pulmonology). As a result, the practitioner must learn to treat patients medically as well as surgically. Otolaryngologists do not need to refer patients to other physicians when surgery is needed and, therefore, can offer the most appropriate care for each patient. The downside is that patients will come to clinic with relatively benign, nonsurgical complaints, such as sore throats. Often, general practicing otolaryngologists refer specialized cases such as cochlear implants, facial cosmetics, revision sinus surgery, or advanced cancer of the head and neck to a subspecialty surgeon within otolaryngology.

In fact, medical students who truly enjoy operating should realize that the majority of otolaryngologic patients are managed medically—not surgically. Compared with other surgical subspecialties, you will perform more diagnostic and therapeutic procedures on patients in the clinic, such as laryngoscopy. However, usually only about one in ten patients evaluated will require a surgical procedure. This proportion varies somewhat depending on the type of practice and on the kind of patients that you are seeing. For example, if referrals come principally from primary care physicians, the percentage of patients who require surgery will be lower than from referrals from other otolaryngologists. Alternatively, if your focus is on pediatrics or head and neck cancer, the percentage of patients who need surgery may also be higher compared with the general patient population. On the whole, however, otolaryngologists usually operate about 1 to 2 days per week. Medical students who wish to operate more often than that may want to consider another subspecialty.

Since the American Academy of Otolaryngology has kept the number of residency training positions relatively stable over the last few decades, otolaryngology is a small field. Practicing within such a narrowly defined surgical subspecialty fosters collegiality. Throughout a career in this specialty, you will quickly recognize the same people, from residency interviews to national meetings and professional education courses. Those familiar faces will be your colleagues during your practice. Choosing a small specialty allows otolaryngologists to network, share ideas, and develop lasting friendships. The downside, of course, is a greater degree of scrutiny from your peers, both in the private practice community and in academic centers.

VARIETY WITHIN A SUBSPECIALTY

Most otolaryngologists would agree that no other subspecialty in medicine allows for so much variety. The patient population includes people of all ages, gender, and socioeconomic strata. The pathology is equally as diverse. On any given day in the clinic, you may begin by using rigid endoscopes to evaluate a patient with sinus complaints. The next patient may have a thyroid nodule requiring fine needle aspiration. Others might complain of hearing loss, necessitating an examination under the otologic microscope. For the symptom of hoarseness, the use of a flexible fiber-optic laryngoscope is rather ubiquitous in the office of any otolaryngologist. Each patient requires a special type of evaluation for which the otolaryngologist must draw upon a variety of skills.

As you can tell, otolaryngology clinic—with its routine procedures—is busy and exciting. You are constantly working with your hands. In addition to interviewing the patient, these specialists are spraying, suctioning, removing, inserting, manipulating, and examining. The list is quite extensive: patients with routine cerumen impaction who need their ears cleaned out under the microscope, hoarse patients who require evaluation with a flexible nasal laryngoscope, sinus surgery patients who need nasal debridement using rigid nasal endoscopes, and much more. Medical students should think of these clinical procedures almost like short operative cases.

In contrast to other areas of the body, the anatomy of the head and neck lends itself to ready examination. Most internal mucosal surfaces are visualized well with the use of flexible and rigid endoscopes. The neck is typically not as difficult to palpate as the abdomen, for example. The ability to evaluate head and neck structures easily is reassuring for both the clinician and the patient because many diagnoses are made upon the initial examination and do not require imaging studies. In other areas of medicine, it is frustrating to have a patient present to clinic only to be sent away for an imaging study that will undergo review during the next visit. The average otolaryngologic patient, on the other hand, receives an expedient answer, and the physician is generally satisfied that he or she has made the correct diagnosis.

You will find that the variety found in operating room is just as significant in the clinic. No other surgical specialty allows the opportunity to operate on both soft tissue and bone, use endoscopic and open approaches, and perform long and short cases all in the same day. The majority of otolaryngologic surgeries performed are ambulatory, which means that patients usually go home on the same day. This contrasts with other surgical specialties, which may require inpatient hospitalization after a procedure. Surgical cases range in complexity from simple tonsillectomies and myringotomies to microsurgery of the ear and skull base, benign and malignant head and neck tumor surgery, reconstructive airway surgery, nasal and sinus surgery, microscopic voice surgery, and even cosmetic facial plastic and reconstructive procedures. At a typical academic medical center, a day in the operating room might include a 90-minute nasal endoscopy (with biopsy of the nasopharynx, direct laryngoscopy, and open neck biopsy), a 3-hour four-gland exploration/parathyroidectomy for hyperparathyroidism, a 30-minute excision of a vallecular cyst, and an hour-long suspension microlaryngoscopy and excision of vocal cord papilloma. The cases may add up to a long day, but nothing is routine. The bottom line is that the variety offered by surgical otolaryngology is virtually unmatched.

Whether in the operating room, intensive care unit, or on the wards, the otolaryngologist is truly the master of the head and neck, as well as the airway. You will be the one providing definitive treatment in the form of emergency tracheostomies, complicated airway reconstruction, resection of acoustic nerve tumors, and resection of tumors encasing the carotid artery or lying at the base of the skull. During residency training, budding otolaryngologists are asked to evaluate and treat acutely ill patients in airway distress. You will need to do something about it—quickly. Are you the kind of person who can handle that kind of situation without losing your cool? While it is true that most otolaryngologists do not encounter as many emergencies as other surgical specialists, when problems arise they can be potentially fatal. Would you like to provide emergency care in such situations? Think carefully, therefore, before choosing otolaryngology.

THE DOCTOR–PATIENT RELATIONSHIP

As surgical consultants, otolaryngologists take care of patients with single, well-defined problems. These physicians see about 30 to 40 patients per day in their clinic, so this specialty is not well suited for medical students who desire minimal patient contact. Although patients are generally healthy (with discrete medical issues), you still have the amazing privilege of near-total strangers sharing their personal stories and entrusting you with their care. Otolaryngologists solve these problems quickly and effectively and produce tangible results. Patients are generally thankful and pleased at the results obtained from undergoing a particular procedure. Despite the fact that most of these patients are referrals, outpatient visits provide an opportunity to form meaningful doctor–patient relationships.

Head and neck surgeons can, however, have long-term relationships with their patients. Pediatric otolaryngologists may see children for years to manage recurrent infections or chronic airway problems. Head and neck oncologists follow patients for the duration of their disease, and then to monitor recurrence following surgery, radiation, or chemotherapy. Otologists maintain long-term relationships to follow hearing loss, chronic mastoiditis, and Ménière disease. Specialists in laryngology may treat patients for many years who have vocal cord paralysis, spasmodic dysphonia, laryngeal carcinoma, or professional voice issues.

In addition, the day-to-day practice allows otolaryngologists to discharge patients from their care after helping them, opening up the chance to see new patients. This style does not mean, however, that the otolaryngologist does not have chronic patients. In reality, though, there are far fewer chronic patients than in most specialties, and the majority of patients are fairly healthy. Otolaryngology patients typically have finite problems. They come to see these specialists for a particular issue—not with a laundry list of complaints. It is up to the otolaryngologist to address that single issue. Once that problem is solved, your job is generally done.

HOW TO BE A GOOD OTOLARYNGOLOGIST

While there is no single personality type best suited for otolaryngology, the specialty, like most, appeals to individuals with common characteristics. In fact, studies tend to support the notion that otolaryngologists share similar personality traits. Colleagues often refer to these specialists as "gentlemen surgeons," "nice people," and physicians with "unassuming personalities." These surgeons are extremely bright, amiable, easygoing, and, for the most part, humble. Otolaryngologists are often meticulous perfectionists with a preference for tackling medical issues that can be solved quickly rather than chronic conditions. They enjoy seeing immediate results. Like most surgeons and procedural subspecialists, they tend to be action oriented. Intense, curious, and inquisitive, yet generally good natured, otolaryngologists are often characterized as "aggressive, without being rude."

Beyond a good personality and inquisitive nature, surgical, as well as clinical, otolaryngology requires excellent manual dexterity and a firm understanding of the numerous tools in our armamentarium. At their disposal, they have microscopes, lasers (handheld, fiber optic, and standard), microdebriders, drills, coblators, balloons, surgical laryngoscopes, rigid endoscopes, rigid bronchoscopes, optical forceps, flexible scopes, and, even in some cases, the surgical robot. Mastering these tools and instruments requires familiarity and ease with technology. To stay on top of the game, they must also keep abreast of new technological advancements.

Meticulousness is also a key. The surgical anatomy of the head and neck is incredibly complex. Although any surgical specialty requires a firm grasp of anatomy, no other specialty requires working knowledge of so many essential anatomic structures in as small of a space. Precision is critical—there is not much room to spare! Whether dissecting out the facial nerve during a parotidectomy, performing an ossicular chain reconstruction in the middle ear, excising vocal cord masses, performing endoscopic sinus surgery, or dissecting out the recurrent laryngeal nerve during a thyroidectomy, avoiding mistakes requires a great deal of concentration and patience.

LIFESTYLE CONSIDERATIONS AND PRACTICE OPTIONS

Compared with other surgeons, otolaryngologists enjoy a relatively balanced lifestyle between life and work. Their colleagues often joke that ENT really stands for "every night tennis." This may be an exaggeration, but most otolaryngologists have regular working hours that allow them to go home and pursue other activities at the end of the day. This flexibility is largely because the general acuity of otolaryngology patients is not high, that is, there are few emergencies that require immediate attention. In fact, the average otolaryngologist spends about 5 hours compared with other subspecialties. Also, most patients (except those with extensive head and neck cancer) who undergo surgery are relatively healthy and procedures are performed on an outpatient basis. This combination of factors makes call nights and clinical days less grueling without the worry about emergencies and acutely ill patients. Common emergencies that do require timely intervention include posttonsillectomy bleeds, epistaxis, infections including peritonsillar and neck abscesses, and airway difficulty requiring tracheotomy. Regardless, otolaryngology is still regarded as a family-friendly surgical subspecialty.

A typical day in the clinic begins at 8:00 AM and ends at 5:00 PM. Otolaryngologists usually see about 90 patients per week during their 3 to 4 days in the clinic. Unlike other surgical subspecialties, the clinic is where most otolaryngologists generate the majority of their income. In fact, some physicians see patients in the clinic exclusively and refer them to other otolaryngologists for surgical treatment. Operating room time is 1 or 2 days per week. Since most patients are discharged home after surgery, the amount of time spent on the hospital wards seeing patients is minimal. The average otolaryngologist spends roughly 2 hours per week making hospital rounds, so if you enjoy rounding on patients in the hospital setting, otolaryngology may not be the best match. Obviously, the nature of your service depends on your specific subspecialty. Head and neck oncologists perform incredibly complex surgical cases. Accordingly, they have longer hours than their colleagues and operate on sicker patients. These patients stay in the hospital longer than other cases and are generally associated with more serious complications.

It used to be that after finishing residency, most otolaryngologists were given a choice between a career in private practice or academics. Today, there are far more career options for the graduating specialist to consider. The small number of otolaryngologists also ensures a steady demand for their services. Positions for otolaryngologists are plentiful and nearly all residents are guaranteed a job after completion of training. The traditional options—private practice or a full-time academic appointment—remain the most popular choices. However, there are also "clinical" academic appointments, which offer otolaryngologists the opportunity to teach residents while maintaining a private practice. Other career options include consulting for pharmaceutical companies, medical equipment manufacturers, and other private industries. Some otolaryngologists elect to leave the clinical world entirely and delve into the administrative side of medicine, either by working for an organization such as the American Academy of Otolaryngology—Head and Neck Surgery or for health care establishments.

VITAL SIGNS

MEDIAN COMPENSATION

Otolaryngology $365,171

Data from American Medical Group Association.

FELLOWSHIPS AND SUBSPECIALTY TRAINING

Advanced surgical training in the subspecialties of otolaryngology is available to graduating residents, although most do not pursue fellowships. A minority of residents wish to focus their practice on a particular subspecialty. While a specialty focused on the "head and neck" may already seem fairly specialized to medical students, fellowship training can be particularly valuable for those who wish to pursue an academic practice. Some residents seek additional credentialing to boost their referral rate, particularly in urban settings where the market is often more saturated. In some cases, residents complete fellowships to balance out a residency experience that emphasized certain procedures over others. Nonetheless, most graduating residents are more than capable of performing most or all procedures performed by fellowship-trained otolaryngologists. A fellowship should not be viewed as a prerequisite for performing certain types of otolaryngologic surgery. Applications for these fellowships—most of which are 1 year in duration—are due during the third year of training.

Facial Plastic and Reconstructive Surgery

Fellowships in facial plastic surgery provide focused experience on the cosmetic, functional, and reconstructive surgical treatment of the head and neck. The fellowship generally covers cosmetic procedures such as blepharoplasty (eye jobs), rhytidectomy (facelifts), rhinoplasty (nose jobs), Botox use, chemical and laser dermabrasion, and many others. Some programs focus more heavily on reconstructive plastics procedures, such as the Mohs procedure, microneurovascular anastomoses, tissue transfer techniques, and facial reanimation. A small subset of reconstructive fellowships focuses on the bony facial skeleton. Applicants in these areas will receive training in cleft-lip and plate surgery, various orthognathic procedures, and congenital cranial defects.

Facial plastic and reconstructive surgery (FPRS) requires extreme meticulousness in the surgical suite or operating room, and a special ability to deal with demanding patients. Procedures involve extensive soft-tissue dissection techniques and a working knowledge of the intricacies of the facial nerve. The field also requires a familiarity with geometric shapes and angles, especially in the case of head and neck reconstruction. The vast majority of facial plastic surgeons enter into a private practice at the end of their training.

This is an extremely competitive fellowship to obtain. According to the San Francisco Matching Program, the 2005 Match rate for 38 positions was about 74%.

While it is also possible to become board certified in FPRS by doing a certain number of index cases and being elected into the subspecialty, the majority of board-certified FPRS surgeons have completed fellowships. Certification in this subspecialty requires successful completion of a clinical fellowship followed by passage of the rigorous written and oral facial plastics–reconstructive surgical board examinations.

Otology, Neurotology, and Skull Base Surgery

Neurotologists and otologists deal with congenital disorders of the ears including microtia (small or deformed ears) and atresia (failure of the external auditory canal to develop). These conditions sometimes require complex reconstruction in several stages. Surgical options for infectious disease and their complications range from tympanostomy tube insertion to tympanomastoidectomy. The otologist performs reconstruction of the tympanic membrane (tympanoplasty) as well as the ossicular chain (stapedectomy, ossiculoplasty). He or she also performs cochlear implants, which have recently become popular for the treatment of certain types of profound hearing loss. As an aside, it is quite a gratifying experience to witness a deaf person regain hearing. Tumors treated by the neurotologist and skull base surgeon include acoustic neuromas, facial schwannomas, and neuroendocrine tumors. These cases sometimes

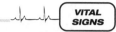

VITAL SIGNS

OTOLARYNGOLOGY 2011 MATCH STATISTICS

- Number of positions available: 283
- 323 US seniors and 62 independent applicants ranked at least one otolaryngology program
- 98.9% of all positions were filled in the initial Match
- The successful applicants: 96.1% US seniors, 1.1% foreign-trained physicians, and 0% osteopathic graduates
- Mean USMLE Step I score: 243
- Unmatched rate for US seniors applying only to otolaryngology: 11.8%

Data from National Resident Matching Program.

RESIDENCY TRAINING

Residency in otolaryngology requires 5 years of postgraduate training. There are currently 103 accredited residency programs. All residents complete 1 year of general surgery internship before training in otolaryngology. It is possible to tailor the internship year to include rotations that closely overlap with future training, such as plastic

(continued)

surgery and anesthesiology. Within the 5-year residency, up to 6 months may be used for research. Some programs allow residents to add up to 2 years of protected research time to their total training. Residents work long hours and take frequent overnight call, but the amount of in-house call decreases with each successive year. In many programs, residents begin taking "home call" as early as their second year. Call nights are more difficult in programs with significant facial and neck trauma exposure. The complexity of cases and patient responsibility— culminating in the fifth year (chief residency)—increases dramatically. Clinical exposure includes rotations in the four major areas of this specialty: facial plastics, head and neck surgery, otology and neurotology, and pediatric and general otolaryngology. Most programs require at least 3 months of research during the residency. Completion of basic residency training allows you to practice pediatric and adult general otolaryngology, head and neck surgery, facial plastics, and otology. For individuals who wish to pursue advanced training, opportunities exist for fellowships in subspecialty areas.

THE INSIDE SCOOP

require cooperation with neurosurgical colleagues. In the clinic, commonly encountered conditions include otitis media and externa, hearing loss, vertigo and other balance disorders, and tinnitus.

Like other subspecialties, neurotology, otology, and skull base surgery require great patience and precision and the ability to work with a broad patient population. It also requires a unique set of surgical skills, including expert use of the drill as well as the ability to perform meticulous two-handed surgeries. This subspecialty also offers many exciting opportunities for research and is well suited to those inclined toward basic science. Many neurotologists perform research in addition to clinical duties, and as a result, most have an academic practice. In fact, the majority of the basic science research conducted in the field of otolaryngology is focused on hearing loss.

A fellowship in otology, neurotology, and skull base surgery focuses on disorders of the outer, middle, inner ear, and the skull base. The fellowship lasts from 1 to 2 years. Otology is an unaccredited 1-year clinical fellowship. Neurotology and skull base surgery, on the other hand, is an accredited 2-year program leading to board certification after an oral and written examination. In neurotology, there is more focus on skull base and acoustic tumors, although the vast majority of the cases performed by neurotologists and otologists are the same.

Head and Neck Surgical Oncology

This fellowship (which does not lead to board certification) takes 1 year to complete and provides training in the surgical treatment of advanced cancer of the salivary glands, endocrine glands, and aerodigestive tract. Common procedures performed by the head and neck surgeon include thyroidectomy, parathyroidectomy, cervical lymphadenectomy (neck dissection), parotidectomy, surgical resection of the primary cancer site, as well as microvascular reconstruction. The head and neck oncologist has the option of closing of the soft-tissue defect created by surgery by himself or herself, or working with a reconstructive surgeon. In most academic centers, two separate teams perform the entire reconstruction.

Oncologic resection and reconstruction cases can be quite long (6 to 12 hours or more!) and involve several surgeons. Salivary gland surgery (parotidectomy, submandibular gland resection, etc) and thyroid/parathyroid surgery also involve similarly intricate surgical techniques to preserve the facial nerve or the laryngeal nerves, respectively. The variety of head and neck surgical cases, the challenge of resection and reconstruction to preserve speech and swallowing function, and the many opportunities for research (especially the tumor biology and genetics of squamous cell carcinoma) make this subspecialty attractive to many graduating residents.

Head and neck surgeries are generally not well suited for the physician who wants to get in and out of the operating room quickly, or who prefers working solo. Rather, cases are often long and require sharing responsibilities with a surgical team. Head and neck surgeons should also be prepared for new techniques and advances to emerge in the coming years. Traditionally, head and neck fellowships trained individuals using open surgical techniques. Fellowships now include training in minimally invasive endoscopic techniques. For instance, many advanced laryngeal cancers are now being resected intraorally with lasers and sinonasal tumors are now frequently excised endoscopically. These developments make for a rapidly changing surgical practice.

Pediatric Otolaryngology

These 1- to 2-year fellowships offer specialized training in rhinologic, head and neck, otologic, and laryngologic procedures in the pediatric and adolescent patient population. Conditions often encountered by the pediatric otolaryngologist include chronic tonsillitis, sinusitis, otitis media, hearing loss, congenital cysts and masses, aspiration and swallowing disorders, and upper airway obstruction/sleep apnea. Common surgical procedures include adenotonsillectomy, myringotomy with pressure-equalization tube placement, removal of foreign bodies of the upper aerodigestive tract and ear canals, upper airway endoscopy, tracheotomies, resection of branchial cleft or other congenital cysts/masses, endoscopic sinus surgery, and otologic surgery including tympanoplasties and mastoidectomies. The degree of fellowship training in cochlear implantation, laryngotracheal reconstruction, and cleft lip/palate repair varies by program.

Obviously, the pediatric otolaryngologist needs to enjoy working with children. Remember, however, that in most cases you will not be dealing directly with the children, but rather their parents. These subspecialists have to feel comfortable dealing with the concerned parents of small children, who often require a great deal of reassurance throughout the course of treatment. Pediatric otolaryngology is ideal for the person who seeks a steady supply of routine surgical cases, such as adenotonsillectomies and ear tubes, supplemented by a diverse mix of other procedures.

Rhinology—Allergy and Sinus

Sinus surgery and rhinology deal with the medical and surgical aspects of nasal and sinus disease, as well as disorders involving the anterior skull base. Common problems include nasal obstruction and smell disturbances, chronic sinusitis and rhinitis, allergies, proptosis, and medical and surgical disease involving the anterior skull base. The advent of surgical endoscopes and modern video imaging, coupled with advancements in 3D CT scan–guided surgical scopes and instruments, has revolutionized this very popular surgical subspecialty, which formerly depended on more invasive open surgical approaches with less cosmetically appealing results.

Functional endoscopic sinus surgery and septoplasty are the bread and butter of most rhinology practices. Rhinology fellows also become comfortable handling challenging surgical cases such as endoscopic approaches to tumors of the sella turcica (such as pituitary adenomas), orbital decompressions, frontal sinus surgery, repairs of cerebrospinal fluid leaks in the anterior skull base, and oncologic resection of sinonasal tumors. Due to their complexity, most general practice otolaryngologists will refer such cases to a rhinology specialist.

At present, the patients with rhinologic complaints are significantly more likely to receive surgical treatment than any other subspecialty within otolaryngology (insert numbers, citation). Given the comparatively high number of operative candidates, rhinology is an appealing practice for those who want to maximize their time in the operating room. Rhinology is also a good choice for those who enjoy the use of specialized equipment and technology. Technological advancements are flooding the discipline of rhinology, as newer minimally invasive endoscopic techniques and image-guidance surgeries are becoming increasingly popular.

Laryngology

Laryngeal fellowships are typically 1 year in duration and have become increasingly popular, especially for concentrated training in advanced microsurgical techniques of the larynx and management of the professional voice. The laryngology fellow becomes expert in the fascinating functional anatomy of the voice box, or larynx, and the disease processes that affect this organ system. Typical complaints encountered by the laryngologist include hoarseness (dysphonia), problems with swallowing (dysphagia), vocal cord weakness and paralysis, management of the professional voice, vocal cord polyps and masses, neoplasms of the larynx, and upper airway stenosis and obstruction. Recent advances in fiber optics and imaging technology coupled with sophisticated rehabilitation techniques have revolutionized this field.

Laryngology fellows become experts at flexible endoscopy, laryngeal stroboscopy, and electromyography. Specialized surgical cases handled by laryngologists include endoscopic and microsurgical evaluation and dissection of laryngeal polyps, nodules, and other lesions; laser surgery of laryngeal lesions and webs; permanent medialization procedures for vocal cord paralysis; and resection of laryngeal cancer, both endoscopically and via the neck in larger tumors. Many of the procedures performed in this discipline are office based and include temporary medialization of the paralyzed vocal cord and Botulinum toxin injections for spastic vocal cords.

Laryngology is primarily an office-based practice that tends to have more repeat customers than other subspecialties of otolaryngology. Professional singers, politicians, and others who use their voices on a daily basis provide for an interesting clientele. Laryngologists should also be open to working as a team, as many laryngologists see patients in tandem with a speech and language pathologist, who can assist in the initial fiber-optic evaluation of the upper aerodigestive tract and larynx.

Sleep Medicine and Surgery

Of all fellowship training options following otolaryngology training, these are relatively newer. They are 1- to 2-year fellowships offering specialized training in all aspects of medical and surgical sleep medicine. Fellows receive comprehensive clinical multidisciplinary exposure to sleep disorders, and receive intensive training in diagnostic and surgical advanced techniques. The full spectrum of sleep disorders is covered, ranging from those unique in infancy and childhood to those found in adulthood and aging, as well as translation of common sleep disorders as they manifest differently in children and adults. Sleep medicine and surgery fellowships are unique in that they are open to multiple specialties. They are designed for board-eligible physicians who have successfully completed an accredited residency training program in a relevant discipline (ie, neurology, psychology, internal medicine/pulmonary, pediatric pulmonary, or otolaryngology).

WHY CONSIDER A CAREER IN OTOLARYNGOLOGY?

Despite its highly specialized focus, otolaryngology requires a broad range of clinical skills in order to take care of the diverse patient population. With the exception of patients suffering from head and neck cancer, most patients are generally healthy and need outpatient surgical procedures. Of course, the anatomy of the head and neck region is challenging, complex, and thoroughly engaging. The intricate procedures in this specialty require a mastery of precise examination skills, hand–eye coordination, and manual dexterity. At the same time, otolaryngologists are also well-rounded professionals who enjoy teaching and conducting research, while still finding time to enjoy their lives outside of the hospital. For those medical students who are up to the challenge, otolaryngology is a specialty that will provide years of intellectual stimulation, technical challenges, and personal satisfaction.

ABOUT THE CONTRIBUTORS

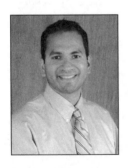 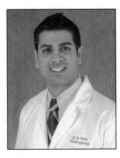

Drs Arjun Joshi and Neil Tanna completed residency training in otolaryngology—head and neck surgery at the George Washington University Hospital in Washington, DC.

Dr Joshi is assistant professor of surgery at The George Washington University. He graduated with honors from Cornell University. He attended medical school at the State University of New York—Upstate in Syracuse, where he was a member of the AOA honor society. Following his otolaryngology residency, Dr Joshi completed fellowship training in head and neck surgical oncology and microvascular reconstruction at the University of Alberta. He enjoys spending time with his wife and children and his personal interests include biking, camping, and international travel. He can be reached by e-mail at ajoshi@mfa.gwu.edu.

After completing otolaryngology training, Dr Tanna completed a plastic surgery residency at University of California, Los Angeles (UCLA). He also obtained fellowship training in microvascular and advanced reconstructive surgery at New York University (NYU). He received his medical and undergraduate degrees through an accelerated program at Rensselaer Polytechnic Institute and Albany Medical College. His clinical interests include reconstructive and aesthetic surgery. Dr Tanna is very grateful for the inspiration and support of his wife, family, and friends. He may be reached by e-mail at ntanna@gmail.com.

25

PATHOLOGY

Lisa Yerian and Edmunds Z. Reineks

Why would anyone want to become a pathologist? After all, their patients are already dead! For most people, pathology conjures up images of morgues, dead bodies, and jars of formaldehyde. Although forensics and autopsies are important elements of pathology, this specialty encompasses a much wider array of investigative arenas. Pathologists use the oldest diagnostic techniques (gross examination) while also developing the newest (multiplex real-time polymerase chain reaction or liquid chromatography–tandem mass spectrometry). By combining these clinical insights and laboratory advances, they remain at the forefront of diagnostic tools and medical discovery.

Pathology is exciting, multidimensional, and fundamental to medicine. Its limited patient interaction makes pathology an often-misunderstood field. Until recently, popular culture has not taken to glamorizing this medical specialty, which has led to pathology's rather low profile within society. No one writes novels about the heroic pathologist who spends hours poring over slides searching for cancer cells lurking under a lymph node capsule or searching for a compatible unit of blood for a patient with many antibodies from prior transfusions. Movies and television shows never portray the pathologist who saved a man's life by detecting a deadly sarcoma in a seemingly routine gangrenous toe specimen, or who identified a rare form of bacteria in a sputum specimen and averted a hospital outbreak. This is, in fact, what pathology is all about.

THE STUDY OF DISEASE AND ILLNESS

The practice of pathology involves the detection, analysis, and understanding of disease processes. As the only branch of medicine considered both a basic science

WHAT MAKES A GOOD PATHOLOGIST?

✓ Likes precise scientific evidence.
✓ Has excellent management and organizational skills.
✓ Is an independent, studious, and inquisitive person.
✓ Likes serving as a consultant to other physicians.
✓ Enjoys the challenge of difficult cases.

THE INSIDE SCOOP

and a clinical specialty, pathology is somewhat unique. By studying tissues, cells, and fluid samples, pathologists unravel the mysteries of how a particular disease arises and develops. To do so, they draw on a variety of methods, ranging from microbiology to molecular biology. All diseased tissues in the body express themselves through symptoms, signs, and laboratory abnormalities. Without the information provided by pathologists, most physicians would have difficulty interpreting their patients' clinical presentation and managing the progression of their illness.

The practice of pathology is divided into two primary areas—anatomic and clinical. *Anatomic pathologists* examine organs, tissues, and cells to diagnose or further characterize a disease process. They make exact diagnoses on specimens from sources including biopsy, fine-needle aspiration, body-fluid analysis, exfoliation, autopsy, and surgery—and the information they provide in the pathology report is used for patient prognostication and management. Anatomic pathologists typically love delving into gross and light microscopic examinations, immunohistochemistry, electron microscopy, and even molecular analyses in pursuit of the best diagnosis. Anatomic pathologists always have to be vigilant in their work. Each day, there is the possibility of discovering unexpected disease processes, and the ever-present risk of missing or misinterpreting an important abnormality.

Clinical pathologists analyze blood, body fluids, or other patient specimens. They are experts in the scientific principles and techniques of laboratory medicine as well as the administrative aspects of overseeing a laboratory. Most serve as laboratory directors at a hospital or independent laboratory, where they are also involved in issues of management and quality assurance. Clinical pathologists analyze quality control data to determine the sensitivity and specificity values of new diagnostic tests and serve as an important contact for clinicians seeking recommendations on the best test to confirm or exclude a particular diagnosis and how to interpret test results. To provide accurate and informative answers, clinical pathologists need a good understanding of how each laboratory test works and the pathophysiologic processes that can result in abnormal findings.

Pathologists, however, are more than experts on the abnormal—they are also intimately familiar with the normal state of health. Consider the following example: to detect cellular aberrations within a section of thyroid gland, pathologists mentally compare the specimen with their thorough understanding of normal thyroid morphology. Knowing healthy anatomic structure well is the most accurate way to recognize diseased states (and even yet-to-be-described pathologic conditions). Medical students interested in pathology, therefore, should focus their efforts during the biochemistry, cell biology, genetics, gross anatomy, and histology courses in order to develop a strong knowledge base in these areas, which provide the necessary framework on which pathologists expand their knowledge of human disease.

It is not always easy to achieve the noble goals of diagnosis, description, and advanced understanding of disease. A pathologist requires an exhaustive command of the current medical literature. They have to stay on top of the latest advances and make every effort to assimilate new information. For this reason, pathology tends to attract individuals who never feel satisfied that they know (or will ever master) enough medicine. You must be committed to a lifetime of learning. Most good pathologists are copious readers because they need to know more than just the common disease entities. Their medical colleagues expect them to be ready to discern zebras—unexpected or unusual findings—and the associated clinical implications. "Pathologists have to know just about everything there is to know about disease," commented a senior resident. This requirement makes pathology intellectually demanding, yet extremely rewarding.

AUTOPSY AND MICROSCOPY: TO SEE FOR ONESELF

In pathology, understanding is power. If you are the type of person who always asks "why," then you should definitely consider a career in pathology. Pathologists do not only rely on textbooks, journal articles, or dictated reports. Instead, they want to see for themselves exactly what is going on inside the body—deep in the tissues, within individual cells, in DNA, RNA, and proteins. This curiosity explains the emphasis on gross dissection (autopsy) and microscopic examination (histology). Using these skills, pathologists investigate a patient's disease process or the events leading to his or her death. They work methodically and diligently until a puzzle is solved and then move on to the next clinical enigma with great energy.

To appreciate disease for themselves, pathologists engage in a lot of hands-on analytical work. They handle diseased body parts, specimens, and pieces of tissue.

They dissect bodies, carefully section and examine organs, and select the best sections to be processed and made into slides for histologic evaluation. In fact, you may be surprised to discover that pathologists function just like all other physicians. They obtain patient histories (by reviewing medical records, police reports, and communications from other colleagues), perform internal and external physical examinations (on bodies and specimens), and order additional tests (including radiologic, genetic, toxicologic, and laboratory studies). These investigations yield multiple pieces of information that are integrated into the final diagnosis.

Pathologists like to solve problems by analyzing increasingly detailed levels of information. In an autopsy, the pathologist reviews the clinical history and then performs the postmortem gross examination. There are many reasons why pathologists study patients after their deaths. Many people die without a known reason; others have a primary diagnosis, but the exact cause of death remains a mystery. In a study of autopsy data, it was found that 48.8% of deceased patients were clinically misdiagnosed.[1] Over half (58%) of these clinical errors were major diagnoses that had been missed—if detected before death, a change in treatment may have lead to cure or prolonged survival. As the "ultimate measure of quality control in medical practice,"[2] the autopsy is essential for determining the extent of disease and the effectiveness of treatment. Autopsies enable physicians to evaluate diagnostic and therapeutic procedures so that they can prevent similar deaths and improve clinical outcomes. Of course, forensic autopsies also provide valuable information used to pursue justice. Medical examiners interpret the physical evidence to determine criminal causes of death (accidents vs homicides or suicides).

It is fascinating and humbling to see a human body inside and out. But this specialty has a greater scope than dissecting bodies in the morgue. Most of the anatomic pathology completed today, in fact, deals with tissues and specimens from people who are alive. Thanks to modern laboratory tests and imaging studies, many illness can be diagnosed clinically (ie, for diseases such as congestive heart failure). But many diseases do require a tissue diagnosis. This is why pathologists are also experts at microscopic analysis of specimens. For instance, they closely examine tissues sent directly from the operating room (frozen sections) to determine the presence of malignancy. When looking at cells under the microscope, one resident commented that "the best part about pathology is the minute in which you go from staring blankly at a field of pink and blue to suddenly 'reading' what is going on in the specimen and, therefore, in the patient's body." Combined with the autopsy, these techniques yield amazing insight into human anatomy, microscopic structure, biochemistry, and physiology.

MAKING CONFIDENT DECISIONS THAT CHANGE LIVES

Every day in hospitals across the country, pathologists make critical decisions that impact patient care. Their reports dictate the direction of a patient's treatment plan and, thereby, his or her life. The assessments are often difficult because pathologists grapple with a multitude of tough questions: Could the histologic pattern represent a follicular lymphoma or just a reactive lymph node? Does this child's bone marrow show evidence of acute leukemia, or are the cells simply immature lymphocytes (hematogones) normally present in a young patient? Are those malignant tumor cells sitting in a lymphatic channel or within an artifactual space? Is this electrolyte measurement "real," or does it represent a specimen handling error? How does one know if this result is correct?

Thoroughness, accuracy, and painstaking attention to detail are all essential to the practice of pathology. Keep in mind that the final pathology reports have huge consequences for the patient. Their conclusions determine, for instance, whether a teenager undergoes a risky bone marrow transplant or whether a middle-aged man loses his prostate gland. After consulting with the pathologist, an oncologist may decide to initiate chemotherapy, a neurosurgeon may stop operating on a brain tumor, and a general surgeon may completely remove a patients' colon. Misdiagnoses lead to unnecessary disability, increased morbidity, and sometimes even death.

Making these diagnostic decisions can be extremely difficult. Despite their poise and confidence, most pathologists humbly recognize their clinical limitations. They have to balance their own level of uncertainty with their desire to provide as much useful information as possible. Many times, they refrain from making a diagnosis (benign vs malignant, positive vs negative) if the specimen material is less than adequate. In these situations, under- or overdiagnosing a suspected lesion could yield catastrophic results for the patient. When additional information, such as new stains or antibody testing, becomes available, pathologists then adjust their diagnoses accordingly.

To provide the best patient care, pathologists regularly read, study, and know when to ask for help. When examining a specimen, they systematically think of every diagnosis a given abnormality could represent, from horses (common) to zebras (rare). They also have to determine whether a tissue sample is truly negative versus being nondiagnostic—two terms with distinct meanings and different consequences. Adding to this pressure, pathologists have to be certain that the patient's clinician understands all of the implications surrounding a diagnosis. For those interested in a career in pathology, expect some sleepless nights: "Did I make the right diagnosis?" "Did I undercall (or overcall) this biopsy?" "Did I miss anything?"

The true answer to the clinical question accompanying a specimen is not always clear. Sometimes, surgeons and other clinicians identify an expected diagnosis and try to compel the pathologist to make an unwarranted conclusion. Often this type of pressure occurs even when there is no evidence supporting the preferred diagnosis. Self-confidence is highly valued by surgeons, while recognition of one's limitations keeps patients (and pathologists) safe. Just because a clinician believes that a patient has a given disease does not mean that the pathologist has evidence to support its diagnosis. In the interest of patient care, pathologists stand firmly by their professional opinions, even in the face of disgruntled physicians and surgeons. They have to protect the patient from therapeutic interventions before firmly establishing a diagnosis (or lack thereof). In these cases, pathologists act as advocates for the patient.

On the flip side, a pathologist must be extremely careful if the clinician's preferred diagnosis fails to correlate with laboratory data or clinical differential diagnoses. For instance, mental alarms go off when histopathology appears inconsistent with radiologic or gross impressions, or when laboratory values do not correlate with clinical signs and symptoms. In these cases, pathologists proceed with caution. In the field of bone pathology, for example, this type of clinico-pathologic correlation is essential. Bone lesions have characteristic appearances on radiographic films, and many textbooks and experts therefore recommend that histologic diagnosis on bone lesions should never be rendered in isolation from the radiologic impression. During an intraoperative bone consultation, an accurate determination of benign versus malignancy could mean the difference between local resection and amputation!

PATHOLOGISTS AS CONSULTANTS

Pathologists do not spend their entire days holed up in laboratories and morgues. As experts on disease processes, they are routinely communicating with their colleagues. Whether in person, on the telephone, through a written report, or at a conference, pathologists discuss their patients with other physicians all the time. Every specimen arriving in the pathology department carries an accompanying clinical question, and a pathologist receives telephone consultations from doctors inquiring about the meaning of a lab value or pathologic finding. Whether the patient has an unusual neck mass or a surprising laboratory result, clinicians turn to pathologists for the answer. Sometimes the questions are not clear, and pathologists have to sort out the relevant clinical inquiry. Is it cancer? What type, grade, and stage? Are there additional features that help assess the patient's prognosis and potential response to therapy?

The famous physician Sir William Osler once referred to the pathologist as "the doctor's doctor." Every aspect of their clinical care is essentially a consultative service. Because of this advice-giving role, good communication skills (both oral and written) are of utmost importance. While making the best diagnosis, pathologists often struggle to state their findings in a clear, concise manner. They formulate comments that convey the relative significance of individual findings but never under- or overstate their degree of certainty. It is a challenging art form. "Communication skills are my currency with the clinicians," a senior faculty member in pathology remarked. "Other doctors cannot tell how good a pathologist is diagnostically. They only judge us on what they can—on our ability to communicate with them."

Because of this consultative role, pathology is a perfect specialty for medical students who appreciate precision in written and spoken language. Pathologists have to produce the most accurate and clearly written reports. They have to dictate each observation succinctly and in the proper format. For cases in which a diagnosis cannot be made, they must enumerate the relevant findings and the significance of each. If a possible diagnosis exists, the pathologist has to be cautious, never overstating their conviction. Like all fields of medicine, pathology is fraught with gray areas. Thus, in some cases, pathologists walk a fine line between under- and overinterpreting the findings. It is quite a challenge to submit final reports that are clinically useful yet do not overimply diagnostic certainty. Word selection and order become critical factors. As such, pathologists tend to be good writers, striving to develop precise and accurate reports.

THE DOCTOR–PATIENT RELATIONSHIP

Like other hospital-based physicians, such as those in radiology and anesthesiology, pathologists are anonymous, behind-the-scenes doctors. After all, most pathologists do not meet, talk with, or examine their patients in vivo. It is an unsuitable specialty for medical students wishing to meet patients, perform thorough history and physicals on their patients, and have intimate doctor–patient relationships. Although there are rare exceptions—bone marrow biopsy, fine needle aspiration, and plasmapheresis—in general, pathologists have little to no patient contact. Instead, pathology is perfect for those immensely satisfied by providing other physicians with the best thing possible—the most carefully considered, sweat-over, thoroughly analyzed, complete and accurate diagnosis.

Despite this lack of patient contact, pathologists are real doctors who always care about people. Indeed, many pathologists relate their personal need for distance from the patient as a reason for choosing pathology—because they are at risk of becoming *too* emotionally involved. Although seemingly invisible to their patients, their unique role allows them to make a big difference in patients' lives. One residency program director reiterated why pathologists are some of the most caring doctors around:

When I was in medical school, one of my patients died during a surgical procedure that I, pressured by my attendings and residents, advised the patient to have. After that point, I decided that never again would a person die because of something I said.

Although she wanted to avoid making life-or-death decisions in medicine, she ironically chose a specialty—breast pathology—where she makes these decisions every day. She pores over cases late into the night and through weekends, searching for foci of tumor invasion and double- and triple-checking resection margins to verify if the surgeon completely removed the tumor. A diagnosis of invasive malignancy sentences a patient to a dangerous and traumatic course of surgery, chemotherapy, and radiation. In fact, this pathologist cares about patients so much that she turned to a specialty in which she would not have to go through the emotional pain of directly interacting with patients, their fatal diseases, and their families. Many pathologists relate similar experiences and claim they chose pathology because they care "too much." They are so pained by the suffering of their patients that they cannot practice effectively. For many, pathology provides much needed distance from the emotional demands of patient interactions.

QUESTING FOR KNOWLEDGE: PATHOLOGY RESEARCH

In all fields of medicine (and especially pathology), the current textbooks are slightly behind and medical literature barely keeps up with the growing amount of clinical and basic science information. There is always much more to discover and learn. And the pathologist holds an ideal position to ask and answer probing questions about disease processes. Every day, pathologists are examining gross, histologic, cytologic, chemical, and molecular alterations. They have daily access to clinical material and are in regular direct communication with clinicians. Because of the integration of basic science and clinical consulting, pathologists have a distinct advantage in the area of translational research. As physician–researchers, pathologists maintain a special ability to identify the tissue, diagnosis, and cells in question. Today, with an ever-increasing number of molecular tests and techniques, researchers can detect subtle changes in human tissues and cells with ever-increasing levels of sensitivity and precision.

Pathologists advance our understanding of disease by studying tissues, cells, receptors, proteins, and genes, and their roles in disease. They analyze unusual findings, recognize patterns of disease, and make new connections between abnormal observations. They take new developments from laboratory bench research and test them for bedside utility. They develop new diagnostic tests and procedures, identify gene mutations and new disease entities, and study the pathogenesis of disease. In doing so, many pathologists either conduct their own research or collaborate with other researchers (MDs or PhDs). Through articles in scientific journals, together they bring the latest techniques to the forefront of clinical use. For these reasons and more, pathologists hold an optimal position to pursue descriptive and experimental research.

LIFESTYLE CONSIDERATIONS AND PRACTICE OPTIONS

A day in the life of a pathologist is difficult to describe, given the variation between different areas of specialty. For anatomic pathologists, a typical day includes performing gross evaluation of resection specimens, interpreting slides, writing (or dictating) and editing pathology reports, and communicating with clinicians on a formal and informal basis. For clinical pathologists, a typical day includes tasks related to overseeing clinical laboratory operations in addition to speaking with colleagues. For both types of pathologists, an academic setting also includes varying amounts of teaching and research. In general, though, the practice of pathology entails relatively controllable working hours. Compared with other specialists, pathologists have more employment opportunities that provide a good lifestyle for family and outside interests. Pathologists are rarely called into the hospital at late hours, and most practices employ a rotating "on-call" system with a designated individual carrying an institutional pager on a rotational basis with other pathologists in that hospital or practice group. The pathologist on call will provide after-hours consultation, answering questions, handling urgent laboratory issues, and reviewing specimens.

In anatomic pathology, intraoperative consultations (frozen sections) require a surgical pathologist to give an immediate tissue diagnosis. In the past that required the pathologist to go to the hospital, but an increasing number of practices

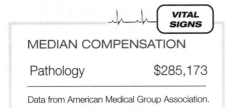

are employing telepathology to allow pathologists to interpret slides off-site. Most surgeries for which an intraoperative consultation is anticipated are scheduled as elective cases during the day. Sometimes, however, a late-night, weekend, or emergency surgery requires a pathologist to interpret the frozen section. In clinical pathology, high-priority overnight calls come in the form of urgent laboratory values that must be reported to the clinician who ordered the test. At other times, pathologists may have to confirm an abnormal finding that requires prompt therapeutic intervention, such as leukemic blasts in peripheral blood smear. Other late-night calls may involve rush advice on the best test to rule out a particular diagnosis, the best way to obtain a particular specimen, or administrative and managerial issues.

Pathologists can pursue a variety of practice options. Most work in private pathology practices, either at community hospitals or stand-alone laboratory centers. Clinical pathologists typically serve as laboratory directors, consulting to clinical services on challenging cases and making clinicopathologic diagnoses. Others work in regional or local independent laboratories. Some pathologists are employed directly by nonpathology group practices of physicians that perform many biopsies and have in-office laboratories (ie, urologists, gastroenterologists, and dermatologists).[3,4] A significant number, particularly those dedicated to careers in research and teaching, become faculty at medical schools and university teaching hospitals. Forensic pathologists typically work in city or county medical offices. Government, military, pharmaceutical, and biotechnology organizations make up the remaining group of employers. There are many exciting opportunities for pathologists in all avenues of practice. Some professional pathology organizations have forecast a shortage of pathologists for the future, but this view is controversial.[5] Other reports suggest a decline in private practice opportunities and a commoditization of pathology services by nonpathology physicians and/or large corporate labs.[6] This situation may have arisen due to an oversupply of pathology trainees.[7] Recent reports indicate that a substantial portion of fellows have difficulty obtaining jobs near the end of their training.[8] Medical students with an interest in pathology should investigate the employment landscape during their pathology rotation(s) through contact with many residents and fellows to base their impressions on primary evidence rather than biased sources or anecdotal reports.

FELLOWSHIPS AND SUBSPECIALTY TRAINING

Blood Banking and Transfusion Medicine

Blood banking specialists make sure that patients in the hospital receive safe blood products. Packed red blood cells, cryoprecipitate, and single donor platelets are some of the products under the expertise of the transfusion specialist. These pathologists oversee blood donation, pretransfusion testing of compatibility and blood-related antigens and antibodies, and selection of blood for transplant. Therapeutically, they manage transfusion reactions, plasmapheresis, exchange transfusions, and peripheral stem cell harvests. From kids with leukemia to adults with anemia, these pathologists have opportunities for patient contact and work closely with clinicians. In most hospitals, they often act as immunohematologists, procuring and processing blood products and tracing the causes of transfusion reactions.

Clinical Chemistry

Did you particularly enjoy biochemistry class? These pathologists draw on their expertise of biochemical processes to diagnose, confirm, and monitor a patient's disease status. They use sophisticated tests that quantify levels of many inorganic substances in body fluids—electrolytes, gases, glucose, proteins such as tumor markers and cardiac biomarkers, and hormones. Clinical chemists apply this biochemical data to understand the cause and progress of disease in the human body. Toxicology is also an important part of chemical pathology, including therapeutic drug monitoring and detection of illegal drugs or poisons. As supervisors of laboratory technicians, clinical chemists assure timely and accurate measurements through a tight system of quality control.

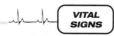

VITAL SIGNS

PATHOLOGY
2011 MATCH STATISTICS

- Number of positions available: 518
- 289 US seniors and 487 independent applicants ranked at least one pathology program
- 91.2% of all positions were filled in the initial Match
- The successful applicants: 56.5% US seniors, 30.5% foreign-trained physicians, and 7.1% osteopathic graduates
- Mean USMLE Step I score: 226
- Unmatched rate for US seniors applying only to pathology: 3.4%

Data from National Resident Matching Program.

Cytopathology

Rather than examining whole tissue sections, cytopathologists study individual cells obtained from fluid samplings, secretions, fine-needle aspirations, scrapings, and mucosal brushings. In the pursuit of a diagnosis, these specialists draw on techniques of cytochemistry, immunocytochemistry, and molecular techniques in addition to standard light microscopy. They look closely at the nucleus, cytoplasm, cellular adhesion and architectural features, and the background material (mucin, colloid, debris, etc). The Papanicalou test ("Papsmear")—the shining star of cytopathology—still remains the best cancer-screening tool ever invented. These pathologists must also stay current on molecular techniques, which are playing an increasing role in this field. Cytopathologists examine thousands of cervical screening tests and save many women's lives.

Dermatopathology

Dermatopathologists are experts in diagnosing diseases of the skin. Certification in this subspecialty is under joint responsibility of the American Board of Pathology and the American Board of Dermatology. Dermatopathologists may undergo residency training in dermatology or in pathology, and as dermatopathology fellows, they become specially trained in various forms of microscopy (light, electron, and fluorescence). Dermatopathologists work closely with their colleagues in dermatology to diagnose infectious, inflammatory, and malignant processes, and many dermatopathologists actually see patients.

RESIDENCY TRAINING

Residency programs in pathology vary in length, depending on whether one chooses to complete training in anatomic pathology (3 years), clinical pathology (3 years), or both (4 years). There are currently 151 accredited programs, mainly in combined anatomic and clinical pathology. Pathology does not require a medical or transitional internship year. During residency, physicians typically do not take in-house call, but rather go home every night and return to the hospital during the night if needed. Much of the training emphasizes

(continued)

Forensic Pathology

Every day, in the hospital, at home, in the workplace, in public places, and on the streets, people die. Some deaths are expected, while others are unexplained, occur under suspicious circumstances, or may be secondary to trauma, homicide, or

suicide. The role of the forensic pathologist is to properly classify deaths as natural or unnatural, and if unnatural, as
accident, homicide, or suicide. They establish the cause of death through gross
inspection, microscopy, toxicology tests,
and crime laboratory methods. In addition to performing autopsies and writing
the official report, they also testify in court.
In some cases, the forensic pathologist
even visits the crime scene to conduct an
investigation. Many forensic pathologists
serve as chief or deputy medical examiners of a city or county.

Hematopathology

Hematopathologists draw on an extensive array of techniques to examine a

reading and self-study. Typical
anatomic pathology rotations
include surgical pathology,
cytopathology, autopsy, and
forensic pathology. Typical clinical
pathology rotations include clinical
chemistry, microbiology, transfusion medicine, hematopathology,
coagulation medicine, and
immunology. Fellowships in
pathology last 1 to 2 additional
years and many fellowship
programs lead to a special
qualifications certificate.

THE INSIDE SCOOP

specimen. These specialists are experts in diseases of the lymph nodes and bone
marrow, such as leukemias and lymphomas. They examine bone marrow samples from patients and review abnormal blood smears for malignancy, infection,
and anemia. They integrate gross and microscopic examinations with information derived from clinical hematology, flow cytometry, immunohistochemistry,
cytogenetics, and molecular laboratories. Hematopathologists work closely with
their colleagues in medical hematology–oncology. Together, they integrate laboratory testing and clinical data in the diagnostic workup and disease monitoring
of patients with leukemias, lymphomas, and bleeding disorders.

Informatics

Informatics is a newer specialty, with only a handful of fellowships currently
available in academic pathology departments. The official recognition of the
specialty, known as "Clinical Informatics," was announced by the American Board
of Medical Specialties in October, 2011. It is projected that the certification will
be available through the American Board of Pathology as well as the American
Board of Preventive Medicine. This specialty is a natural fit for pathology, since
in many hospitals, the laboratory information system (LIS) provides the bulk of

the data in the patients' electronic medical records in the hospital information system (HIS), consisting of pathology reports and laboratory test results. In the genomic era, the ability to organize, store, retrieve, and interpret vast amounts of data and apply it appropriately for clinical purposes is likely a valuable skill for pathologists to establish and maintain.

Medical Microbiology

Enjoy looking at bacteria, viruses, parasites, and fungi? Medical microbiologists strive for efficient isolation and accurate laboratory diagnosis of infectious diseases. They are trained not only in the principles used to establish diagnosis but also in the correlation of culture results with the clinical setting. In addition to culturing and classifying organisms, microbiologists also utilize in vitro antimicrobial susceptibility testing. Also, molecular testing has increasingly become a useful tool in virology and microbiology studies. Microbiologists also participate in epidemiologic studies and hospital infection control procedures, and they may be called upon to review the significance of a particular isolate and treatment recommendations.

Molecular Genetic Pathology/Cytogenetics

If you like the latest, coolest techniques in molecular biology as they apply to human disease, this is the subspecialty for you. These pathologists apply molecular methods, such as fluorescent in situ hybridization, polymerase chain reaction, and gene sequencing, to analyze abnormal cells at the level of DNA and RNA. Tests offered by the molecular diagnostics laboratory include virus and bacterial detection and identification, mutational analysis for genetic counseling, and evaluation for clonality and translocations. Cytogeneticists study chromosomes to look for abnormal number and structure for primary diagnosis and to monitor disease status. Prenatal, constitutional, and cancer cytogenetic analysis provide information that is widely used in many fields of medicine.

Neuropathology

Neuropathologists specialize in the study of diseases of the central and peripheral nervous systems and their related tissues. They also often review muscle biopsies in the workup and diagnosis of myopathies, neuropathies, and neuromuscular disorders. Much of their work centers on gross and histologic examination of specimen material. Yet, in the complete workup of a case, neuropathologists may review MRI and CT scans and employ immunohistochemistry, molecular testing, and electron microscopy.

Pediatric Pathology

Pediatric pathologists specialize in the diagnosis and study of diseases of the developing human embryo, fetus, and child. This broad area of pathology encompasses disorders of early development (including embryology, placentology, and teratology), gestational and perinatal diseases, inherited diseases, and diseases of childhood. They often practice both surgical and autopsy pathology, reviewing surgical biopsy, prenatal, and autopsy specimens.

Surgical Pathology

Surgical pathologists make histologic diagnoses based on tissue sections from biopsy and surgical resection specimens. As a consultant to clinicians, their most acute role occurs during the urgent, intraoperative frozen section. Freezing the tissue permits thin sectioning so that microscopic analysis can be performed within minutes while the patient is in the operating room. Surgeons need these pathologists to answer a variety of questions: What is the diagnosis? Is it cancer? Should we perform a more extensive resection? Are lymph nodes involved? Is the malignancy totally excised? Have we obtained enough tissue to complete the diagnostic workup? A key skill is the pathologist's ability to recognize or determine the key questions to be answered with every frozen diagnosis requested. Most surgical pathology work is done via "routine" (not frozen) tissue analysis. In addition to tissue diagnostics, surgical pathologists develop new classification systems, describe new disease entities, and test prognostic and diagnostic markers. Surgical pathology offers a variety of fellowship opportunities in virtually every organ system: neuropathology, dermatopathology, hematopathology/lymphoma, gastrointestinal/liver pathology, breast pathology, lung, cardiac pathology, head and neck pathology, bone and soft tissue pathology, renal pathology, genitourinary pathology, obstetric–gynecologic pathology, and endocrine pathology. Subspecialty training in an area of surgical pathology provides additional time to study, refine diagnostic skills, and pursue research.

WHY CONSIDER A CAREER IN PATHOLOGY?

Consider a career in pathology because you are prepared to have patients' diagnoses—and consequently treatment—rest in your hands. Choose pathology because you like to be precise in your words and exacting in your diagnoses. Choose pathology because you are vigilant in your work and tireless in your commitment to arriving at the best diagnosis for your patient. Choose pathology because you want to help each patient by guiding his or her care with your knowledge, experience, and wisdom. Choose pathology because you feel inspired rather than intimidated by the vast amount of knowledge you must acquire and continue to have at your fingertips throughout your career. Choose pathology because you want an intellectually rigorous specialty. Choose pathology because you want to use your knowledge to make observations, to ask questions, and, in doing so, to contribute to medical knowledge.

Pathology is a fundamental discipline of medicine, requiring a broad mastery of basic and clinical sciences. The practice of pathology requires you to retain your knowledge of pathophysiology from medical school education and build upon that knowledge to understand disease processes at ever-increasing levels of complexity. As physicians, consultants, and researchers all in one, pathologists contribute to patient care by making diagnoses and guiding therapeutic intervention. They are educators who impart their knowledge and understanding to their colleagues. Pathologists are real doctors who are simply fascinated by disease and its cellular processes.

One pathologist commented, "pathology is a versatile specialty that may not have been 'found' by many. Certainly those who have found it love it."[2] If you enjoy delving into scientific mystery and prefer the science of medicine over direct patient care, then consider becoming a part of the select group that have found their niche within this specialty.

ABOUT THE CONTRIBUTORS

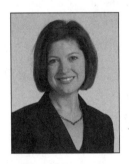 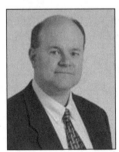

Dr Lisa Marie Yerian recently completed pathology residency training and fellowship in gastrointestinal and liver pathology at the University of Chicago Hospitals. She is now a gastrointestinal and liver pathologist at the Cleveland Clinic. Dr Yerian earned her BS in biology at the University of Notre Dame and attended medical school at the University of Chicago—Pritzker School of Medicine. In her free time, Dr Yerian enjoys trail running and cooking (the kitchen is her second laboratory). She can be reached by e-mail at yerianl@ccf.org.

Edmunds Reineks, MD, PhD, earned his BS in physics and served as an engineering division officer in the US Navy aboard the USS California (CGN-36). He then completed premed coursework at the University of Washington (Seattle) and pursued medical and graduate studies at Case Western Reserve University (Cleveland). He completed pathology residency training at University Hospitals of Cleveland and a fellowship in clinical chemistry at the Cleveland Clinic. He works at the Cleveland Clinic as medical director of the automated chemistry lab and point-of-care testing.

REFERENCES

1. Bayer-Garner, I.B., Fink, L.M., et al. Pathologists in a teaching institution assess the value of the autopsy. *Arch Pathol Lab Med.* 2002;126:442–447.

2. Walsh, M.J. Pathology: The "unloved" specialty. *Can Med Assoc J.* 1993;149(8):1078–1079.

3. In Office Pathology. Accessed January 9, 2012; http://www.iopathology.com/agreements.php.

4. Pernick, N. (ed.). Pathology Outlines. Accessed January 9, 2012; published March 2011; http://www.pathologyoutlines.com/management/vachette201103b.html.

5. College of American Pathologists. Accessed January 9, 2012; published February 26, 2011; http://www.cap.org/apps/docs/pathology_residents/pdf/joint_session_presentation_slides.pdf.

6. Pernick, N. (ed.). Pathology Outlines. Accessed January 9, 2012; published March 2005; http://www.pathologyoutlines.com/management/ness200503.html.

7. The Student Doctor Network. Accessed January 9, 2012; http://forums.studentdoctor.net/showthread.php?t=868089.

8. Rinder, H.M., Wagner, J. *2011ACSP Fellowship and Job Market Surveys: A Report on the RISE, FISE, FISHE, and TMISE Surveys*; Available online at http://www.ascp.org/PDF/Fellowship-Reports/2011-ASCP-Fellowship-Job-Market-Surveys.pdf.

26
PEDIATRICS

Aaron J. Miller

In nineteenth-century England, before the advent of pasteurized milk, immunizations, intravenous hydration, or antibiotics, half of all children died before reaching their fifth birthday.[1] George Armstrong, a prominent physician of this time, described in his *Account of the Diseases Most Incident in Children* (1808) how the specialty of pediatrics was quite literally still in its infancy, with many doctors simply afraid to take care of infants and children:

I have heard an eminent physician say, that he never wished to be called in to a young child; because he was really at a loss to know what to order for it. Nay, I am told, that there is nothing to be done for children when they are ill.[1]

Clearly, the medical care of children has come a long way. In addition to the primary care and preventive medicine of general pediatrics, pediatricians can choose to focus on acute problems requiring immediate treatment (critical care, neonatology, emergency medicine) or a wide range of technical procedures (cardiology, pulmonology, gastroenterology). With such a wide variety of career options, considering a career in pediatrics starts with one not-so-simple question: Do you like kids?

CARING FOR CHILDREN AND YOUNG ADULTS

Pediatrics is the specialty of medicine that focuses on the comprehensive care of children—beginning from birth and continuing through the adolescent years. Yes, kids are cute, innocent, and fun, and most will get better. But children also rarely explain their symptoms, know several ways to soil your clothing, have parents who can be frustrated and angry, and sometimes, sadly, do not get better. It is important

WHAT MAKES A GOOD PEDIATRICIAN?

✓ Has a particular interest in children.
✓ Enjoys extensive patient contact.
✓ Is a laid-back, sensitive, and good-natured person.
✓ Likes working with his or her mind.
✓ Prefers taking care of a healthier patient population.

THE INSIDE SCOOP

to note that caring for kids is not just about treating their physical and medical problems. Every good pediatrician also addresses the mental and emotional health of his or her patients, which is equally as important as organic disease.

Most pediatricians practice general pediatrics, which particularly involves a lot of health maintenance and preventive medicine. It is your crucial job to make sure the child is developing appropriately, reaching each milestone, and otherwise healthy. Without you catching if there is anything wrong, the child could have serious health problems as an adult. In the outpatient setting, the emphasis is on growth, development, diagnosis of acute and chronic illness, parent education, and child advocacy. The inpatient setting also covers a wide range of medical and social issues, from respiratory distress in preemies to head trauma in adolescents.

General pediatricians enjoy the challenge of being proficient in a wide range of topics. Many diseases of adulthood first present in infancy and childhood with just a few vague symptoms, and the general pediatrician must know the initial workup and then when to consult subspecialists. For example, a patient who is not gaining weight has a wide differential diagnosis including gastroesophageal reflux, celiac disease, Hirschsprung disease, inflammatory bowel disease, congenital heart disease, hypothyroidism, cerebral palsy, neglect, cystic fibrosis, tuberculosis, HIV, urinary tract infection, renal disease, metabolic disease, eating disorders, collagen vascular disease, and malignancy. The pediatrician keeps the wide differential diagnosis in mind when taking the first steps, obtaining consults when necessary, and making sure that every last test and lab result is being followed up. During sick visits, your skills in diagnosis are critical as you decide which kids will improve on their own and which kids are truly sick and need further attention.

HOW TO BE A GOOD PEDIATRICIAN

The keys to caring for children and enjoying the field of pediatrics do not always come naturally. Medical students with any interest in kids should take full advantage of their core clerkship and learn as much as they can from the residents and attending physicians. By getting an inside glimpse into the skills required to care for children, you will quickly figure out whether or not pediatrics is the right match.

For both office visits and admissions to the hospital, all pediatricians first have to establish a good rapport with the child and his or her parents. A rushed introduction keeps the child and parents on edge, making the examination difficult and harder to gain their trust. From the moment you walk in to the room, set the tone by going straight to the child and introducing yourself with your first name. Kids are usually apprehensive about meeting doctors, and if you introduce yourself to the parents first, it reaffirms their fear that the physician is there to talk about "something bad" that is going on. You then look at the child and parents to gauge their level of anxiety and worry. Especially if the diagnosis or prognosis is unknown, pediatricians have to use more concrete reasoning—with a focus on the facts—with both parent and child.

After introductions, it is important to convey empathy for what the child and the parents are experiencing. Even a simple affirmation—"you guys must be exhausted"—goes a long way toward helping both parties feel like their concerns, anxiety, and needs are well understood. If the situation is not too tense, pediatricians look to break the ice by asking the child to "give a high-five" or asking the teenager about their career aspirations. When children perceive that their doctor is a fun, laid-back kind of person, they feel much more relaxed and at ease.

After obtaining a complete history, pediatricians begin the second important part of their evaluation: the physical examination. Often this starts by taking a minute to observe how the child looks in a parent's arms or in his bed. A child can convey a great deal of subtle clinical information to the physician in these moments of quiet and tranquility. For example, a toddler admitted for a cough might cry at a rate of 28 breaths per minute (which is normal) but may be loud enough to conceal abnormal findings such as wheezes and rhonchi. Giving this child a few minutes to calm down, however, could reveal a breathing rate of 50, indicating respiratory distress. In this case, pediatricians often wait until the patient has relaxed (and does not have those large breaths or that surge of adrenaline helping her) before an examination.

Pediatricians are very careful to make sure that they obtain an accurate physical examination. To help keep a scared child at ease, they playfully hand children their stethoscope, or have their mother put it on their chest. Especially when examining infants and toddlers, pediatricians know to check their ears and throat last. Any initial cooperation quickly dissolves as soon as the doctor grabs that otoscope and tongue depressor. This is important because pediatricians, as excellent diagnosticians of abnormal heart sounds, must always listen carefully to the child's heart. After all, 1% of children are born with major congenital heart lesions, including atrial and ventricular septal defects, obstructive lesions, and cyanotic heart disease.[2] Because nearly half of all children will have a murmur at some point in their life, your cardiac examination skills play a crucial role in diagnosing sick children and, likewise, in preventing many needless referrals.[3]

When discussing the options for treatment, pediatricians have to assume the role of educator. They not only explain the potential therapy choices to the parents but also have to draw on their creativity to explain it to the child in an understandable way. Children and their parents come to their pediatrician in their most vulnerable moments—physically and emotionally—and they need someone who places their issues into perspective and explains why a certain plan of action is best.

WORKING WITH CHILDREN AND THEIR PARENTS

Medical students often wonder about the special relationship between children's parents (the "second patient") and their pediatrician. At certain times, you will grow frustrated because you are dealing with parents who have become overly demanding. In the inpatient setting, there is little difference between pediatric patients and adult patients—both will have family members whose anger will test your patience. In the outpatient setting, where most kids are healthy, you will have fewer of these encounters, but each one will still require you to understand the bigger picture.

Although the parents of sick children can become frustrated or angry, pediatricians can still help alleviate their concerns. The parents' anger is mostly based on a fear of the unknown, often made worse due to exhaustion from being up all night, and the fear that they are not being listened to or are not being informed of the current plan of diagnosis and treatment. All pediatricians know that a few minutes spent listening intently and acknowledging their experience will bring a strong sense of relief and trust.

Although the pediatrician–parent relationship can be challenging at times, there is nothing quite like the privilege of caring for their children. It takes more than just liking kids to be a good pediatrician. Because children are often hesitant to explain their symptoms, you must be able to approach them on their level to connect with them. Kids are fun. Their energy and enthusiasm are very refreshing. After settling the pressing medical issues at hand, at least for the moment, pediatricians look for any opportunity to make the child smile. Kidding around and being playful is just a part of your job. Have fun with it. And at the end of the day, when you are tired from having dealt with this battle and that, there is nothing quite as fulfilling as knowing that you have helped a young, innocent child.

Not everything, however, about pediatrics is easy, fun, and rosy. It is particularly tough to cope with the death of one of your young patients. Unlike adults, who sometimes can accept death if they have "lived a complete life," a child's death is always sad. Your heart goes out most to the family, because you know that the loss you are feeling is only a fraction of the loss that is hitting them. It is a time of quiet and reflection. Your empathy and patience will help in being the foundation as they begin their process of grieving and healing. Although some kids do not get better from their illness, fortunately very few children die. In fact, the overall mortality rate of children in the United States, from birth to 19 years, is 0.07%.[4] The neonatal and pediatric intensive care units, where deaths most frequently occur, draw physicians who are strong enough to deal with the loss of a patient on a regular basis.

BEING AN ADVOCATE FOR CHILDREN

In every field of medicine, physicians act as advocates for their patients. This role is especially important in pediatrics, where your patients are only beginning to find their voice. With every new issue, pediatricians are always asking themselves, "What is it that brought this child here?" and more specifically, "What are the family dynamics at home and the living conditions that may have contributed to this issue?" Whether taking a careful history when a child suffers a burn, working with community leaders to make homes safer, or just asking about environmental exposures for a child with asthma, pediatricians are always looking for answers that will make a real difference in a child's life.

The American Academy of Pediatrics (AAP), which has always advocated on children's behalf, was originally founded in response to the government's inadequate policies on child health. Under the Sheppard-Towner Act of 1921, the federal government aimed to reduce infant and child mortality by creating matching grants for states to provide teaching to new mothers and frequent health visits for their newborns. As one of the first movements to provide health care for the poor, the program was seen as "an imported socialistic scheme" by certain members of the American Medical Association (AMA) and the government. In 1929, the law was repealed, and tensions rose. Seeing that the needs of children were being neglected, a group of pediatricians split away from the AMA in 1930 and formed the AAP.

Pediatricians today have many avenues to focus their energy. Clinical research, community involvement, acute care settings, and the office all provide opportunities for pediatricians to find their own niche to do what they do best: care for children.

LIFESTYLE CONSIDERATIONS AND PRACTICE OPTIONS

In general, pediatricians lead busy but manageable lives. However, the hours worked and amount of call taken vary greatly among practice settings and pediatric subspecialists. General pediatricians in ambulatory settings work 4 or 5 days a week and are on call for parents' phone calls on a regular basis. Some of the middle-of-the-night phone calls can become tiring over time, but pediatricians who spend more time educating their anxious parents during office visits will end up sleeping much better.

Private practice is a great setting for those who like to make the big decisions about where, when, and how a practice will run. Going into solo practice is still possible, but many pediatricians choose to join a group practice. The group can hire you as a general employee, or you can be hired for a partnership track. This track usually consists of working for them for a year, then, if it goes well, buying into the practice. Being a partner adds another layer of challenges, but allows more freedom. You will have equal say in every issue, from leasing office space and hiring support staff to deciding which insurance plans you will accept and which lab tests should be run in your office.

The majority of childhood illnesses can be handled during office hours set aside for sick visits. If the child needs more attention, however, your role in the emergency department (ED) remains very important. Many EDs today are staffed by pediatricians, allowing you to take part in the patient's progress on the phone and arrange for prompt follow-up. In some suburban and rural hospitals, however, the ED is staffed by adult physicians who do not feel comfortable performing procedures such as lumbar punctures on newborns. Pediatricians sometimes have to come in during the middle of the night to perform these procedures. In addition, you may also be called in to attend cesarean section deliveries. Although most hospitals have nurse practitioners or

VITAL SIGNS

MEDIAN COMPENSATION

Allergy and immunology	$195,973
Cardiology	$244,944
Endocrinology	$185,901
Gastroenterology	$236,700
General pediatrics	$202,832
Hematology–oncology	$205,099
Infectious disease	$199,165
Neonatology	$265,000
Nephrology	$217,767
Neurology	$209,955
Critical care	$256,913

Data from American Medical Group Association.

residents to cover all deliveries, some rely on private pediatricians to take regular call.

In a group practice, all physician members take alternate turns going to the hospital to round on the group's inpatients. The morning starts in the nursery, meeting new babies and their families, and then moves to the general floor. Rounds usually finish before noon, in time for you to go back to the office and see afternoon appointments.

Hospital-based clinics and health maintenance organizations (HMOs) are good positions for pediatricians who do not want to deal with every last detail of the business side of a practice. These offices are just as fast-paced as private offices. Many contracts with hospital-based clinics require the pediatrician to spend 1 month per year as the attending on the hospital's general floor. This month serves as a nice break from the day-to-day work of the office and offers an opportunity to work with a wider circle of colleagues and learn more about how to handle certain disease processes.

As the entire field of medicine has specialized, more hospitals have begun hiring pediatricians to be the full-time attending of service on the general pediatric floor. They are known as hospitalists. This position is especially good for those who enjoy a more acute setting where kids are sicker and need more immediate workups to diagnose their illness. Many cases can be handled by you, the general pediatrician. In a tertiary care center, where patients have many more chronic and complex conditions, the general pediatricians then assume the role of the team leader, working with specialists on a daily basis and learning from their input the important information that will help make a diagnosis and treat the sick child.

VITAL SIGNS

PEDIATRICS 2011 MATCH STATISTICS

- Number of positions available: 2482
- 1988 US seniors and 1819 independent applicants ranked at least one pediatrics program
- 98.2% of all positions were filled in the initial Match
- The successful applicants: 72.5% US seniors, 16.7% foreign-trained physicians, and 9.3% osteopathic graduates
- Mean USMLE Step I score: 221
- Unmatched rate for US seniors applying only to pediatrics: 2.5%

Data from National Resident Matching Program.

RESIDENCY TRAINING

Residency in pediatrics requires 3 years of postgraduate training. There are currently 199 accredited programs (excluding combined programs with other specialties). Residency programs are offered by both academic medical centers and community hospitals. The training includes experience in both general pediatrics and subspecialty areas. It is a rigorous program, requiring in-house overnight call every third to fourth night while on an inpatient rotation. Rotations in general pediatrics, subspecialties (consults and clinic), intensive care (pediatric and neonatal), nursery, and emergency medicine are required. Because of the current emphasis on primary care, one-third of the residency curriculum must take place in an ambulatory setting. All residents spend one-half day per week in a continuity clinic where they manage their own panel of patients over the course of 3 years. The decision to subspecialize and apply for fellowships typically occurs during the second year of residency.

THE INSIDE SCOOP

FELLOWSHIPS AND SUBSPECIALTY TRAINING

The many subspecialty areas within pediatrics are great for those physicians who want to know everything about a particular focused topic. In the past decade, there have been multitudes of advances in scientific research. In particular, doctors and scientists are studying the early childhood roots of many chronic adult illnesses, providing plenty of exciting new prospects for early diagnosis and treatment. Many pediatrics subspecialists eventually choose to stay in an academic setting, where their time is split between clinical work, teaching, and research. A growing number of subspecialists, however, are taking their skills into private practice.

Except where noted, each of the following fellowships requires 3 full years and leads to official board certification. In general, the first year is full of clinical work—with long hours spent on the wards—and the last 2 years are mostly research based with the occasional overnight call.

Adolescent Medicine

This subspecialty is a great field for those who want to become advocates and give advice to an age group that really needs it the most. For most teenagers, these years are the healthiest ones in their lives. They have outgrown many childhood illnesses and their body is years away from starting to wear out—but they still struggle with many important issues, including school performance, sexuality, substance abuse, sexually transmitted diseases, pregnancy, depression, and more. For many of your patients, you will be the only adult with whom they feel comfortable talking about their issues. Every encounter with them is an opportunity to validate their feelings and experiences, letting them know they are sane for feeling as they do, and that they should still aim high and chase after their dreams.

A fellowship in adolescent medicine can be entered from both pediatrics and internal medicine. The pediatrician is more familiar with how they got where they are, and the internist is more familiar with where they are headed. Either way, you will become an expert in helping young adults to achieve their full potential.

Allergy and Immunology

This subspecialty offers a relaxed practice setting in which you apply the concepts of immunology to real patient problems. You will be consulted to evaluate infants and children with disorders such as eczema, unexplained episodes of anaphylaxis, frequent sicknesses or rare diseases, failure to thrive, and vomiting or diarrhea that has not responded to initial treatment. This field also offers leading areas of research, where almost every day new forms of immunotherapy are coming forward to help treat immune-mediated disease. A fellowship in allergy and immunology lasts 2 years and qualifies the subspecialist to treat both adults and children.

Cardiology

Cardiology is a busy, exciting field in which you gain expertise in a wide range of technical skills. To diagnose complex congenital heart disease, these subspecialists perform many echocardiograms (an ultrasound of the heart) and cardiac catheterizations (threading catheters into the heart to define its anatomy through fluoroscopy). They also manage pacemakers and cardiac arrhythmias. Of all pediatric subspecialists who remain at an academic medical center, cardiologists often have the longest hours, working closely with cardiac surgeons and pediatric intensive care unit staff to manage complex cardiac disease. For those who maintain more of an office setting, referrals come in for evaluation of new murmurs, chest pain, syncope, and palpitations. Although many times these symptoms end up not being related to the heart, there will be a significant number of children you will diagnose with arrhythmias such as the Wolff–Parkinson–White syndrome and structural abnormalities such as patent ductus arteriosus.

Child Abuse Pediatrics

Child abuse pediatrics, is an intense field in which the pediatrician becomes a medical expert on questions of abuse and neglect. You learn the intricacies of interviewing a child who might reveal a story of molestation, while being careful not to ask leading questions. You act as a consultant to lawyers and are occasionally called to testify in criminal or family court. The medical side of this subspecialty includes evaluating fractures, intracranial and retinal hemorrhages, sudden infant death syndrome, burns, ingestions, sexually transmitted infections, abnormal genitalia, rashes, and Munchausen syndrome by proxy. Many child abuse pediatricians also have interests in researching the incidence and mechanism of accidental injuries in children, which can be mistaken for abuse, and work with leaders in the community to find more effective ways to make homes safe and avoid harmful injuries.

Critical Care Medicine

Critical care medicine is the perfect fit for pediatricians who prefer an acute fix-it-now-type setting. These subspecialists perform lots of procedures such as placing chest tubes, central lines, and endotracheal tubes. They are the experts of physiology and medicine as managers of the ventilators, ventriculostomies, and invasive heart monitors. The ability to think quickly is of paramount importance as they assess and treat patients suffering from head trauma, postoperative cardiac surgery with complex physiology, sepsis, severe asthma, end-stage cancer, and more. Critical care pediatricians also must have a great deal of compassion, sympathy, and the ability to speak with families when their child is dying. The death of a child is especially sad, and parents cope with this tragedy with fear, anger, and frustration. Your empathy and patience help serve as the foundation for their process of grieving, healing, and coming to terms with the loss they are about to experience.

At academic centers, critical care specialists are on service about 2 weeks per month and sometimes need to stay long hours when there are very complicated cases. Other institutions are structured with shift work, allowing very predictable hours.

Developmental–Behavioral Pediatrics

Specialists in development and behavior have a keen eye for subtleties in child behavior. With infants, they first rule out any concurrent medical causes for a given delay and then perform a careful assessment so that appropriate referrals for speech, occupational, or physical therapy can be made. Infants who are at risk for delays should also be referred to developmentalists, including those born prematurely, who had congenital heart disease or meningitis, or who experienced any other event that may have temporarily impaired oxygen flow to the brain.

Older children with learning issues in school can also benefit from seeing a developmentalist. Although the general pediatrician should feel comfortable diagnosing and treating attention-deficit hyperactivity disorder, some children may have receptive or expressive deficits at the root of their problem that, if diagnosed, could lead to more effective strategies for therapy. Currently, a fellowship in developmental pediatrics lasts 3 years. In the near future, this fellowship will become part of a 6-year residency leading to triple board certification in pediatrics, neurology, and development.

Emergency Medicine

Emergency medicine attracts those who enjoy the challenge of a totally undiagnosed patient needing immediate attention. They must be comfortable knowing every type of disease presentation and form of trauma. After stabilizing the patient's airway, breathing, and circulation, the physician moves immediately to diagnosis and treatment. With patients who are more stable, the pediatrician must have strong clinical skills to assess how ill a patient truly is, and whether it is safe for them to go home. When a patient is nonverbal, this decision can be difficult. Similar to adult emergency medicine, this subspecialty carries a higher rate of malpractice lawsuits. These suits come more often from frustration and occur less often with physicians who take a quick minute to sit down during the history taking, helping the parents feel that they are receiving the doctor's full attention.

One of the advantages of emergency medicine is the flexibility in work schedule. If you are a mother or father and only want to work part time, you can earn a very good salary working just two or three 12-hour shifts per week.

Endocrinology

Endocrinologists love hormones. On a daily basis, they focus on the biochemistry of the human body and how it relates to thyroid function, calcium deposition, menses, extreme obesity, genital ambiguity, secondary sex characteristics, insulin-dependent and insulin-resistant diabetes mellitus, short stature, and more. With so much groundbreaking research in medicine today happening at the biochemical level with cell receptors and manipulation of DNA, endocrinology has become a field rich with opportunity for research and development.

Gastroenterology

From infants who are failing to thrive to teenagers with possible signs of in-flammatory bowel disease, the gastroenterologist plays an integral role in tough cases where a diagnosis is not known. Upper and lower endoscopy is your tools to visualize the disease process within the patient's gastrointestinal (GI) system and to biopsy the tissue for help in discerning between immune-mediated, infec-tious, and neoplastic etiologies. For instance, with infants, you use pH probes to help see whether chronic vomiting is gastroesophageal reflux alone or also due to a milk protein allergy. A significant number of children with chronic med-ical issues and problems gaining weight need a gastric feeding tube, and you will learn to insert this tube percutaneously aided by endoscopy. Emergencies needing a consultation from a pediatrics gastroenterologist, such as upper GI bleeding, occur less often with kids than adults, which allows for regular working hours.

Hematology–Oncology

Because hematology and oncology encompass such a wide variety of diseases and treatments, many subspecialists eventually concentrate on one of these two fields. Both areas are extremely interesting because an initial abnormality in white blood cells, hemoglobin, or platelets can end up having a wide range of causes, includ-ing genetic, infectious, immune mediated, ingestions, metabolic, and neoplastic. Diabetes, cancer, and several unknown factors put some children at higher risk for thrombotic events. They show up in the emergency room with an acute episode, which means that this subspecialist takes on the challenge of finding the cause and initiating anticoagulation. Many of the patients in your office will be children suffering from complications of sickle cell anemia or iron-deficiency anemia that did not respond to iron therapy.

Pediatric oncology attracts physicians who have a strong desire to always be there for their patients and family during tough and scary times when no one knows whether the child will be able to grow up and have a healthy life. Fortunately, with the latest therapies, we are approaching the point where 80% of all cancer in children and adolescents can be cured.[5] Research in genetics and tumor angiogenesis provides even more hope on the horizon.

A fellowship in pediatric hematology–oncology is very intense. As an attend-ing, your months on inpatient services will be very busy. However, hematology–oncology patients receive most of their care as outpatients, which means months not spent on service will be very manageable.

Infectious Disease

Stubborn bugs and new-fangled drugs make up the world of infectious disease. Along with understanding the physiology and defenses of the human body, subspecialists in this field enjoy knowing all about bacteria, viruses, parasites, fungi, and the critters that host them and pass them on to children. In the inpatient setting, these pediatricians are consulted for advice on treating infections with resistant bacteria and patients with complex medical issues. Many specialists in pediatrics infectious diseases take care of children who are HIV positive. They provide regular medical care, follow their CD4 antibody count and viral load, and spend time talking with the child and helping ensure that he or she will be compliant with medications.

Neonatal/Perinatal Medicine

Neonatologists deal with a wide range of medical issues, from lung immaturity and intraventricular hemorrhage in preemies to infectious issues and congenital defects in full-term infants. Perinatal is often added because it emphasizes how neonatologists work in close conjunction with obstetricians in cases of preterm labor or when a fetal abnormality has been diagnosed by ultrasound or amniocentesis. Advancements in technology and medical understanding have lowered the minimum age of viability of newborns to 22 to 23 weeks of gestation. Along with these advancements have come many ethical and philosophical questions about quality of life and how much should be done. Neonatologists, therefore, pay close attention to the desires and dynamics within the infant's family, spending time with them to help them cope and understand what lies ahead.

Depending on the hospital where these specialists choose to practice, most maintain predictable working schedules in the form of shifts. In academic medical centers, they are more likely to serve as the attending physician for month-long blocks at a time, available by phone every night to discuss cases with the fellow or nurse practitioner.

Nephrology

Pediatric nephrologists have a vast understanding of human physiology and the body's shifts in fluids, electrolytes, and acid–base disturbances. They diagnose and treat a wide range of diseases: renal artery stenosis, poststreptococcal glomerulonephritis, diabetes insipidus, and chronic renal failure. From the time they perform the renal biopsy, through the process of peritoneal dialysis, nephrologists build strong relationships with their patients who have chronic disease. During a morning clinic, they might see referrals for hematuria or proteinuria that was not explained by the initial workup of the general pediatrician. In the afternoon, they make rounds on the inpatient ward to manage, for example, the high-output renal failure of a child who has just received a new kidney. Residents and attendings always seem to be picking their brains during interesting cases at morning report—their insight is always quite helpful.

Neurology

Pediatric neurologists are very patient, caring individuals who spend most of their time with children who suffer from diseases of the nervous system. These problems can range from benign headaches, seizures that disappear in late childhood, and attention-deficit disorder to severe and progressively fatal diseases such as Duchenne muscular dystrophy, progressive seizure disorders such as infantile spasms and tuberous sclerosis, and various congenital brain malformations such as Dandy-Walker syndrome and pachygyria. Their careful examination skills help to find focal deficits, leading to quicker diagnosis and appropriate treatment. Many find this field frustrating because it seems like symptoms are only controlled and patients are rarely cured. But pediatric neurologists are drawn to their field because they know their interventions can improve their patient's quality of life. A fellowship in pediatric neurology is usually part of a combined residency (2 years of pediatrics, 1 year of general adult neurology, and 2 years as a fellow in pediatric neurology).

Pulmonology

Almost every disease process can affect a child's breathing and lung function, making pulmonology a very busy and exciting field. With infants, the pulmonologist helps to determine whether repeated wheezing episodes are from environmental triggers or due to aspiration from a swallowing dysfunction or gastroesophageal reflux. For toddlers, they get to use bronchoscopes to remove small Lego pieces that have been aspirated and polysomnograms to diagnose sleep apnea. Children of any age acquire complicated pneumonias that may form loculated pleural effusions needing a chest tube for drainage. When a child has asthma severe enough to cause more than one admission to a hospital, a pulmonologist is consulted and continues to see them as an outpatient, providing important education and treatment that will help save the patient's life.

Rheumatology

Pediatric rheumatologists have a gift for taking vague symptoms of aches and pains and rashes, and finding a diagnosis and treatment that can drastically improve a patient's quality of life. In the mysterious world of immune-mediated diseases, clinical and bench research are revealing that children and adolescents suffer from a set of diseases that is distinct from adult diseases. Juvenile rheumatoid arthritis, for instance, is falling out of vogue because it is not simply rheumatoid arthritis in a small person. Rather, the various juvenile inflammatory arthritides have distinct characteristics that need to be taken into account when deciding on a plan of action. Other diseases pediatric rheumatologists diagnose and treat include Lyme disease, the various forms of lupus, and dermatomyositis. Treatments for most rheumatologic diseases (anti-inflammatories and immunosuppressants) are not curative, but they are very effective in helping children live healthier, happier lives.

Certificate of Added Qualifications

After completing a residency in pediatrics, the following 1- and 2-year training programs are available to provide further training and expertise:

Hospice and palliative medicine: 1 year
Medical toxicology: 2 years
Neurodevelopmental disabilities: 2 years
Pediatric transplant hepatology: 1 additional year after completing 3-year pe-
    diatric gastroenterology fellowship
Sleep medicine: 1 year
Sports medicine: 1 year

WHY CONSIDER A CAREER IN PEDIATRICS?

Pediatrics offers many different avenues in which a physician can find his or her personal niche: long-term health issues, acute critical care, and specialties that emphasize anything from physiology to psychosocial skills. A career in pediatrics also provides balance, because you continually educate both children and their parents. By building long-term relationships, pediatricians get to see kids when they are doing well, not just when they are sick. In the same day that you meet an infant who may not be growing properly, you will also give words of encouragement to a teenager, inspiring him to set goals for his future, and talking to him about sex, drugs, and rock and roll.

At the most fundamental level, of course, all pediatricians simply love working with kids. Forming special connections, they can understand and communicate with children when other doctors may not. While building a great deal of trust, pediatricians help kids reach their potential and be the best they can be. Medical students considering this specialty should make the most out of their clerkship and determine whether spending time with infants, children, and young adults is something that they enjoy. If you come away even a little more energized, with a feeling of gratification from having helped a child, then perhaps pediatrics is the career for you.

ABOUT THE CONTRIBUTOR

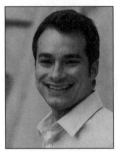 Dr Aaron Miller is a pediatrician in New York City. After growing up in Indianapolis, he did his undergraduate work at Goshen College and attended medical school at Indiana University School of Medicine. Dr Miller completed his residency in pediatrics at New York Pres-byterian Hospital–Cornell Medical Center and later became board certified in child abuse pediatrics. Dr Miller is currently director of the Lincoln Child Advocacy Center at Lincoln Medical and Mental Health Center and is chair of New York City Health and Hospital Corporation's Comprehensive Evaluation and Treatment of Child Abuse and Neglect (CETCAN).

REFERENCES

1. Colon, A.R. *Nurturing children: A history of pediatrics*. Westport, CT: Greenwood Press; 1999.

2. Bernstein, D. The cardiovascular system. In: Behrman, R., Kleigman, R. (eds). *Nelson textbook of pediatrics*. Philadelphia, PA: Saunders; 2000:1362.

3. Etchell, E., Bell, C., et al. Does this patient have a systolic murmur? *JAMA*. 1997;277:564–571.

4. Federal Interagency Forum on Child and Family Statistics. *America's Children: Key National Indicators of Well-Being, 2002*. Federal Interagency Forum on Child and Family Statistics, Washington, DC: US Government Printing Office; 2002.

5. Cone, T.E. *History of American pediatrics*. Boston, MA: Little Brown and Company; 1979.

27

PHYSICAL MEDICINE AND REHABILITATION

Vicki Anderson

Surprisingly, many students have completed several years of medical school before they finally learn about "physical medicine and rehabilitation (PM&R)" and what this specialty entails—the restoration of function using physical modalities. PM&R is based on the philosophy that addressing physical and cognitive impairments due to injury and disease will decrease disability. Physicians who specialize in PM&R are known as physiatrists.

PM&R is an underrecognized specialty, that even today, remains misunderstood by some in the medical community. If you tell someone you are interested in physiatry, you will undoubtedly get many questions: Did you say psychiatry? You are going to become a physical therapist? Are there really residency programs in PM&R? How long has this specialty been around? Although under appreciation of this burgeoning field is still common, this is changing as demand for the specialty grows and as patients continue to make amazing physical and cognitive gains while under the care of a physiatrist. Today more medical students have an opportunity to rotate with a physiatrist either as a brief portion of a neuroscience or ortho rotation. More interested students can choose to do an elective rotation in PM&R, which are more available in many institutions.

AN OVERVIEW OF PM&R

PM&R is the discipline concerned with preventing, diagnosing, and treating a variety of neurologic, musculoskeletal, and cardiopulmonary disorders through rehabilitative measures. A typical patient base can include, but not limited to, those with conditions such as strokes, spinal cord injuries, traumatic brain injuries, burn injuries, postchemotherapy and cancer deconditioning, sports injuries, multiple sclerosis, amyotrophic lateral sclerosis, and, in children, cerebral palsy, spina bifida, muscular dystrophy, and postoperative orthopedic procedures. Because of the vast spectrum of disease, physiatrists can focus on one (or more) of these medical problems. For instance, in many practices, there are physicians who subspecialize in pediatric rehabilitation and take care of only these younger patients. The practice of one physiatrist can look vastly different than her colleague she trained with based on the patient population.

Physiatrists coordinate the rehabilitative care of people with physical impairments and disabilities using a multidisciplinary approach. They prescribe pharmacologic agents to treat conditions such as spasticity, musculoskeletal pain, and neurologic pain. The physiatrist becomes quite adept at integrating the rehabilitation program in light of the patient's medical conditions, for example, determining precautions during physical therapy and monitoring medical stability. Physiatrists formulate specific regimens including physical, occupational, and speech therapy, as well as coordinating care from other professionals, such as, psychologists, neuropsychologists, dieticians, respiratory therapists, vocational counselors, orthotists, prosthetists, rehabilitation equipment engineers, sports/fitness trainers, and doctors of other medical specialties. Every regimen is tailored to prepare the patient to meet a particular goal or set of goals.

It is the physiatrist, with the help of the rehabilitation team, who sets goals for the patient. With the PM&R specialist as team leader, they meet at appropriate intervals during a patient's hospital stay to discuss the patient's progress, goals, and any pertinent social or psychological issues. The team also includes the patient and his or her family, with whom the physician also meets to ensure open lines of communication. Education of both patient and family is essential to increase the likelihood that the patient's physical and social needs are met. Ultimately, this means a successful integration into society.

Other essential responsibilities include prescribing assistive technology and adaptive devices to augment the patient's level of functioning: a wheelchair or walker to increase mobility, a communication device, or hand-operated reacher to allow greater independence in performing activities of daily living. To do so, physiatrists assess the difference between a person's functional level and the functional level required to perform a specific task. Physiatrists, along with other professionals of the team, evaluate whether a wheelchair is of the appropriate size, cushion is made of right material, and the seat is positioned correctly. There are many factors to evaluate in order to leverage a patient's physical capabilities in order to optimize performance. They are the experts at determining the energy expenditure required of patients with orthotic and prosthetic devices and prescribe these devices accordingly. Critical research in the most recent advances in prosthetic devices has originated due to the contributions of research physiatrists.

In rehabilitation care, the patient's basic neurologic and musculoskeletal function is essential, as well as the many psychosocial issues that affect the patient's participation in the community. This includes a program that attempts to solve the social and economic problems that may interfere with the patient's recovery.[1] As public policy and education advocates, physiatrists play a major role in public awareness of safety. In this specialty, therefore, you will find many opportunities to fight for patients' rights.

Physiatrists as consultants are able to recommend rehabilitation, what type of rehabilitation and to what extent. A physiatrist has the right and responsibility to withhold inpatient rehabilitation from ineligible patients, such as hospice patients who are not expected to regain much function before the end of their lives. As you can tell, an entire array of possible ethical situations can confront a physiatrist. But just like any other area of medicine, patients are free to obtain second opinions. Conceivably, one physiatrist may not accept a patient for rehabilitation while another deems him or her an appropriate candidate.

The physiatrist as consultant can offer different input depending on the consulting specialty and the patient's needs: anything from wound care recommendations to electrodiagnostics to pain medication management. There are so many facets of care that PM&R doctors learn to address doing their training. One concept that is learned is to offer the consulting doctor input that will allow the patient to transition to the next steps of rehabilitation.

Other ethical issues physiatrists face include concerns of distribution and access to health care resources. Like primary care physicians, they may find themselves spending increasing amounts of time convincing an insurer that physical rehabilitation will benefit the patient and it will ultimately save money and resources. Of course, in many of these instances, the bottom line is the incentive to cut costs, but perhaps the idea of spending resources on those with disability also plays a role. As human rights and the dignity of the human being overcome archaic prejudices and economic priorities, new legislation will be passed to assist the disabled and the handicapped to take their rightful place in society.[1]

Unfortunately, physicians can spend much time and effort fighting for human rights through paperwork, telephone conversations, and lobbying. For those involved in this struggle, this time-consuming advocacy work has been largely successful and quite rewarding. This advocacy has contributed to the fruition of equal rights acts such as the 1990 Americans with Disabilities Act. Disabled people now have greater access to public places and transportation making possible greater functioning at home and work. Physiatrists, along with other advocates, lobbied to propel these issues to the forefront and influence the political system. Ultimately, they sought to better meet the needs of people by promoting health and quality of life. There are several professional organizations for PM&R, and its subspecialties, that remain active in lobbying and advocacy work. Physiatrists do not just treat patients with severe disability, the field of PM&R has also attracted many who are interested in sports medicine—working with trained athletes and performers, such as musicians and dancers. Sports medicine doctors can become athletic team physicians. There is a branch of PM&R, few are experts in, regarding performing arts rehabilitation. The goals of care for the professional athlete and the performer are obviously different than for a patient who has moderate to severe disability. In these cases, the physiatrist is focused on enhancing performance or is treating an injury, for instance, due to repetitive movements. For both the athlete and performer, PM&R specialists are trained in dynamic interventional techniques that can enhance balance and proprioception and increase range of motion and strength.

REASONS WHY PHYSIATRISTS LIKE PM&R

Do you like knowing what happens to patients after stabilizing an acute medical event? Are you interested in how people adapt in the aftermath of a major medical condition? Do you feel dissatisfied with the loss of contact with your patients when they are discharged from your care? If so, then PM&R may be a satisfying career for you. Ask yourself these questions before, during, and after your core clerkships in surgery, internal medicine, and pediatrics.

Dr Howard Rusk, a pioneer in the field of rehabilitation medicine, identified three phases of medical care: preventive, curative, and rehabilitative. He insisted that the last phase should not be "passive convalescence" but active training to regain function and achieve greater independence and quality of life.[2] It is the attending physiatrist who prescribes physical and occupational therapies and coordinates goals among the multidisciplinary

WHAT MAKES A GOOD PHYSIATRIST?

✓ Enjoys caring for chronic problems.

✓ Can be satisfied by small successes (possibly over long periods of time).

✓ Is a creative, hopeful, easy-going person.

✓ Can lead an interdisciplinary health care team.

✓ Likes being heavily involved in patients' lives, initially and sometimes ongoing

THE INSIDE SCOOP

teams. The patient population consists of people with both chronic and acute medical conditions requiring rehabilitation: orthopedic patients after a hip or knee replacement, patients who have suffered strokes, or patients with major injuries leading to paraplegia and tetraplegia. The PM&R specialist can also be involved in managing transplant patients and cardiopulmonary rehabilitation. PM&R doctors can treat both the young and the old, for this type of care is needed among all people, regardless of age. However, most physiatrists are able to tailor their practices based on their interests and training.

Unfortunately, many misconceptions about rehabilitation medicine exist. "Early in my career, I found it disconcerting that many other physicians didn't know very much about my specialty," commented a university-based physiatrist. "Over the years, I have found it rewarding to educate others about my career, especially because I enjoy my career so much." Patients are often transferred to "rehab" by internists and surgeons as part of discharge planning without fully understanding or appreciating the purpose of this care. Rehabilitation hospitals that provide inpatient programs are not simply "dumping grounds" after an acute hospitalization. At times, it can be rather frustrating to deal with this misunderstanding among colleagues. However, in most circumstances, cooperation from both parties, the physiatrist and the referring physician, can be negotiated. You are the one imbued with the power to decide if and when it is appropriate for a patient to begin a rehabilitation program. All physiatrists, therefore, value the virtue of patience when educating others about the importance of rehabilitation medicine. Their decisions are ultimately based on clinical expertise and their patients' best interests.

There is room for many different interests and practice types in physiatry—all of which focus on coordinating rehabilitative care and addressing each physical impairment or disability. For instance, sports, spine, and interventional pain—which requires many fluoroscopically guided spine and joint injections to manage pain—is an ideal subspecialty for those interested in a lot of hands-on work. Physicians who choose this field often want to do physical work, without the intensity or time pressure of major surgery.

PM&R is a specialty with great variety. Some say that PM&R's organ system is the musculoskeletal system. However, rather than focusing on one organ system, the physiatrist collectively evaluates and treats deficits in function that result from one or more anatomical or physiological abnormality. One physiatrist commented that she liked the fact that PM&R "is not limited to any one organ system—it is not even limited to the body—but includes the psychosocial aspects of the patient's care."

THE DOCTOR–PATIENT RELATIONSHIP

Are you inspirational? Would you like to build long-lasting relationships with your patients? The doctor–patient relationship is a valuable and rewarding part of a career in PM&R. You meet patients at their baseline or after an acute decline of functional status and help them overcome their limitations, thus building long-term connections. One of the many rewards in physiatry is the enormous sense of fulfillment and purpose in day-to-day activities. Although clinical improvement may be slow in many instances, small gains over time in a patient's function and quality of life make it worth all the effort.

We know from data that a patient under the care of a rehabilitation doctor has a higher chance for significant functional improvement from a recently acquired physical impairment. The earlier you establish this relationship, the better the outcome. The PM&R doctor is a constant source of stability and encouragement. Many patients prefer to see only their physiatrist for medical care. Their clinics are usually more accessible to people with disabilities, and patients may feel greater acceptance by the clinic staff. Most people naturally believe that their overall level of functioning has a great influence on their physical health. A physiatrist is more likely to delve deeper into these issues by inquiring about the specifics of their patients' daily functioning.

A career in PM&R also means that you must feel comfortable discussing many personal—often intimate—issues. For instance, patients with disabilities, especially spinal cord injuries, may be concerned about sexual functioning as well as reproductive problems. These concerns must be addressed with care and sensitivity, which is part of what being a good physician is all about.

Many physicians who choose this specialty have been influenced by personal experience with disability, either their own or of someone they know. What is your own interest in working with people who have disabilities? Do you feel comfortable in their presence? If you ask PM&R specialists why they chose this specialty, the overwhelming response is that they "like taking care of people." Their responsibilities, therefore, are twofold: clinical work, in which they take care of patients with physical impairments, and advocacy work, in which they fight on behalf of people with disabilities.

HOW TO BE AN EXCELLENT PM&R PHYSICIAN

A superb understanding of neuroanatomy, neurophysiology, and the musculoskeletal system serves as the basis for your daily practice when evaluating patients and discussing rehabilitation plans with colleagues. A good physiatrist can execute the neurologic examination as good as any neurologist and the musculoskeletal examination as skillfully as any orthopedic surgeon or rheumatologist. As directors of an interdisciplinary team, physiatrists are also adept at coordinating people and tasks.

In an inpatient rehabilitation facility, the physician manages many chronic medical issues, such as controlling blood sugars in the diabetic patient, continuing antihypertensive medicines for the stroke patient, and administering cardioprotective agents for the post–heart-attack patient. Other medical complications that may occur under a physiatrist's care include neurogenic bladder and bowel, autonomic dysreflexia, and spasticity. A PM&R doctor must be adept at managing acute situations, too. When preventive measures fail, the rehabilitation doctor must either handle an acute scenario or delegate the responsibility to the appropriate party. Moreover, a good PM&R specialist is astute at determining when a previously stable patient is becoming acutely ill. Another piece to this skill is knowing when a patient needs to see another type of practitioner or specialist. In fact, coordinating the care of patients within the health care system is an important part of the job.

THE TYPICAL DAY OF A PHYSIATRIST

The daily responsibilities of a physiatrist vary due to variations in practice types, patient populations, and subspecialty. In PM&R, the types of conditions you will treat encompass a variety of functional impairments. For example, an older patient population provides more opportunities to work with stroke rehabilitation and hip and knee replacements. A younger population, on the other hand, may present with more traumatic injuries, such as those suffered in sporting accidents, motor vehicle collisions, or work-related injuries, for example.

Practice settings are varied and include an inpatient rehabilitation hospital, day rehabilitation center, and outpatient clinic. Many physiatrists have the responsibility of caring for patients at two or more types of locations. The type of daily work will depend on geographic region (whether at an academic center or in a private practice group), subspecialty interest, and referral base.

In an inpatient rehabilitation setting, there are three areas crucial to a patient's health. A PM&R specialist is first responsible for managing any acute medical issues, such as hypertension, diabetes, and infectious disease. Second, you address medical concerns uniquely related to rehabilitation. These include pressure ulcers and problems related to proper bowel and bladder function. You may find yourself placing urinary catheters, measuring urinary bladder volume, dis-impacting bowels, or debriding ulcers at the bedside. Third, there are functional rehabilitation issues to consider. In an acute rehabilitation setting, patients stay in rooms with beds much like other hospitals, but there are also physical therapy gyms and other therapy spaces where small miracles take place daily. A PM&R physician might also want to evaluate patients during their therapy sessions. For instance, a physical therapist might demonstrate a patient's limited flexibility for the physiatrist so that he could, in turn, prescribe or recommend other exercise or modalities to enhance the patient's range of motion. Interdisciplinary team rounds are also an important part of PM&R. In this group, various allied health professionals share information about patient progress and, as needed, revise their goals for patient care. These comprehensive rounds enable PM&R specialists to get the whole story on the progress and treatment of their patients.

In some cases, day rehabilitation centers are often the next setting to which a patient with a complex disability, traumatic brain injury, or stroke will be dis-charged after inpatient rehabilitation. "Day rehab" supports the notion that each comprehensive rehabilitation program can be tailored to suit the specific needs of each individual patient. The model focuses on patients who could benefit from a longer, more intense outpatient rehabilitation than would be prescribed with just one outpatient therapy alone. Therefore, these patients participate in various disciplines, usually two or more, and may include physical therapy, occupational, or speech therapy 3 to 5 days per week. In addition, there are vocational rehabilita-tion counselors and measures to determine functional capacity for work. At these facilities, there are physiatrists who manage the patients' rehabilitative medical care while monitoring functional gains.

Outpatient practice in PM&R is as important as inpatient rehabilitation. These clinic visits allot time to determine new goals, evaluate patient progress, and troubleshoot issues along the way. However, there are a host of physiatrists whose primary practice is all outpatient, so if their patient requires inpatient, acute, or rehabilitation care, they will fall under another physician's care/service. This physiatrist will likely treat more common conditions such as osteoarthritis, back pain, myofascial pain, and musculoskeletal injuries. Outpatient physiatrists are more sports, spine, and musculoskeletal oriented. They take care of patients with both subtle and severe impairments and may become more involved in worker's compensation cases. Keeping patients motivated to perform their home exercise program is an important part of the continuum of care. They may also find time in their schedule to perform more interventional work, such as facet joint injections, spinal injections for discogenic pain, or hip injections.

Prevention

Physiatrists encourage their patients to live safely, maintain safe homes, and wear helmets and proper equipment when participating in sports and recreational activities. In an effort to reduce the probability of injury, for example, a physiatrist who is the physician for a sports team makes judgments as to whether it is safe for a player to continue participating. In general, education plays a key role in the effort to prevent both initial injury and disease and the complications that result from injury and disease.

Diagnostics

The history and physical examination are essential tools in this specialty. Often patients are referred to PM&R specialists after receiving an initial diagnosis (and in some cases, after the initiation of treatment). The physiatrist must then reevaluate the situation and bring new, creative solutions to the table. The patient history allows the physiatrist to focus on the patient's premorbid functional level and set appropriate goals. They ask questions such as, "How many stairs do you have at home?" and "What types of things can you do for exercise, before and now?" Physical examinations are often repeated during the care of a rehabilitation patient. The ability to remain objective, pay attention to details, and compare physical examinations to chart progress is invaluable to this specialty. Often physiatrists are the first people to recognize a subtle spinal cord injury, spasticity of the limbs, or musculoskeletal abnormality in patients referred by other physicians. In accordance, the physiatrist can measure these deficits and initiate a medical plan of care that is most appropriate in treating the condition and its associated comorbidities.

To help define disease and its progression, all physiatrists make use of laboratory and radiologic studies. They perform electromyography (EMG), nerve conduction studies, and evoked potential studies — diagnostic modalities that residents in both PM&R and neurology are trained to use. Using these high-tech tools can help to differentiate between motor neuron disease, radiculopathies, peripheral neuropathies, and myopathies, for instance. These studies, therefore, complement each other and supplement the clinical history and physical examination in diagnosing a neuromuscular disorder.

Physiatrists, depending on their particular focus or subspecialty, become astute at interpreting diagnostics such as radiological imaging, so that a spinal cord injury doctor will become familiar with spinal MRIs and the sports specialist in interpreting musculoskeletal images. However, still relying on our colleagues for their expertise in the final official interpretation.

Therapeutics

Therapies used by PM&R physicians include physical therapy, ultrasound deep heat, transcutaneous nerve stimulation, high-voltage galvanic stimulation, biofeedback, phonophoresis, and microwave diathermy. Physiatrists also perform intramuscular and intra-articular injections. Because of the wealth of treatment options, the specific ones you choose depend on your preferences. For instance, someone who trained at an institution heavily involved in biofeedback research and treatment is more likely to use this technique. PM&R specialists who trained at a school that emphasized interventional procedures may tend to turn to injections and other minimally invasive techniques. Ultrasound-guided musculoskeletal injections are relatively new in the practice of PM&R and is being integrated into the PM&R residency training curriculum.

LIFESTYLE CONSIDERATIONS AND PRACTICE OPTIONS

Physiatry is a rewarding profession that allows the practicing physician to develop continuity of care with patients. This is especially true if you have a more general practice or focus on pain management for patients who require life-long health care. Some physiatrists start solo practices, join medical groups with other physiatrists or a multispecialty practice, work in free-standing rehabilitation facilities, or remain in academics. For instance, a group of orthopedic surgeons may prefer having a PM&R specialist provide care for postoperative patients following hip and knee arthroplasty. Or a physiatrist in this group may care for patients who are not surgical candidates but have orthopedic-related medical problems. In this situation, physiatrists use their expertise to prescribe a program as part of the solution.

Taking a closer look at some of the statistics, you will see that there will always be a need for specialists in PM&R. Many elderly patients require rehabilitation to reclaim lost strength and function after being hospitalized for a short period of time or during their stay at a nursing home. Every year, thousands of people are born with cerebral palsy or sustain severe traumatic brain injuries, from which more people are surviving than ever before. As the population ages and the rate of survival from previously fatal accidents and illnesses continues to increase, the number of disabled people continues to rise.[3] By 2020, it is estimated that 9 to 14 million people older than 65 years will have moderate to severe disability.[4]

Because there are now only 7000 physiatrists in the United States, expanding this specialty and training more physicians are the only ways to treat all these

patients with chronic disabilities. Although some analysts predict an oversupply of physicians in various medical specialties, the demand for PM&R specialists will only increase. One study projects
that the demand will exceed the supply of
physiatrists until 2015.[5] Because PM&R
is a referral-based specialty, the need for
more physiatrists will only increase fur-

VITAL SIGNS

MEDIAN COMPENSATION

Physical medicine
and rehabilitation $236,800

Data from American Medical Group Association.

ther as the medical community better understands and appreciates their skills
and knowledge. Medical centers are now making a concerted effort to introduce
PM&R to those students who may be interested in caring for people with acute
and chronic disabilities.

Physiatrists' patient population overlaps with those of several other specialists:
nonsurgical orthopedic practitioners (who treat sports medicine and work-related
injuries), neurologists (who treat pain, spasticity, neurological disorders), and anesthesiologists (who provide chronic pain management services). Both neurologists
and physiatrists perform thorough neurologic physical examinations, make use of
EMG in diagnosis, and interpret neurologic imaging studies. But future PM&R
physicians should not be overly concerned about competition within the health
care marketplace. Although neurologists and physiatrists see many of the same
medical conditions, they care for patients at different points in the medical time-
line and vary when it comes to patient goals, treatment plans, and therapeutic
modalities. In fact, some argue that they are actually part of a multidisciplinary
team spanning practice boundaries. Ideally, neurologists and physiatrists should
cooperate and share their knowledge and skills to help the patient achieve the
best possible medical care. In many instances, you will work closely with the
neurology service and share information and teachers.

FELLOWSHIPS AND SUBSPECIALTY TRAINING

Some prominent figures in the field are proponents of PM&R as more of a primary
care practice. They believe that residency programs in physiatry should train
graduates to become primary care physicians for patients with disabilities. Not
surprisingly, there is some disagreement within the profession as to what this
role would actually mean for the practice of PM&R. Advocates for a primary
care model maintain that subspecialization detracts from a primary care focus,
whereas others believe that the current movement toward subspecialization will

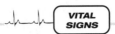

PHYSICAL MEDICINE
AND REHABILITATION
2011 MATCH STATISTICS

- Number of positions
  available: 373
- 212 US seniors and 367
  independent applicants
  ranked at least one PM&R
  program
- 96.5% of all positions were
  filled in the initial Match
- The successful applicants:
  50% US seniors, 16.1%
  foreign-trained physicians,
  and 29.7% osteopathic
  graduates
- Mean USMLE Step I score:
  214
- Unmatched rate for US
  seniors applying only to
  PM&R: 8.2%

Data from National Resident Matching
Program.

strengthen, stabilize, and validate this discipline. For instance, today there is a great need for physiatrists who perform interventional techniques, such as injections for back pain, tenosynovitis, bursitis, arthritis, and myofascial pain syndrome. Not only are reimbursements for these procedures more lucrative but the delivery of health care also has shifted to outpatient services to conserve expenses and control costs.

Should you consider completing a fellowship? In some instances, residency training more than adequately prepares you to practice in a subspecialty area of interest. After all, on-the-job experience as a practicing physiatrist can be enough to mold a physician into a "subspecialist." A physiatrist at a rehabilitation center agreed, "If you are hired into a position— for instance your first attending job— where you are doing mainly spinal cord injury or traumatic brain injury, then you will become an expert in those areas." In fact, the first practice position you select after residency training could be more important to your career than obtaining a fellowship position. Pursuing formal subspecialty training, therefore, is an individual decision based on personal and professional objectives.

Clinical fellowships in PM&R typically last 1 to 2 years, where the 2-year fellowships are more research oriented. Subspecialty training allows the resident to become an expert in an area of rehabilitation before actually having to treat patients as an attending physician. In addition, fellowships continue, where residencies left off, to promote learning of evidence-based practice of rehabilitation medicine. There are many recognized fellowships but only a few that are officially accredited by the ACGME. You can become board certified in these areas following successful completion of the subspecialty examination.

At the current time, the American Board of Physical Medicine and Rehabilitation does not offer certificates of special or added qualifications for the remaining subspecialties.

Spinal Cord Injury Rehabilitation Medicine

Patients who have suffered trauma to their spinal cord have special medical issues related to the level and severity of injury. Physiatrists trained in this subspecialty learn how to manage acute problems such as autonomic dysreflexia or hyperreflexia, as well as chronic complications such as urinary incontinence, wound care, infertility, and sexual dysfunction. They have to be able to respond to psychological factors, such as patients' fear of reinjury and its effect on their disability. Spinal cord injury fellows not only become experts in the clinical care of acute traumatic spinal cord injured individuals but they also treat nontraumatic spinal cord injuries, such as those caused by multiple sclerosis, cancer, or amyotrophic lateral sclerosis.

Pain Management

Fellowships focusing on treating patients with chronic pain syndromes are primarily sponsored by the American Board of Anesthesiology; there are 11 PM&R-based programs in the United States.

RESIDENCY TRAINING

Residency in PM&R requires 4 years of postgraduate training. There are currently 79 accredited programs. There are also several positions in combined PM&R programs with additional training in neurology, pediatrics, or internal medicine. All require a general internship year (PGY-1), which can be internal medicine, surgery, or transitional. In a typical program, residents gain experience in both inpatient and outpatient rehabilitation medicine. The amount of work hours varies per individual program. Overnight call—usually only a few times per month—is generally benign. Resident physicians have monthly rotations that provide training in general rehabilitation of neurological conditions, deconditioning, strokes and spinal cord and traumatic brain injuries, as well as pediatric rehabilitation. Many programs have substantial elective time to gain experience in particular areas of interest within PM&R.

THE INSIDE SCOOP

This number has increased over the last 4 years and will likely continue to increase in the number and size of programs. As many physicians know, there is a huge need for pain specialists to manage this special patient population. The daily activities include pain clinic, in which a fellow manages a patient base either medically or via interventional techniques. Some of the simpler procedures include epidurals, facet joint and target point injections, and fluoroscopically guided steroid injections. With its emphasis on procedures, pain medicine has become a lucrative area of expertise due to high reimbursements. Interventional pain management takes a different approach to the patient from traditional PM&R.

Pediatric Rehabilitation

Although physiatrists can work with patients in all age groups, many choose to subspecialize in caring only for children with chronic disabilities whose issues are profoundly different from those of adults. Currently, there are four pediatric rehabilitation medicine programs in the United States. Pediatrics rehabilitation specialists treat kids with cerebral palsy, muscular dystrophy, spasticity, burns, spina bifida, and developmental issues related to prematurity at birth. This fellowship provides additional time for physiatrists to develop their skills in integrating a child into an environment that stimulates development and increases their physical, cognitive, and social functioning. Pediatric rehabilitation is both specialized and diverse, given that the patients vary from infants to adolescents. Pediatric physiatry addresses those disorders potentially affecting children on a long-term basis, often involving multiple organ systems. The emphasis is on helping patients achieve developmental skills and independence in self-care and mobility appropriate to their age. The fellowship also addresses the role of the physiatrist as coordinator of multiple services (medical, social, or educational), as well as the importance of acting as liaison and advocate for the child and family.

Brain Injury Rehabilitation Medicine

Fellowships in brain injury rehabilitation tend to focus on traumatic brain injury but include those of other origins, such as anoxic injuries to the brain. Functional levels range from the comatose to the mildly cognitively impaired in brain injury patients. The fellowships are usually 1 to 2 years based on the length of the research component. These physiatrists learn how to manage brain injury early while the patient is in ICU or neurosurgery service and become experts in managing everything from acute agitation to long-term medical complications associated with brain injury. Caring for brain-injured patients range from prescribing neurostimulant pharmacology, to advancing the brain's plasticity, to establishing behavioral modification protocols. Brain injury patients tend to have longer initial inpatient rehabilitation stays, and therefore this specialist needs to be very comfortable dealing with the day-to-day medical issues that may arise. Outpatient work will likely include spasticity management with botulinum toxins injections, intrathecal baclofen pump management, serial casting, and pain management. This specialist is intimately involved as a liaison to other professional and social services the patient might require for social integration.

Sports, Spine, and Musculoskeletal Medicine

Physiatrists can subspecialize in the diagnosis and treatment of sports-related injuries or musculoskeletal problems. They primarily manage musculoskeletal diseases but are still very knowledgeable in general rehabilitation. These subspecialists also receive training in electrodiagnostic studies, trigger point injections, and fluoroscopically guided spinal injections. Their patients are athletes, workers, or any individuals with a physical impairment, subtle or more involved. They often care for the young patient who may have pain or declining performance in their workouts due to a physical injury. Fellowship will prepare this doctor to become effective and efficient in managing common complaints, such as low back, hip, knee, and shoulder pain, whether related to recreation or occupation activities.

Stroke Rehabilitation

Physiatrists with a special interest in caring for stroke patients can choose to subspecialize in this area of medicine. Stroke fellowships provide additional expertise in treating patients throughout the entire spectrum of recovery from a cerebrovascular accident. This includes management of acute stroke on a consult service, acute rehabilitation, and subacute (less intense) rehabilitation. Stroke specialists receive additional training in neuroradiology and neuropharmacology and work closely with their colleagues in neurology.

Neuromuscular Fellowship

One new fellowship in the last few years focuses on training the physiatrist interested in treating and diagnosing patients with neuromuscular disease. Training is focused on electrodiagnostic techniques.

WHY CONSIDER A CAREER IN PM&R?

PM&R is one of the youngest specialties in the medical profession. It became a member of the American Board of Medical Specialties in 1947 after the veterans of World War II returned home with amputations and other combat-related injuries.[6] The separate disciplines of PM&R became a single entity when two prominent physicians—Howard Rusk (rehabilitation) of New York University and Frank Krusen (physical medicine) of the Mayo Clinic—began collaborating. Through their efforts, with funding from the US Department of Health, Education, and Welfare, opportunities for training in this new field of PM&R began to blossom. Now, more US senior medical students than ever before are choosing careers in physiatry.

This burgeoning field is full of rewards, both for the physician and patient. The doctor–patient relationship is central to medical care, especially because physiatrists evaluate their patients in a holistic manner—involving both the body systems and the external ecosystem. The referral-based practice of PM&R also offers versatility: you can have a solo practice, be part of a multispecialty group practice, or work in academics. There is also a great deal of variety in terms of patient care, from bedside treatment to rehabilitation plans, from educational programs to patient advocacy. Within the small community of physiatrists, there are many opportunities for leadership, both in the public and private sector. PM&R is a perfect specialty for all types of personalities—introverts, extroverts, cerebral, and exuberant individuals alike.

Medical students wanting to make a difference in the lives of patients suffering from acute and chronic disabilities should seriously consider this specialty. As a specialist in PM&R, you will become a beacon of hope for physically impaired and chronically ill patients. These physicians pick up medical care at the point where the internists, surgeons, and pediatricians have left off. For those physicians who entered medicine to help people, there is no better choice than PM&R for a fulfilling medical career.

ABOUT THE CONTRIBUTOR

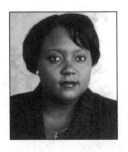 Dr Vicki Anderson is an attending physician at the Milwaukee Veteran Affairs Medical Center and an assistant professor of PM&R at the Medical College of Wisconsin. She was born and raised in Chicago, Illinois. Dr Anderson earned her undergraduate degree in the biological sciences at Stanford University. She then moved back to her hometown to attend medical school at the University of Chicago, where she also earned an MBA and completed residency training at the Rehabilitation of Institution of Chicago, RIC. After completing fellowship training in spinal cord injury medicine in 2008, she has worked mostly with veterans who have had spinal cord injuries.

REFERENCES

1. Flax, H.J. The future of physical medicine and rehabilitation. *Am J Phys Med Rehabil.* 2000;79:79–86.

2. American Academy of Physical Medicine and Rehabilitation Web site. Accessed July 2006 from www.aapmr.org.

3. Ogle, A.A., Garrison, S.J., et al. Roadmap to physical medicine and rehabilitation: Answers to medical students' questions about the field. *Am J Phys Med Rehabil.* 2001;80(3):218–224.

4. Kunkel, S.R., Applebaum, R.A. Estimating the prevalence of long-term disability for the aging society. *J Gerontol.* 1992;97(S2):53–60.

5. Lewin Group. Supply of and demand for physiatrists: Review and update of the 1995 physical medicine and rehabilitation workforce study: A special report. *Am J Phys Med Rehabil.* 1999;78:4777–4785.

6. American Board of Medical Specialties Web site. Accessed July 2006 from www.abms.org.

28

PLASTIC SURGERY

Gregory H. Borschel

What is plastic surgery? Is it Hollywood? Is it nose jobs? Is it silicone?

Although many plastic surgeons perform cosmetic surgery on high-profile patients, this specialty involves much more than Hollywood movie stars and breast implants. The word *plastic* is derived from the Greek *plastikos*, meaning "to shape, change, or mould." The goals of plastic surgery are threefold: (1) to alter surgically the form and function of anatomy—either normal or pathologic; (2) to improve quality of life; and (3) to preserve life itself.

No other surgical specialist draws on a wider base of anatomic knowledge or operates in more regions of the body than does plastic surgeon. It has been said that plastic surgeons operate on "the skin and its contents," alluding to the fact that on any given day, plastic surgeons might find themselves operating on the face, on the hand, inside the cranium, or inside the abdominal or thoracic cavities. The field has developed from the contributions of people from many different backgrounds, including general surgery, orthopedics, oral and maxillofacial surgery, dermatology, neurosurgery, and otolaryngology.

Plastic surgery receives extensive media attention, yet remains poorly understood by the general public—and often by physicians as well. In some ways, it may seem to be a paradoxical specialty. Plastic surgery encompasses all of aesthetic surgery, yet it also deals with clinical problems that are often considered grotesque, including chronic wounds, limb replantation, and head and neck reconstruction. It is considered a surgical subspecialty, yet the fund of knowledge needed for even a basic understanding of the discipline requires a five- to eight-volume text. And although it is a relative newcomer as an organized specialty, some of the first recorded operations were plastic surgery procedures.

THE EVOLUTION OF PLASTIC SURGERY

Although most contemporary plastic surgical techniques were developed only within the last few decades, plastic surgery is actually one of the oldest surgical specialties. Historians believe that the Indian surgeon Sushruta, who took a flap of tissue from the forehead and covered a nasal tip defect, performed the first documented plastic surgery in 600 BC.[1] In the fifteenth century, Western plastic surgeons began using surgical techniques to alter the form and function of the human body.[2] Tagliacozzi, an Italian plastic surgeon, developed a technique to restore tissue to noses lost in traumatic amputations.

Much of the history of contemporary plastic surgery was shaped by war. Early twentieth century plastic surgeons such as Sir Harold Gillies[3] and Vilray Blair[4] served in World War I and helped develop many of the fundamental techniques and principles still used today. World War II and the Korean and Vietnam wars later produced great numbers of complex wounds. Advances in critical care and trauma surgery meant that patients with increasingly devastating injuries could potentially be saved. In this setting, the plastic surgeon earned two relatively new responsibilities. First, it was recognized that acute wound coverage was necessary to prevent secondary infection and subsequent loss of vital structures. Second, the functional and aesthetic demands of patients became a greater priority. Plastic surgeons realized that even if a soldier's life was saved, if he was so disfigured that he could not present himself in public, then he might consider his life not worth living. Plastic surgeons then developed new procedures to maximize function, especially in the case of upper- and lower-extremity reconstructive surgery, and devised more aesthetic facial reconstructive techniques.

In the 1960s, Paul Tessier and others popularized new methods of manipulating the bones of the face and skull, leading to the development of craniofacial surgery. The microsurgical revolution began at the same time. Microvascular anastomotic techniques allowed reliable free tissue transfer (free flaps) for reconstructing complex defects throughout the body. In the 1960s and 1970s, tissue expansion led to innovative methods in breast reconstruction, aesthetic breast augmentation, and reconstruction of large congenital and acquired cutaneous defects. Within the last few decades, other significant advances have come into wide acceptance in plastic surgery, including the use of thin fasciocutaneous flaps for lower extremity and head and neck reconstruction, osteocutaneous flaps for mandible reconstruction, lasers for vascular malformations, advanced means of bony fixation, distraction osteogenesis (bone stretching to produce new bone) for mandibular and long bone reconstruction, suction-assisted lipectomy (liposuction), and the use of engineered tissues.

The goals of the plastic surgeon include restoration of a feeling of wholeness to the patient. All plastic surgeons strive to achieve the best functional and aesthetic result for every patient in order to relieve suffering, both physical and mental. Tagliacozzi himself said, "as plastic surgeons we perform operations not to delight the eye, but also to heal the mind."

THE ALLURE OF PLASTIC SURGERY

There are always many more applicants to plastic surgery programs than positions available. What makes plastic surgery so compelling? Why would conscientious, idealistic new physicians want to go into a specialty that many associate with vanity?

No other surgical specialty—not even general surgery—deals with so many regions of the body. The breadth of anatomy seen within a typical week (or even within a single day) often includes the head, neck, chest, abdomen, lower and upper extremities, breast, and hand. Some may view this as a liability. Most plastic surgeons, however, welcome the variety and tend to become bored if repeatedly faced with the same types of clinical problems. They enjoy the beauty of anatomy, especially that of the more intricate regions, such as the hand and face.

Some plastic surgeons say they find their work particularly rewarding because the results are often so visible. For example, after a cleft lip repair, the surgeon's efforts are publicly evident for the next 80 years or more. One of my now retired mentors, Dr M. Haskell Newman, told me that seeing a parent's smile after their child's cleft lip has been repaired is one of the most fulfilling experiences in all of surgery. I think he is absolutely right. Likewise, when a patient awakens following replantation of a severed limb (or scalp, ear, nose, or even penis) and sees the successfully reattached part, it reaffirms the plastic surgeon's choice of a career.

Physician–patient relationships in plastic surgery can be quite lengthy and involved. Most plastic surgeons find these relationships in particular to be quite rewarding. For example, in the case of congenital deformities, patients often require 10 or more operations prior to reaching adulthood. Families with inherited congenital anomalies, such as Apert or Crouzon syndrome, may have multiple generations followed by the same surgeon. Similarly, many problems in the upper extremity mandate a careful, staged approach to treatment. For example, if a man loses his thumb in a farming accident, he will need a procedure to achieve closure of his initial wound. He will require reconstruction to provide him with useful thumb function, which can sometimes take the form of a toe-to-thumb transfer. The surgery itself is quite involved and rehabilitation is certainly a long-term endeavor. Likewise, patients with facial paralysis (such as with Bell palsy) or brachial plexus injuries may require multiple therapeutic procedures over several years.

WHAT MAKES A GOOD PLASTIC SURGEON?

✓ Prefers working with his or her hands.

✓ Enjoys trying new approaches to the same problem.

✓ Is an independent and creative thinker.

✓ Likes seeing the immediate results of treatment.

✓ Is a perfectionist who pays close attention to details.

THE INSIDE SCOOP

Plastic surgery can be physically demanding. The training is intense, especially during the core surgery years, and the clinical component of most categorical plastic surgery programs lasts 6 years. Some operations are lengthy or technically challenging. Most plastic surgeons, including this author, have participated in operations that lasted more than 24 hours. Some have said that microsurgery, in particular, is a young surgeon's sport. Not only can these procedures be long but the anastomosis of small vessels also can sometimes be quite challenging. However, there are still many microsurgeons—many of them pioneers in the field—who continue to practice today.

BEING THE SURGEON'S SURGEON

It has been said that the plastic surgeon is "the surgeon's surgeon." Colleagues from other surgical disciplines will often refer patients to the plastic surgeon—either to help with a planned reconstructive need or, occasionally, to help with a complication.

For example, neurosurgeons may require assistance in reconstructing defects after removing certain brain and cranial tumors, or after repairing meningomyeloceles. General surgeons routinely consult plastic surgeons for reconstruction after mastectomy, burn care, and abdominal wall reconstruction. Orthopedic surgeons call upon plastic surgeons to help with complex soft tissue reconstruction following fracture fixation, especially in the distal lower extremity. Many orthopedists work in partnership with plastic surgeons during replantations, spine procedures, and reconstructions following sarcoma extirpation. In most centers, oral/maxillofacial surgeons and otolaryngologists often use plastic surgeons in head and neck reconstruction after cancer extirpation. Vascular surgeons ask for assistance in covering exposed prosthetic vascular grafts with muscle flaps. Cardiothoracic surgeons may call upon their plastic surgery colleagues to close sternotomy wounds that have failed to heal, resulting in mediastinitis. Plastic surgeons also work with urologists in complex urogenital reconstructions. They may collaborate with multiple surgical teams during complex congenital cases, such as the separation of conjoined twins. Plastic surgeons routinely team up with dermatologists in the treatment of melanoma and other skin cancers. They often collaborate with other specialists, including speech therapists, physical therapists, occupational therapists, dentists, and orthodontists. Most plastic surgeons find these collaborations enjoyable and productive.

LIFESTYLE CONSIDERATIONS AND PRACTICE OPTIONS

Plastic surgeons generally practice in one of two environments: academia or private practice. Some practices consist of a mixture of the two. Academic plastic surgeons are based in large tertiary care centers. Private practice plastic surgeons may have affiliations with larger hospitals, and they may also treat patients in a number of smaller venues as well. Academic plastic surgeons have usually completed a fellowship in a subspecialty, whereas private practice surgeons may or may not have pursued additional formal training within plastic surgery. Financial opportunities can be substantially greater in private practice. Regardless of type of practice, plastic surgeons are almost always among the highest-paid physicians (along with neurosurgeons and cardiothoracic surgeons).

A plastic surgeon can decide to be on call for emergencies at local hospitals. Most find it important to take call for two main reasons: first, it allows them to develop relationships and referral patterns with other physicians and second, it may bring in a large proportion of income early in a plastic surgeon's practice. It may also be a requirement for admitting privileges in hospitals.

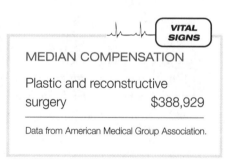

VITAL SIGNS

MEDIAN COMPENSATION

Plastic and reconstructive
surgery $388,929

Data from American Medical Group Association.

As with many specialties, certain regions of North America are overserved. Nearly half of board-certified plastic surgeons are found in the greater New York or Los Angeles metropolitan regions. In these areas, it can be difficult to establish a new practice. Conversely, certain geographic locales—particularly rural ones—are markedly underserved. In these regions, hospitals and clinics are often more willing to pay more for the services of a plastic surgeon. Regardless of practice environment, plastic surgeons have historically described themselves as busy professionally and contented personally.[5]

A plastic surgeon's week is generally devoted to operating, seeing patients in clinic, and rounding on patients on the wards. Much of a plastic surgeon's time is spent in the operating room (usually from 2 to 4 days a week). Most plastic surgeons see patients in clinic 1 or 2 days a week. In addition to rounding on their inpatients, plastic surgeons see inpatients in consultation from other physicians. In an academic environment, 1 or more days a week are often devoted to academic activities, such as basic or applied science or clinical outcomes research.

FELLOWSHIPS AND SUBSPECIALTY TRAINING

Many plastic surgeons choose to pursue additional training upon completing a plastic surgical residency. Microsurgery fellowships are quite popular, as are hand surgery fellowships. There are also programs in craniofacial surgery, aesthetic surgery, pediatric plastic surgery, and burn surgery. Most fellowships last 1 year, although they can be as short as 2 months or as long as 2 years or more.

Aesthetic Surgery

Aesthetic, or cosmetic, surgery involves the manipulation of tissues to enhance appearance. Common aesthetic procedures performed by plastic surgeons include rhinoplasty (reshaping of the nose), facelift, aesthetic eyelid surgery, laser skin resurfacing, botulinum toxin injection, breast augmentation, liposuction, and body lifts.

The field of cosmetic surgery is unique among surgical disciplines. First, aesthetic operations are performed on an elective basis for no truly functional purpose (although it has been argued that the function of the face, eg, is to "look good"). In other words, patients are subjected to all the risks of anesthesia and surgery despite their being physiologically healthy. These patients can suffer all types of complications that are possible with other types of surgery, including nerve damage, hematomas, infections, skin loss, significant scarring, myocardial infarctions, and even death. The aesthetic surgeon must be comfortable knowing that these adverse events will doubtlessly occur at some point despite even the most careful patient selection, perfect surgical technique, and smooth anesthesia.

Aesthetic surgeons must enjoy participating in detailed discussions with their patients about their aesthetic issues and the surgical plan. Honest two-way communication is essential to be sure that patients' aesthetic expectations are realistic. They require much more question-and-answer time than reconstructive patients do. Careful patient selection is critical. Usually, however, the expectations of the aesthetic patient are reasonable, and their response to cosmetic surgery is predictable.

Cosmetic surgery is unlike other fields within plastic surgery because of economic issues. There are no laws dictating the price of a facelift or blepharoplasty. Therefore, surgical fees are determined by supply and demand, and often these fees can be very high—on the order of $10,000 to $25,000 for a facelift alone, not including anesthetic expenses. Not surprisingly, other practitioners with varying degrees of training are performing cosmetic procedures. For example, dermatologists, dentists, oral surgeons, otolaryngologists, and even some ophthalmologists perform facial aesthetic surgery. Likewise, some obstetricians and general surgeons have performed breast augmentation and liposuction. Some states have passed laws preventing nonsurgeons from performing cosmetic surgery.

For those with artistic abilities, aesthetic surgery offers a means of sculpting the human body into living art. And the results can be truly impressive! Patients with facial aging can often be made to look

---

VITAL SIGNS

PLASTIC AND RECONSTRUCTIVE SURGERY 2011 MATCH STATISTICS

- Number of positions available: 108
- 175 US seniors and 36 independent applicants ranked at least one plastic surgery program
- 100% of all positions were filled in the initial Match
- The successful applicants: 91.6% US seniors, 0.1% foreign-trained physicians, and 0.1% osteopathic graduates
- Mean USMLE Step I score: 249
- Unmatched rate for US seniors applying only to plastic surgery: 24.6%

Data from National Resident Matching Program.

---

literally decades younger and more energetic. Likewise, a woman who has had multiple pregnancies resulting in abdominal wall laxity and breast involutional ptosis can be made to look like she has the body of a 20-year-old. A young, otherwise beautiful girl who happens to have a prominent nose or ears can be given more harmonious features. It can be quite gratifying indeed to provide joy to a patient who has been concerned with a cosmetic deformity for years.

Most aesthetic fellowships last 6 months and tend to focus on a specific region—facial aesthetic surgery or body contouring surgery. There is currently no certificate of added qualification (CAQ) or universally accepted board examination for aesthetic surgery.

Residency in plastic surgery requires 5 to 8 years of postgraduate training depending on the pathway chosen. There are currently 90 accredited programs. Typical rotations include plastic surgery, orthopedics, otolaryngology, maxillofacial surgery, pediatric general surgery, neurosurgery, trauma and burn surgery, general surgery, vascular surgery, emergency medicine, anesthesiology, and critical care. Rotations on plastic surgical services include pediatric plastic surgery, microsurgery and general reconstruction, hand surgery, aesthetic surgery, and burn reconstruction. Some programs may have satellite centers including private hospital affiliates or Veterans' Administration medical centers. Residents also devote significant time to patient care and preparation for case presentations and conferences. Most plastic surgery residents publish papers during residency. In light of recent ACGME work hour guidelines, most residents have time for raising families and participating in outside athletic, musical, and artistic interests. Most residents develop collegial, productive relationships with their attendings that continue beyond residency.

THE INSIDE SCOOP

Burn Surgery

One-year fellowships are available to those seeking advanced training in burn critical care, acute surgery, and burn reconstruction. Plastic surgeons often head burn units in North America and elsewhere, although general surgeons also play a major role in burn care. Burn surgeons treat patients with thermal injury, electrical injury, chemical injury, immune-mediated burn-like injuries including Stevens-Johnson syndrome, and cold-related injury. Plastic surgeons often focus on burn reconstruction rather than acute burn care. The care of these patients can be quite challenging and highly rewarding. Much of burn reconstruction requires the use of local flaps, skin grafts, and tissue expansion. However, many cases require multiple stages, strategic planning, and advanced techniques.

Craniofacial Surgery

Craniofacial surgeons treat diseases of the bones and soft tissues of the face and skull. They often work with children, treating such conditions as craniosynostosis (premature fusion of the sutures of the skull), cleft palate, hemifacial microsomia (delayed growth of one side of the face), and conditions such as Apert, Crouzon, Treacher-Collins, and Pfeiffer syndromes. They can also work with adults, treating patients with untreated congenital anomalies, craniofacial trauma, and tumors of the skull base, as well as orthognathic deformities.

A team approach is used in the workup, management, and follow-up of children with craniofacial anomalies. Craniofacial surgeons work closely with neurosurgeons, dentists, speech pathologists, social workers, and pediatricians to plan craniofacial and orthognathic (jaw correcting) procedures. Craniofacial surgeons usually practice within a large tertiary care medical center to generate the case volume necessary for sustaining a standing craniofacial anomalies program. However, many craniofacially trained plastic surgeons find that the volume of craniofacial cases in their practice is less than desired.

Hand and Upper Extremity Surgery

Hand surgeons treat a variety of conditions of the hand and upper extremity, including fractures, tendon lacerations, traumatic amputations/devascularizations, rheumatoid arthritis, nerve entrapment syndromes, tumors, and congenital anomalies. In a single day, a hand surgeon may perform a replantation from an industrial accident, see a newborn with complete syndactyly, and perform implant arthroplasties to restore function in a patient with rheumatoid arthritis. Restoring pain-free function is the top priority in hand surgery. Cosmesis is also a secondary goal once pain and function have been addressed.

Worldwide, most hand surgeons are initially trained in plastic surgery. In the United States, however, plastic surgeons represent only one-third of hand surgeons, with the balance coming mainly from orthopedics. Passing a qualifying examination earns the physician a CAQ, which some centers may require in order to be on call. Hand fellowships are often combined with microsurgical fellowships ("hand–micro" fellowships). There is significant crossover between hand surgery and microvascular surgery training; both usually involve advanced microvascular and microneural techniques specific to the upper extremity. Because hand surgeons often perform procedures involving small vessels and nerves of the upper extremity, a strong microsurgical background is critical. There is currently great demand for hand surgeons, especially those with a plastic surgery background, in both private and academic practice.

Microvascular Surgery

Microsurgeons are trained to manipulate tissues by creating microvascular anastomoses and microneural coaptations. They can, for example, replant a severed digit or extremity by repairing the vessels and nerves under the operating microscope. Microsurgical techniques are also used to perform free tissue transfers (free flaps). For example, if a woman has a mastectomy for cancer and desires an autologous (from her own tissue) reconstruction, then an excellent option is a flap reconstruction in which skin and fat are removed from the abdomen and placed on the chest wall to reconstruct the breast. Similarly, in cases of congenital facial paralysis, the gracilis muscle can be transferred to the face to make facial expression possible.

The microsurgical revolution occurred in the 1970s and 1980s. Demand for surgeons who have completed microvascular fellowships remains high, although perhaps not as high as during the past 20 years. Many plastic surgery programs provide extensive microvascular experience, and many plastic surgeons find that they are able to perform the more routine free tissue transfers without the need for further training. However, for complex reconstructive problems, especially those involving the head and neck and the extremities, advanced microvascular training is valuable.

Pediatric Plastic Surgery

Pediatric plastic surgeons address the specialized plastic surgical needs of children, analogous to the way in which pediatric general surgeons address the general surgical needs of children. Pediatric plastic surgeons are usually based in children's hospitals and are university affiliated. Conditions treated by pediatric plastic surgeons include certain craniofacial anomalies, including cleft lip and palate and velopharyngeal insufficiency (nasal speech); separation of conjoined twins; congenital anomalies affecting the face, ears, hands and upper extremities, trunk, and chest wall; and vascular anomalies including hemangiomas and vascular malformations. In addition, pediatric plastic surgery encompasses pediatric burn reconstruction, soft tissue tumors, and traumatic reconstruction, particularly of the face, hands, and lower extremity. There are several craniofacial fellowships that include aspects of pediatric plastic surgery. However, there are very few fellowships that encompass the entire breadth of pediatric plastic surgery. Most of these last 12 to 24 months.

SO YOU WANT TO BE A PLASTIC SURGEON?

Unlike other surgical subspecialties, there are several paths a medical student can take to become a plastic surgeon. In essence, there are really two models, "integrated" and "traditional." The best—and most highly desired—among them is the integrated model. In this route, the medical student is accepted into a 6-year categorical plastic surgery training program in which he or she is considered a plastic surgery resident from day 1. Integrated residencies are specifically designed to give the resident graduated responsibility and experience in plastic surgery with a tailored foundation in related disciplines, including orthopedics, otolaryngology, maxillofacial surgery, neurosurgery, burn, trauma, and general surgery and sometimes anesthesiology, oculoplastic surgery, and dermatology.

An alternative to the integrated model is the "combined" (or "3 and 3") training model, which is actually a variation of the traditional model, explained later. In a combined program, the resident functions as a general surgery resident during the first 3 years of residency. In fact, most combined programs require matching into a categorical general surgical residency with the implicit understanding that the resident is interested in plastic surgery. In the fourth year, the combined resident switches to plastic surgery training. The amount of time spent on general surgical rotations is generally greater in combined programs than in integrated programs. Residents rarely obtain chief-level operative experience while on general surgery rotations in the combined model. In contrast, residents in integrated programs often function as general surgery chief residents during part of their fourth year. The Match for integrated programs is administered by the National Resident Matching Program (NRMP).

The third pathway is the traditional (or "independent") model. In the traditional model, a resident is taken into a 2- or 3-year plastic surgery fellowship after a general surgery residency, or after completing a program in otolaryngology, orthopedics, urology, neurosurgery, or oral and maxillofacial surgery. Although the majority of plastic surgeons practicing today train in traditional programs, the number of traditional training positions offered is declining as many programs are converting to categorical (integrated or combined) models. The Match for the traditional model is administered by the Plastic Surgery Residency Matching Program (PSMP), a component of the San Francisco Matching Program.

WHY CONSIDER A CAREER IN PLASTIC SURGERY?

The future looks very bright for plastic surgery. On a practical level, this is a field in which it would be nearly impossible to replace physicians with physician assistants and specialty-trained registered nurses (as has already happened in many specialties). Similarly, the physical defects that plastic surgeons repair are caused by problems that will continue to be major public health concerns, including cancer, trauma, burns, and congenital defects. And as long as people have mirrors, the obsession with youthfulness will ensure that there will always be a demand for aesthetic surgery.

On a more cerebral level, the field of plastic surgery offers a variety of clinical problems, many of which have excellent solutions. Others remain unsolved. Just as there is always something that can be done for plastic surgery patients, so too is there room for young plastic surgeons to make valuable contributions to this rapidly advancing field with basic science, applied science, technical innovation, or outcomes research. Plastic surgeons make an immediate impact on the lives of their patients and can profoundly affect how they feel about themselves. It is a wonderful specialty for those who appreciate the beauty of the human body and have a creative imagination.

ABOUT THE CONTRIBUTOR

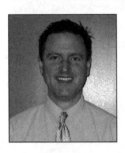

Dr Gregory Borschel completed his plastic surgery residency and research fellowship in tissue engineering at the University of Michigan, followed by a fellowship in pediatric plastic surgery at University of Toronto and The Hospital for Sick Children. He was an assistant professor of plastic surgery at Washington University's St. Louis Children's Hospital. He is now on the faculty at University of Toronto and The Hospital for Sick Children. His clinical focus is on peripheral nerve surgery, microvascular reconstruction, and congenital hand surgery. He also holds a dual appointment in Biomedical Engineering where his research interests include tissue engineering and drug delivery from nerve regeneration. After growing up in Indianapolis, Dr Borschel completed his undergraduate education at Emory University and attended The Johns Hopkins University School of Medicine. Outside of the hospital, he enjoys scuba diving, music, and spending time with his wife, Tina, and his two children. He can be reached by e-mail at gregory.borschel@sickkids.ca.

REFERENCES

1. Thatte, M.R., Thatte, M.L. Venous flaps. *Plast Reconstr Surg.* 1993;91(4):747–751.

2. Micali, G. The Italian contribution to plastic surgery. *Ann Plast Surg.* 1993;31(6):566–571.

3. Rogers, B.O. British plastic surgeons who contributed to the Revue de Chirurgie Plastique and the Revue de Chirurgie Structive (1931–1938): "The big four" in their specialty. *Aesthetic Plast Surg.* 2001;25(3):213–240.

4. Stelnicki, E.J., Young, V.L., et al. Vilray P. Blair: His surgical descendents, and their roles in plastic surgical development. *Plast Reconstr Surg.* 1999;103(7):1990–2009.

5. Morai, W.D, Parker, L. The nonmetropolitan plastic surgeon. *Plast Reconstr Surg.* 1983;72(1):97–103.

29
PSYCHIATRY
Kathleen Ang-Lee

As physicians who treat the mentally ill, psychiatrists have some of the most rewarding long-term relationships with their patients. This is an interdisciplinary specialty, well suited for doctors who wish to use the broadest of all skills—psychosocial, scientific, and clinical. Historically, psychotherapy has always formed the core of psychiatry. But with remarkable advances in neuroscience and drug therapy, this field of medicine has shifted to a more biological-based approach. Now, psychiatrists draw on the latest research in brain imaging, genetics, and psychopharmacology to treat many debilitating disorders.

Most medical students begin their psychiatry clerkship with a preconceived notion of this specialty. You probably imagine that all psychiatrists tell their patients to lie down on their leather couches and talk about their childhood. Or, you may think that these physicians are simply drug dispensers. In reality, the practice of contemporary psychiatry falls somewhere between these two extremes.

THE MEDICINE OF MENTAL HEALTH

Psychiatry is the field of medicine dedicated to the prevention, diagnosis, and treatment of mental illness. The diseases psychiatrists treat include depression, bipolar disorder, schizophrenia, addiction, delirium and dementia, anxiety, and personality disorders.

Psychiatrists meet an essential need within medicine. Psychiatric disorders, which are extremely common in society, often remain undiagnosed. In a given year, nearly 32.4% of all Americans older than 18 years suffer from a diagnosable mental disorder.[1] Like physical diseases of the body, these conditions range in severity. They can cause mild social isolation, severe occupational impairment, or even can be life threatening. Although many patients may not even appear ill, others present with withdrawal, psychosis, or confusion. This wide scope of disease provides intellectual stimulation and daily challenge.

There is no such thing as a typical psychiatric patient. In fact, many students discover that psychiatric patients are even more challenging than those with medical problems. You might be treating a depressed young woman with thoughts of suicide. Your next patient may be someone suffering from panic attacks, obsessive–compulsive disorder, or unusual phobias. Complex cases of schizophrenia, in which the patient presents with extremely distorted views of reality, are de rigueur for the typical psychiatrist. They also manage problems of sexual dysfunction, eating disorders such as anorexia and bulimia, and all forms of substance abuse. If you are interested in working with children, the subspecialty of child psychiatry offers classic cases of attention-deficit/hyperactivity disorder, learning disorders, and other behavioral problems.

Many physicians are initially drawn to psychiatry because of the intriguing combination of medicine, psychology, and the social sciences. This specialty focuses on what makes people tick—how they feel, think, and behave. A psychiatrist in academics explained that "I really enjoyed studying philosophy and psychology in college, and psychiatry seemed to be a way to combine medical science with my background in the humanities and social science."

It is important not to overlook the fact that psychiatrists are, first and foremost, medical doctors. Many medical conditions such as a stroke, thyroid disease, autoimmune diseases, or tumors can cause psychiatric disorders. Psychiatrists need to rule out any possible underlying medical diseases or drug reactions before treating a mental illness. In the hospital, they are called upon as consultants to distinguish between psychiatric causes and other medical causes of patients' symptoms. Every day, psychiatrists see first hand the intricate relationships between mental disorders, emotional illness, and medical diseases of the body. Because psychotropic medications affect other organ systems, psychiatrists must recognize adverse side effects and drug–drug interactions. A strong background in internal medicine and neurology, therefore, is essential for the practice of psychiatry.

If you are planning a career in this specialty, you will get to know well the "bible" of psychiatry—the *Diagnostic and Statistical Manual of Mental Disorders*, or simply, the DSM. Published by the American Psychiatric Association (APA), this mammoth text has undergone several revisions throughout decades of advancements. Based on symptoms rather than etiology, this hefty manual describes and categorizes the operational criteria of all recognized mental illnesses. It does not discuss treatment options. Instead, the DSM serves as a common classification system to which all psychiatrists adhere when assigning diagnoses. Currently, psychiatrists around the world use the fourth edition (text revision) of the DSM. At the time of press, the APA is conducting field trials on the latest update, the DSM-5, and it is expected to be approved in 2013.

THE PSYCHIATRIC EVALUATION: LISTENING TO PATIENTS' STORIES

When evaluating their patients, psychiatrists conduct a specialized psychiatric interview to gather information and initiate treatment. This workup includes a thorough medical and psychiatric history along with a complete mental status examination. Aspiring psychiatrists find that a patient's interpersonal style, choice of subjects, and nonverbal communications—as well as your own emotional reactions to the patient—all constitute valuable data.

There are few mental illnesses for which a definitive laboratory test exists. In psychiatry, the patient interview is often the most important diagnostic instrument. With a complete history and interview, psychiatrists obtain indispensable information that goes beyond mere facts. To succeed well at these endeavors, medical students interested in psychiatry should have good communication and interpersonal skills. It also helps being flexible in your diagnostic thinking and tolerating some degree of uncertainty. Armed with this understanding, psychiatrists make accurate diagnoses and then recommend treatment options.

The doctor–patient relationship is absolutely essential to psychiatry. In this specialty, physicians take time to listen carefully to their patients' personal problems. "I have always been interested in understanding other people and hearing their stories," remarked a psychiatry resident. More than anything, psychiatrists are caring, nonjudgmental, and genuinely interested in what goes on in their patients' lives. Unlike other specialists, they get to spend more allotted time with their patients and maintain good working relationships under difficult circumstances. During these interactions, psychiatrists address the whole patient, including mental, physical, and psychosocial aspects.

As you can tell, this specialty has two intriguing components: the challenging nature of diagnosis and the diverse patients who will share their stories with you. "It's an incredible privilege to have patients let you into their lives. You see and hear things that most people only see in movies or read about in books—this is not mundane medicine," declared a university-based psychiatrist. And, they are

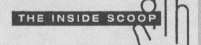
all extremely busy doctors. Mental disorders (particularly depression and alcohol abuse) include seven out of the top ten leading causes of disability in developed countries, with depression projected to be the second leading cause of disability from all health conditions by the year 2020.[2]

This specialty is more than just sitting back and listening to patients' stories. Psychiatrists derive a great deal of personal fulfillment in actively helping patients who have debilitating mental disorders. "There is a sense that you can really change someone's life," one psychiatrist commented. "You don't necessarily have to be a surgeon and operate in order to dramatically alter a patient's life."

THE MIRACLES OF PSYCHOPHARMACOLOGY

Just as many diabetic patients require insulin and heart patients take nitroglycerin, people suffering from a severe mental illness may need a specific type of psychiatric medication. In recent years, the field of psychopharmacology has grown significantly. Treatment with drugs usually ends up being long term, and there are few actual cures. Long ago, mentally ill patients were often placed in public institutions because they were thought to be harmful to themselves or to others. Thanks to the latest drugs on the market, most people today who suffer from a psychiatric illness—even debilitating ones such as schizophrenia—can lead full lives after effective treatment.

What are some of these miracle drugs? Fluoxetine (Prozac), which revolutionized the treatment of major depression in 1987, is probably the best-known example of the class of drugs called selective serotonin reuptake inhibitors (SSRIs), which are relatively safe and have a favorable side-effect profile. These agents not only treat depression but also help manage cases of panic disorder, obsessive–compulsive disorder, and social phobia. Antipsychotic medications also underwent a revolution with the introduction of atypicals (such as risperidone, olanzapine, and quetiapine), which have fewer adverse reactions. Now there are atypical antipsychotics that can be given intramuscularly for acute treatment or in a long-term depot formulation, just like the good old standby—Haldol ("vitamin H"), or as orally disintegrating tablets for faster onset of action. These are just some of the examples of the rapidly evolving psychopharmacology options available to contemporary psychiatrists.

Psychopharmacology involves more than just antidepressant, antipsychotic, and anticonvulsant medications. Now biotechnology and neuroscience are coming together in the new discipline of "pharmacogenomics." This area of drug therapy promises to tailor treatment to each individual in order to improve efficacy and reduce adverse effects. The list of possible medications will now grow even longer.

PSYCHOTHERAPY IN THE TWENTY-FIRST CENTURY

With psychotropic medications increasing in efficacy, specificity, and popularity, many students wonder if there is still a role for psychotherapy in modern psychiatric treatment. In fact, the demise of psychotherapy has been greatly exaggerated. During residency, psychiatrists are trained in many different forms of psychotherapy and it still remains an integral part of this specialty.

What exactly is psychotherapy? It is a systematic method of treatment in which the psychiatrist and the patient discuss troubling feelings, thoughts, and life problems during regularly scheduled meetings. Together, they find solutions to the underlying roots of these issues and help the patient to deal with symptoms. There are many types of psychotherapy, such as those that help patients explore past relationships, discuss repressed feelings, or change thought patterns or behaviors. For most people, psychotherapy conjures up images of Sigmund Freud and classic psychoanalysis. This intensive form of individual psychotherapy involves four or five sessions per week over the course of several years. Psychoanalysts help patients recall and examine past events and memories to help them better understand their present behavior. Other commonly used forms of talk therapy include cognitive therapy, behavioral therapy, psychodynamic psychotherapy, and couples and family therapy.

Whether used alone or in combination with medications, psychotherapy works very well to treat a broad range of mental illnesses and psychiatric disturbances. Thanks to managed care, the stereotype of psychiatrists reclining in their armchairs while listening to patients talk has become outmoded. Today's psychiatrists are not purely therapists. Although they still practice psychotherapy, the modern psychiatrist uses a broader array of treatments—biological, psychological, and social—tailored to the specific needs of the patient. Most psychiatrists consider a combination of medication and therapy to be the most effective solution. A university-based psychiatrist commented that "every interaction I have with my patients is psychotherapy, even when I am only doing 'medication management.'"

As physicians working at the complex interface between mind and body, psychiatrists take advantage of this integrative approach. "You need to have a good understanding of your patients' psychological makeup so you don't attribute biological symptoms to psychological causes, and vice versa," stated one psychiatrist. "The physicians who run into trouble are the ones who only want to look at things as all biological or all psychological, without looking at the big picture." Psychiatrists form therapeutic alliances by listening to patients discuss their illness and how it affects their lives. With this style, psychotherapy becomes intrinsic to pharmacologic treatment.

ELECTROCONVULSIVE THERAPY: TREATING THE MIND WITH ELECTRICITY

When patients struggling with their disease do not respond to mainstay treatment, clinicians sometimes turn to the single procedure available in their therapeutic arsenal: electroconvulsive therapy (ECT). Most people's perception of ECT as brutal and cruel comes from movies such as "One Flew over the Cuckoo's Nest" and "A Beautiful Mind," which depict the early use of shock therapy. During the 1940s and 1950s, psychiatrists in the United States usually performed ECT on the most severely disturbed patients, such as those who suffered from schizophrenia or uncontrolled bipolar disorder. In the early days of the treatment, physicians often conducted ECT at high doses for long periods of time. This method proved harmful to patients, giving ECT its reputation as an abusive treatment that was sometimes used to gain control over unruly patients.

Today, psychiatrists turn to ECT as one of the most effective (and safest) treatments available for major depressive disorder. This therapy can also be extremely beneficial for patients suffering from mania, catatonia, schizophrenia, and other neuropsychiatric conditions. During the procedure, the psychiatrist activates the passage of controlled pulses of electrical current through the patient's brain. The stimulation produces a generalized seizure lasting 25 to 150 seconds. Contrary to popular belief, ECT is a brief, painless procedure. It is always administered under general anesthesia with muscle relaxation. Most patients requiring this course of therapy for depression will undergo roughly 6 to 12 treatments, with one treatment given three times per week.

In practice, psychiatrists either obtain a training certificate to perform electro-convulsive shock therapy themselves or send their patients to an affiliated hospital to receive treatment. In either case, ECT is one of the only nonpharmacologic procedures currently available to treat severe or medication-refractory depression and other psychiatric disorders. It is also effective for patients who cannot take their psychotropic medications for reasons such as underlying cardiac disease. Another promising noninvasive procedure recently approved by the Food and Drug Administration (FDA) in 2011 for treatment resistant major depressive disorder is called repetitive transcranial magnetic stimulation (rTMS). Deep brain stimulation, a surgical procedure, is also being researched for treatment of certain psychiatric disorders. Thus, the therapeutic armamentarium of this specialty is poised to continue expanding in the near future.

REFLECTIONS ON MENTAL ILLNESS AND PSYCHIATRY

Mental illnesses are real diseases that affect a person's brain and change the way a person behaves, thinks, and interacts with others. In medicine, there exists an erroneous belief that diagnosis and treatment within psychiatry has no scientific foundation. The latest research, however, demonstrates strong physiologic and genetic components to most mental illnesses. For instance, neuroscientists have shown that patients diagnosed with major depression have lower levels of certain neurotransmitters, such as serotonin and norepinephrine. And the latest computerized brain imaging techniques can show chemical abnormalities in the brains of those suffering from schizophrenia and other psychiatric disorders. "As psychiatry becomes more and more biologically based, and we continue to increase our understanding of the biological basis of behavior, psychiatry will eventually become more integrated with medicine," declared one psychiatrist in academia.

Despite this shift in focus to biological models, prejudice and discrimination against the mentally ill persists, no matter the type of disease. Some people mistakenly believe that mental illness is caused by personal weakness, poor upbringing, or a defect in character. They think that sufferers of psychiatric disorders should just "snap out of it." Yet the agitated homeless man talking to himself on the street and the chronic alcoholic who cannot quit drinking both suffer from pathophysiologic derangements. Just like conditions such as diabetes or high blood pressure, psychiatric disorders are biochemically based and require long-term treatment.

Many colleagues in medicine who do not look highly upon psychiatry consider its treatments less effective than those in other areas of medicine. The evidence refutes this misperception. With its wide array of powerful drugs, treatment in modern psychiatry surpasses conventional therapies found in other areas of medicine. In a study by the National Institutes of Mental Health, the success rates (defined as "substantial reduction or remission of symptoms") in treating mental illness were superior to certain medical procedures. It looks like psychiatrists have the edge over cardiologists: the success rates for treatment of depression (60–65%), schizophrenia (60%), and panic disorder (80%) were significantly higher compared with acute coronary syndromes treated with angioplasty (40%) and atherectomy (50%).[3] In a similar study, the success rates of therapy for addictive disorders, such as alcoholism (50%) and cocaine dependence (55%), were on the same level as chronic medical diseases such as asthma, diabetes, and hypertension.[4] In addition, much of the morbidity of other illnesses can be traced to behavioral or mental health issues that impair a patients' desire and/or ability to participate in their own health care. Therefore, psychiatric intervention can also significantly improve the outcome of other medical conditions.

Despite this evidence, psychiatrists and other professionals who care for the mentally ill traditionally have not received much respect from their peers. Psychiatry, with its earlier emphasis on psychodynamic and social models, has been seen as fluffy and nonscientific. Ignoring the biological basis of behavior, most physicians perceive psychiatry as less scientific and prestigious than other medical specialties. Nearly half of all psychiatrists agreed that other medical specialists view them as less than important.[5]

Unfortunately, this negative attitude carries over to medical students, who, just like their mentors, perceive psychiatry as a minimally important specialty. In a recent survey, entering first-year medical students believed that psychiatry had less prestige, satisfaction, and intellectual challenge than most other specialties.[6] They felt that the medical community, and the public in general, does not respect psychiatrists' skills and knowledge. Whether based on ignorance or misunderstanding, the persistently low ranking of psychiatry indicates that many continue to perceive it as outside the mainstream of medical practice.

Yet as new developments shift the focus of psychiatry to a biological approach, psychiatrists are beginning to garner more respect from the medical community. After all, they take care of extremely challenging patients most doctors would prefer to avoid. "You can't be thin-skinned to be in this field," a resident remarked. "But psychiatrists get their satisfaction from the knowledge that they have an incredibly important and interesting job—one that can really make a difference in patients' lives." If you are considering a career in psychiatry, do your best to disregard any mocking comments from those who fear treating patients with mental illness. These patients need your care and attention. Every day, they will provide intellectual satisfaction and personal fulfillment.

SCOPE-OF-PRACTICE ISSUES: PSYCHIATRISTS VERSUS PSYCHOLOGISTS

Today, physicians across all specialties are forced to share certain duties with competing non-MD mid-level health care providers. Managed care and its push for cost containment, however, have hit psychiatry unusually hard. Medical students considering a career in psychiatry often wonder about competition from other mental health professionals, such as clinical psychologists, social workers, and nurse practitioners. Many of these professionals can perform psychotherapy. In some states, particularly rural ones, nurse practitioners are often the first-line health providers evaluating and treating psychiatric patients.

In particular, the issue of psychologists being allowed to prescribe psychiatric drugs is currently a matter of hot debate. Clinical psychologists do not have the education or experience to use powerful drugs in treating mental disease. Yet, in 2002, New Mexico made national headlines when legislators passed a law granting prescription-writing authority to psychologists. It became the first state to do so. In this case, psychologists argued that large rural areas of the state do not have enough psychiatrists for prescribing psychoactive medications. They have won a battle lost in other states. In the past decade, about 17 state legislatures rejected similar bills after considering the data and risks of placing potent drugs into the hands of people without medical education. Since 2002, only one other state, Louisiana, has passed a similar law allowing psychologists to have prescription privileges.

Nearly all psychiatrists (and many psychologists) agree that this ill-advised decision in New Mexico and Louisiana has significant potential to harm patients with mental illness. Because only those with the proper education should practice medicine, the medical community seriously questions whether psychologists can prescribe effectively and safely. Clinical psychologists, who hold masters or doctoral degrees, are trained only in psychotherapeutic principles to treat mental disorders. The New Mexico and Louisiana laws grant prescription-writing privileges only to psychologists who take a crash course on psychopharmacology and pass a certification examination. But no quick workshop in drug prescribing, especially when reportedly designed and administered by psychologists, can substitute for the knowledge and skills earned from medical school, postgraduate training, and rigorous clinical experience.

Psychiatrists have extensive training in differential diagnosis, complex psychopharmacology, and the ability to evaluate whether symptoms are related to drugs or new medical problems. Whether or not they prescribe medication, psychiatrists, with their comprehensive understanding of both mind and body, always bring medical evaluation into their interactions with patients, even in psychotherapy sessions. As one academic psychiatrist observed,

As we increasingly understand how the rest of medicine can affect behavior, you must have a strong medical background in order to provide the best care. For instance, I had a patient who was seen by a psychologist who called him 'profoundly depressed with extremely latent speech.' When I saw him, I was able to immediately see that he was actually aphasic, and obtained a CT scan which showed a large brain mass. When you don't have a wide base of medical training, you miss things. This is not just about a power struggle between the psychiatrists and psychologists; it's just about good patient care.

As this example illustrates, there are still many unanswered questions regarding patient safety and psychologists' ability to recognize their own limitations and knowledge gaps (which should prompt a referral). The implications for medication errors and patient safety raise significant concerns. Unfortunately, there remains a lack of consistent empirical evidence for the safety, feasibility, and cost-effectiveness of psychologist prescription laws.

The first psychologists to train under the new law in New Mexico finished their academic and practical preparation at the end of 2003. Will this mark the beginning of a fundamental change in how mental illness is treated in the United States? It is still too soon to tell. Health insurance priorities have already shifted toward drug treatment over psychotherapy. If more states adopted such legislation, it might lead to more patients on psychiatric medications and less insurance reimbursement for psychiatrists' fees. Currently, no other similar bills in state legislatures have passed, but Oregon nearly passed such a law in 2010 (it was vetoed by the governor) and other states are still trying to bring similar bills to their legislature.

Regardless of the outcome, the current debate should not discourage medical students who are interested in psychiatry. Psychiatry is still a specialty that is short of physicians. The huge unmet demand for psychiatrists has been well established.[7,8] Most psychiatrists worry about the quality of patient care under the new law—not their jobs. They are not threatened in any way by competition from other mental health professionals. Remember, for the past several decades, primary care physicians and other nonpsychiatrists have written the majority of prescriptions for psychoactive medications. "We will still be the specialists in the field, seeing the most challenging—and interesting—psychiatric cases," stated a psychiatrist in private practice. The special education and medical experience of psychiatrists make them uniquely qualified to provide both psychotherapy and medication management.

LIFESTYLE CONSIDERATIONS AND PRACTICE OPTIONS

As in specialties such as family practice and general internal medicine, psychiatrists deal with mostly chronic illnesses that require long-term pharmacologic and therapeutic management. They work with adults, children, families, or a combination of all three. You can decide if you want to concentrate more on psychotherapy in your practice or on medication management. Psychiatric hospitalization is now shorter and more focused than in the past, with a greater emphasis on outpatient management and prevention. Managed care guidelines used to commonly limit the number of patient visits to a psychiatrist, but the mental health parity legislation that passed in 2008 has required insurers to apply the same treatment and financial limits to psychiatric and substance abuse treatment that are equivalent (or better) than what they allow for medical and surgical care. This has greatly benefitted outpatient psychiatric treatment, allowing more patients to receive the regular psychotherapy and medication management they need to best manage their psychiatric disorders.

You have a wide variety of practice options in this specialty. Psychiatrists typically see patients in outpatient, inpatient, or emergency room settings. In the hospital, they often work as the part of a team that tailors a wide range of biological, psychotherapeutic, and psychosocial treatments to specific patient needs. Psychiatrists lead a group that may include clinical psychologists, social workers, psychiatric nurses, mental health counselors, and occupational and recreational therapists. Outpatient psychiatrists may have solo or group practices in clinics or community mental health centers. Here, they have the flexibility to set their own hours. They may also work in residential programs, VA hospitals, nursing homes, correctional facilities, and state hospitals. Many outpatient psychiatrists choose to work in a combination of these settings. "There is such a wide range of things you can do in psychiatry," affirmed a psychiatrist in private practice. "You can be flexible in this field and create a niche for

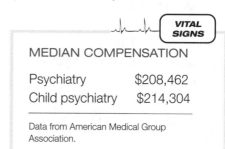

VITAL SIGNS

MEDIAN COMPENSATION

Psychiatry $208,462
Child psychiatry $214,304

Data from American Medical Group Association.

yourself both in terms of your interests and management of your time." The many subspecialties within psychiatry offer additional career opportunities, and the end of the national generalist initiative has created many new jobs for graduating residents. Because of the variety of practice opportunities, psychiatrists generally lead a comfortable lifestyle. Call is minimal to nonexistent, emergencies are few and far between, and office hours are regular. Sound appealing?

FELLOWSHIPS AND SUBSPECIALTY TRAINING

At this time, five psychiatry fellowships are approved by the Accreditation Council for Graduate Medical Education (ACGME) and have their own subspecialty examinations leading to official board certification. Additionally, each fellowship lasts for 1 additional year of training, with the exception of child and adolescent psychiatry (2 years).

There are also several emerging subspecialties within this diverse field, such as emergency and disaster psychiatry, psychopharmacology, neuropsychiatry, and research. Formal fellowships are likely forthcoming. You can also choose to specialize in various psychotherapies by further training at a psychoanalytic or behavioral therapy institute.

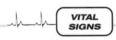

**PSYCHIATRY
2011 MATCH STATISTICS**

- Number of positions available: 1101
- 714 US seniors and 1279 independent applicants ranked at least one psychiatry program
- 97.3% of all positions were filled in the initial Match
- The successful applicants: 60% US seniors, 14.4% foreign-trained physicians, and 10.6% osteopathic graduates
- Mean USMLE Step I score: 214
- Unmatched rate for US seniors applying only to psychiatry: 3.7%

Data from National Resident Matching Program.

Addiction Psychiatry

According to a recent survey by the National Institute on Drug Abuse, approximately 3.5 million Americans are addicted to illicit drugs and 8.2 million fit the diagnosis of alcoholism. Based on these growing numbers, more specialists are needed to work in this critical area. Psychiatrists who specialize in addiction psychiatry are at the forefront of battling this epidemic. When managing disorders of addiction, they draw on their knowledge of pharmacology and physiology. Drugs such as cocaine, alcohol, heroin, nicotine, and methamphetamine have profound, and usually devastating, effects on all organ systems. Addiction psychiatrists are also trained to recognize comorbid psychiatric and substance use disorders.

Child and Adolescent Psychiatry

The child psychiatrist serves as the advocate for the best interests of their young patients. According to the APA, an estimated 7 to 12 million youths in the United States suffer from a diagnosable psychiatric disorder. But only a very small proportion actually receives some form of mental health service. For the most comprehensive medical care, they need the expertise of a specialist in child and adolescent psychiatry.

The mental, behavioral, and developmental problems that affect children and teenagers include autism, attention-deficit hyperactivity disorder, learning disorders, bulimia and anorexia, behavioral disorders, and emotional disturbances. In their diagnostic examinations, child psychiatrists look at many components, from physical to cognitive and from genetic to emotional. They take an integrative biopsychosocial approach and consult with physicians and professionals from schools, social agencies, and juvenile courts. Working with kids challenges your creativity and imagination. And they need you, too—there is currently a national shortage of qualified child psychiatrists. By 2020, the demand for these specialists is expected to increase by nearly 100%.[9] Although this fellowship requires 2 years of additional study, residents usually begin training after their third postgraduate year and complete both residency and fellowship within 5 years.

Forensic Psychiatry

This subspecialty is ideal for physicians who wish to apply their psychiatric training to legal matters. Forensic psychiatrists are not lawyers. Instead, they translate their medical knowledge of mental health into useful advice for the legal system. Forensic psychiatrists serve as clinical consultants to attorneys, victims, perpetrators, courts, or other parties involved in litigation. Through actual court testimony, they offer evaluations of criminal matters, patient competency, malpractice, mental disability, involuntary treatment, child custody, and the insanity defense. Although typically paid by attorneys to serve as expert witnesses, forensic psychiatrists try to avoid bias by focusing on the evidence within their area

RESIDENCY TRAINING

Residency in psychiatry requires 4 years of postgraduate training. There are currently 184 accredited programs. During the first year, residents typically rotate through 4 months of inpatient internal medicine and 2 months of inpatient adult neurology. Depending on the institution, some programs heavily emphasize pharmacology and biochemistry, whereas others focus on psychotherapy. Many residency programs have weekly training groups ("T groups") in which residents provide peer support, teach each other, and help run the residency. The typical monthly rotations include adult inpatient service, consultation–liaison psychiatry, geriatrics, child and adolescent psychiatry, outpatient clinics, addiction psychiatry, emergency psychiatry, and psychotherapy. Residents also can become trained in performing ECT.

THE INSIDE SCOOP

of expertise. Like other legal professionals, they draw heavily on their writing, research, and analytical skills. They review records, interview people, and consult with lawyers and other physicians. Most forensic psychiatrists continue to see patients in a clinical setting in addition to legal consultations.

Geriatric Psychiatry

Elderly patients often present with a set of psychiatric disorders that are more prevalent among their age group, including dementia, delirium, and depression. Geriatric psychiatrists specialize in the biological and psychological components of the normal aging process. They manage the psychiatric effects of acute and chronic physical illness, such as cancer, heart attacks, renal failure, or osteoarthritis. Taking into account the physiologic changes unique to the elderly patient, geriatric psychiatrists use pharmacology to treat primary psychiatric disturbances of old age.

Psychosomatic Medicine or Consultation–Liaison Psychiatry

This subspecialty deals with the diagnosis and treatment of psychiatric disorders in complex medically ill patients. These specialists treat patients with acute or chronic medical, neurological, or surgical illness in which psychiatric morbidity affects their medical care. They also care for patients who may have a psychiatric disorder that is a direct consequence of a primary medical condition.

Psychosomatic medicine represents the interface between psychiatry and the rest of medicine.

WHY CONSIDER A CAREER IN PSYCHIATRY?

Although this specialty is one of the oldest in medicine, World War II marked the beginning of modern psychiatry. At that time, hundreds of recruits were found psychiatrically unfit for induction, sparking a renewed interest in mental health. The federal government devoted massive resources toward the field, particularly with the establishment in 1949 of the National Institute of Mental Health. Medical students of the 1960s, who viewed psychiatry as a means of social change, flocked into the specialty. But while becoming more biologically oriented, psychiatry lost much of its resources due to the nation's desire to produce more generalist physicians. Combined with encroachment from managed care and competition from other mental health care providers, recruitment among graduating medical students began to decline.[10] In fact, the total number of US seniors entering psychiatry reached a low of 428 (52% of all applicants) in 1998.[11] The trend, however, is now rapidly reversing as the need for specialists increases. The number of psychiatrists is far short of the current need, with preliminary estimates placing the shortage at around 45,000 psychiatrists.[12] All signs indicate that this shortage will worsen in the future, since the demand of psychiatric services is increasing significantly due to population growth, greater evidence for the treatability of mental illness, more efficacious medications, and social acceptability of mental illness conditions.[13]

In addition to the flourishing job market, psychiatry has a promising future as a frontier area that overlaps considerably with neurology. During the 1990s (the National Institutes of Health's "Decade of the Brain"), psychiatrists were major players in the remarkable advances in neuroscience, brain imaging, and psychopharmacology. These developments have led to exciting and effective new methods in diagnosis and treatment. Psychiatrists now have new drugs, new high-tech neuroimaging modalities, and the forthcoming DSM-5.

Most students who enter psychiatry have a strong background in humanities and seek the intellectual challenge of dealing with people's minds. This profession provides all of that and more. It blends biology, psychology, and sociocultural aspects together with clinical medicine. You get to know your patients well and strive to restore their mental and physical well-being. You use powerful medications to change lives. You find yourself engaged in challenging and rewarding work: bringing hope to patients suffering from troubling and disabling illness.

ABOUT THE CONTRIBUTOR

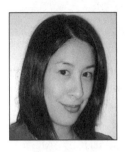

Dr Kathleen Ang-Lee received her BS in anthropology-zoology from the University of Michigan and earned an MD from the University of Chicago—Pritzker School of Medicine. She completed a psychiatry residency and a fellowship in addiction psychiatry at the University of Washington Hospitals. She currently works as a general and addiction psychiatrist in private practice in Seattle, Washington.

REFERENCES

1. Kessler, R.C., Chiu, W.T., et al. Prevalence, severity, and comorbidity of twelve-month DSM-IV disorders in the National Comorbidity Survey Replication (NCS-R). *Arch Gen Psychiatry*. 2005;62(6):617–627.

2. Murray, C.L., Lopez, A.D. *The global burden of disease*. Cambridge, MA: Harvard University Press; 1996.

3. National Advisory Mental Health Council. Health care reform for Americans with severe mental illnesses. *Am J Psych*. 1993;150(10);1447–1465.

4. O'Brien, C.P., McClellan, A.T. Myths about the treatment of addiction. *Lancet*. 1996;347(8996):237–240.

5. Berman, I., Merson, A., et al. Psychiatrists' attitudes towards psychiatry. *Acad Med*. 1996;71:110–111.

6. Feifel, D., Moutier, C.Y., et al. Attitudes toward psychiatry as a prospective career among students entering medical school. *Am J Psych*. 1999;156:1397–1402.

7. US Department of Health and Human Services. *Mental Health: A Report of the Surgeon General*. 1999.

8. US Department of Health and Human Services. The President's New Freedom Commission on Mental Health. *Achieving the Promise: Transforming Mental Health Care in America*. 2004.

9. Oldham, J.M., Riba, M.B. *Review of Psychiatry*, Vol. 13. Washington, DC: American Psychiatric Press; 1994.

10. Sierles, F.S., Taylor, M.A. Decline of U.S. medical student career choice of psychiatry and what to do about it. *Am J Psych*. 1995;152:1416–1426.

11. *Data and Results—National Resident Matching Program*. Washington, DC; 2002.

12. Carlat, D. 45,000 more psychiatrists, anyone? *Psychiatric Times*. 2010;August 3:1–4.

13. DeMello, J.P., Deshpande, S.P. Career satisfaction of psychiatrists. *Psychiatr Serv*. 2011;62(9):1013–1018.

30

RADIATION ONCOLOGY

Stephanie E. Weiss

O nce one of the best-kept secrets in medicine, radiation oncology has become one of the most competitive residencies in the field. Centered around the physician–patient relationship, radiation oncology is an intellectual and evidenced-driven discipline. Its strength and appeal lies in the multidimensional approach to treating cancer patients.

Although a popular field for training these days, it still remains poorly understood even by physicians in other disciplines. Radiation oncologists are a fundamental component of the interdisciplinary practice of cancer treatment and may act as both consultants to referring physicians and primary oncologist to patients. Using a broad oncologic fund of knowledge, the radiation oncologist approaches the treatment of cancer with meticulous application of his/her technical expertise. If their knowledge base and relationship to the patient is like that of the medical oncologist (doctors who prescribe chemotherapy), the approach is more akin to the surgeon. Every cancer patient offers an individual challenge.

RADIATION AS CANCER TREATMENT

Radiation oncology is the specialty of medicine that uses radiant energy for treating usually malignant and occasionally benign disease. For most folks, it is easy to intuitively grasp why we try to surgically remove tumors from a patient, or to think of prescribing a medicinal substance in terms of so many milligrams of a drug orally or intravenously as with chemotherapy. Yet it is not as obvious to conceptualize radiation as a prescription too. Radiation is invisible energy. It is not typically administered by vein or mouth (there are exceptions) but rather by complicated equipment that may not even touch the patient's body.

Like chemotherapy, radiation, usually in the form of photons and electrons, works therapeutically on the molecular level. Chemotherapy kills cells via the administration of chemical substances into the body geared against various cellular targets; radiotherapy inflicts similar damage through radiation. Specifically, radiation works by damaging DNA and thus interfering with the cell's ability to reproduce successfully. It takes advantage of the fact that normal cells can repair radiation-induced DNA damage in-between daily small-dose treatments, whereas a cancer cell cannot.

It is the responsibility of the radiation oncologist to prescribe the proper dose of radiation to the appropriate anatomic field on the patient. Measured in the unit of Gray, the amount of radiation administered is based on the tumor's radiosensitivity as well as the specific tolerance of nearby normal tissues to radiation. Treatment is adjusted accordingly to cause maximum damage to cancer cells while keeping normal tissue within its tolerance. Doctors change the daily dose or overall length of treatment to optimize clinical benefits. The difference in susceptibility to radiation between normal cells and cancer cells is called the therapeutic index. A skilled radiation oncologist manipulates various treatment factors for each plan to take full advantage of this parameter.

THE TYPICAL DAY OF A RADIATION ONCOLOGIST

Those unacquainted with this specialty often make the mistake of equating the radiation oncologist's role to that of a technician. If you choose to practice radiation oncology, get ready for all manner of button-pushing witticisms. Radiation oncologists do not press buttons any more often than our medical oncology partners stand over a Bunsen burner brewing up their concoctions. Specialized trained therapists actually deliver the daily radiation treatment and hold their own special position in the care of cancer patients, which is quite separate from that of the physician.

For a radiation oncologist, the care of a patient typically begins with the referral for consultation often from another member of the interdisciplinary treatment team. For instance, an otolaryngologist who resects a malignant mass from a patient's neck may send that patient to you for further treatment. Medical oncologists refer many of their patients with lung cancer or other malignancies to radiation oncologists for cooperative management. Radiation oncologists rarely receive patients directly from primary care physicians. This is mainly because a patient must first have an established diagnosis relevant to the radiation oncologist before they get to you. Sometimes, the way to your clinic is even more serpentine, in part because radiation oncology simply remains a bit of a mystery even to other physicians. Some patients tread a tortuous path before they find their way to the radiation oncologist, which illustrates the value of having a learned referral base. Because many patients will either need several modalities to treat their disease, or because they have a choice of modality, each with its own risks and benefits, a patient will ideally have met with all the physicians that they need to see prior to the initiation of definitive treatment.

At the initial consultation, you will perform a full history and physical examination. Radiation oncologists need to be fluent in their diagnostic skills to identify sites at risk for disease or toxicity. Special care is taken to assess for sequelae of disease and effects of treatment. Cancer patients are quite prone to a host of systemic problems from the outset. Because patients receive treatment in clinic every day, usually for several weeks, the radiation oncologist is often the diagnostician for many medical problems during this time and a high level of diagnostic acumen is a must.

WHAT MAKES A GOOD RADIATION ONCOLOGIST?

✓ Likes fast-evolving technology.
✓ Wishes to practice evidenced-based medicine, yet likes the challenge of customizing approaches for individual cases
✓ Enjoys an intellectual environment with an emphasis on scientific literature.
✓ Can cope with treating patients who are terminally ill.
✓ Enjoys being part of an interdisciplinary team.
✓ Has an amiable personality.

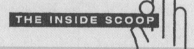

THE INSIDE SCOOP

During the consultative appointment, emphasis is placed not only on the particulars of the patient but also on prior or planned therapy and other diagnostic information. The radiation oncologist must become well versed in relevant surgical procedures, interpreting radiographic images, and in understanding the pathologic variants of disease. At consult, radiation oncologists have a considerable amount of information to correlate to achieve a complete clinical picture and come up with a cogent treatment plan: Was there a total gross resection? Were the margins microscopically positive or was tumor trailing along a nerve bundle? Was there an operative tumor spill? Is there involvement of other organs? In order to design a technically appropriate treatment plan, the radiation oncologist must consider anatomic involvement as defined at surgery and then compare it with findings from diagnostic imaging.

Further testing and clinical investigations are an important part of practicing radiation oncology. Radiation oncologists are involved in directing the overall plan for their patient by ordering relevant additional diagnostic studies. Comprehensive skill at diagnostic techniques, therefore, serves you well in this specialty. In particular, the ability to interpret radiographic and nuclear images and to incorporate the information in your planning and follow-up is vital. Radiation oncologists are concerned with what the surgeon saw, and then have to scan for the presence of radiographic disease occult to the surgeon's eye but is important to encompass in a radiation port. Knowing how a given cancer behaves counts too. For instance, you see a lung mass on computed tomography (CT) scan. Is that all tumor which needs to be treated, or perhaps there is associated consolidation, which could represent an area of lung that your treatment might spare for this frail patient? For the medical oncologist, this procedural aspect may not affect their treatment plan. But for the radiation oncologist, it is of significant import. You will use your knowledge of radiology and nuclear medicine to assist you. You perhaps will order a metabolic imaging scan such as positron emission tomography—a way to look at metabolically active (and likely tumor-related) cells. Before initiating any radiation treatment, you may also suspect the presence of metastatic disease. Appropriate investigations, therefore, will confirm or rule out your suspicions and impact your plan. Radiation oncologists need to understand the clinical behavior of the disease so that they can give the most appropriate treatment.

Radiation oncologists also require a solid understanding of the histology and pathology of cancer. Endometrial cancer, for example, is one of the common malignancies these physicians treat. For this disease, knowing the pathologic difference between high- and low-grade tumors could determine whether a patient should receive any radiation therapy. The expression of particular genetic markers and the depth of lymphatic or vascular invasion—two important diagnostic contributions from pathologists—may also guide the radiation oncologist's protocol. All of this diagnostic and treatment-related information, plus any findings on physical examination, figure prominently in the decision whether to subject a patient to radiation treatment.

PLANNING RADIATION TREATMENT

The resulting treatment is an individually designed plan. Just as surgeons think about how they will approach an operation, radiation oncologists synthesize a great deal of information to come up with the best therapeutic regimen.

The first step in a radiation planning is a mapping procedure called simulation or "sim." Departmental imaging techniques such as fluoroscopy and CT scanning are used to localize the particular target of interest. This region is then referenced to external points so that the patient can be set up for daily treatment. The relationship to normal and sensitive tissue structures is analyzed so that they may be protected. Because tissues in the body all have a limit to the lifetime dose of radiation they can safely receive, treatment plans must always take normal tissue tolerance into account. This is where diagnostic imaging, pathology, and the surgeon's narrative come into play. All of these variables are incorporated by the radiation oncologists as they come up with a treatment plan.

Because radiation oncologists expose the patient to radiation, the goal of therapy is to optimize the beam arrangement so that the prescribed dose reaches the tumor while minimizing exposure to normal tissues. One way in which this can be achieved is by delivering the radiation through multiple beams each approaching the target from different directions. Each beam contains a fraction of the strength that would be needed if only one single beam were used. Thus, as these multiple weak beams pass through normal tissue to their target, the healthy tissue is spared. However, at the point at which all the weak beams converged at the target, the therapeutic dose is delivered.

Radiation oncologists work side by side with professional dosimetrists, optimizing the treatment plan. By applying special filters and changing the relative weights of individual beams, the plan is tailored to meet the physician's specifications. One can loosely think of the dosimetrist's role as parallel to that of pharmacists in medical oncology. They make sure that the correct dose gets to where you prescribe it. In addition, physicists are also on hand to verify the plan and delivered dose as prescribed.

For a very complex plan, the process can take several days. In the event of an emergency such as spinal cord compression or superior vena cava syndrome, a simple plan can be achieved for the sake of expediency. Once on the treatment table, the patient is ready to be set up in the same position as at simulation. The therapist aims the collimator (the tube which shapes the beam of radiation as it exits) and takes a port film. The port film images the patient's anatomy, ensuring that the field in the beam's pathway is the same as planned during simulation. Evolving techniques such as image-guided radiotherapy allow increased accuracy and flexibility in planning and treatment. If the radiation oncologist perceives there is any deviation in setup during treatment, she directs the therapist to shift the patient in the appropriate direction. Once optimized, treatment is given. Radiation oncologists become quickly reacquainted with gross anatomy.

RADIATION THERAPY: DO NOT KNOW MUCH ABOUT BIOLOGY OR PHYSICS?

Undergraduate English majors who managed to wend their way through the premedical curriculum should not feel intimidated by the representation of two of the basic sciences in the course of study of radiation oncology. Radiobiology is the study of the biologic and molecular basis of radiation therapy, for instance, the cellular response to radiation exposure in differing conditions and time schemes. A practicing radiation oncologist uses this information to select the appropriate modality for treatment, choose appropriate energies, and calculate the daily and total dose delivered to a patient. You will become familiar with a variety of isotopes used in the oncology clinic. In training, radiobiology is a discrete area of study that focuses on the practical aspects as it pertains to the clinician.

Physics is also important for the radiation oncologist. It is important not to let a bad experience with premedical physics discourage you from taking a closer look at this specialty. The body of knowledge in both physics and radiobiology required for the radiation oncologist is not overwhelming, nor does it require a particular knack for the physical sciences. Like radiobiology, radiation physics focuses on the practical aspects as it pertains to treatment. The most vexing part of radiation physics is simply that what is unfamiliar may be daunting to undertake for the first time. An intimate background with physics is hardly necessary for medical students prior to entry into this specialty. Residency programs teach the required medical physics program during the course of training. The material that you will learn is a discrete body of knowledge that is rather more conceptual than mathematic and not likely to be overwhelming for anyone who's passed the premedical requirements.

For medical students with a bent toward physics basic science or translational research, radiation oncology is a peach. For the techies, the opportunities are apparent. The development of new technology and the evolution and application of new techniques are rapid. Interestingly, while older techniques are rarely rendered obsolete, the rapidity of change is analogous to what you see in the current era of computers in general. "New" is a relative term. At the time of printing of the last edition of this book, several "boutique" therapies have become standard. Image guidance was a buzzword then and now is operational in most centers. Proton therapy, which offers more precise dosimetry but has been hampered by prohibitive size and cost, was only available at Massachusetts General Hospital and Loma Linda. By 2011, seven other US hospital-based centers are offering protons with others due online in 2012. Innovative techniques such as arc therapy have become widely available. The student who is comfortable with technology can actively partake in research in radiation physics and dosimetry.

Radiation oncology as a field is well organized in terms of running practice-defining clinical trials. These trials test the efficacy of combination therapy, tumor vaccines, cell sensitizers, and normal tissue protectors. There is a considerable presence of academic radiation oncologists in both basic bench-side research and translational work. Translational medicine is a conceptual way of thinking about research so that issues of practical clinical interest are identified, studied in the lab, and brought back to the bedside. It is currently and will remain a practical and very productive area of study that has already led to rapid changes in clinical practice. The routine use of radiosensitizers on the one hand and radioprotectors that preferentially protect normal tissue over cancerous tissue from radiation on the other are direct results of this research. New drug development such as the rational design of vascular endothelial growth factor inhibitors and PARP inhibitors are a result of translational study as are novel therapies such as nanotechnology, hyperthermia, and oxygen enhancers that can be added to radiation treatment to improve outcomes. There are several avenues of entry for a radiation oncology resident interested in research. Certainly, radiation oncology has a relatively high per capita representation of MD and PhDs in the field. However, those who develop the interest a little later down the road have plenty of opportunity available to them.

Most residency programs will have at very least the opportunity for clinical investigation through departmental resources. Departmental resources differ site to site. Just as different surgical programs may offer variable training in select techniques, so too will areas of study differ in radiation oncology. Some places will offer a strong pediatrics experience; others might shine in physics or radiobiology. Thus, your training will have a different flavor depending where you end up and offer different areas of research.

The most basic levels are retrospective chart reviews. These types of studies typically seek relationships between variables and outcomes. They are important because they help guide nuanced clinical decision making that larger studies cannot address and identify patterns that might be evaluated in more definitive studies. Residents are frequently involved in retrospective chart reviews because they are fairly straightforwards, offer good training in the fundamentals of conducting clinical research, and are relatively quick to do.

Less commonly residents will engage in prospective trials. These trials are considered higher quality research and may involve answering new questions or even evaluating new therapies. They typically take much longer to do than retrospective work both because of administrative issues and mainly because patients need to be enrolled over time (often years).

To facilitate prospective studies, there are several cooperative and multi-institutional groups of radiation oncologists. One of the largest is the Radiation Therapy Oncology Group (RTOG). Many academic centers with residency programs are a part of one or many of them and provide a good avenue of entry into major clinical research for a senior resident.

Highlighting the commitment of leaders in radiation oncology toward training a new generation of serious researchers, in 1999, the American Board of Radiology (the certifying body in radiation oncology) introduced the Holman Research Pathway. The Holman Pathway is a residency-level initiative designed to foster interest in careers of basic science and clinical research. Lab scientists within radiation oncology, medical oncology, and molecular biology all welcome medical students interested in partaking in bench research and advancing the field of cancer treatment. No PhD is necessary to apply.

A HIGH-TECH SPECIALTY FOR HIGH-TECH DOCS

Why are more medical school graduates seeking positions in radiation oncology. It has always been a well-paid, good lifestyle field, but these factors alone cannot explain the new interest. The specialty's surging popularity among students may have something to do with the fact that over the last decade and a half, the first generations of doctors raised during the computer revolution have graduated medical school. Many technology-savvy medical students have grown up with both a compelling interest in and familiarity with technology and are drawn to the high-tech nature of radiation oncology.

There are many ways in which advances in technology have a direct effect on patient care in radiation oncology. Improved technology allows us to better manipulate radiobiological differences in normal and tumor cells by altering fractionation. Fractionation is the treatment method that takes advantage of the healthy cell's ability to repair a small amount of radiation damage (whereas a tumor cell is susceptible to destruction). In the 1930s, a group of French physicians observed that a single dose of radiation necessary to sterilize a ram caused prohibitive damage to the skin of the scrotum. By giving smaller doses of radiation for several weeks, they found that they could achieve their objective (sterilization) without producing any unacceptable skin damage. On the basis of these and later studies, scientists postulated that tumor cells were very similar to fast-growing germ cells and applied this model to cancer treatment in humans. Using software algorithms only feasible with modern computing coupled with precision delivery systems, radiation oncologists today treat their patients with increased efficacy and safety. This in turn has led us to alternative fractionation schemes previously unthinkable.

Much of the technical advances seek to exploit the therapeutic ratio—killing tumor cells while leaving healthy tissue intact. A generation ago, technology was limited to easy-to-plan simple opposed beams of radiation. As alluded to before, the older methods are not necessarily retired. They are still common, useful, and practical today particularly for urgent cases. However, developments in bioengineering are increasing our flexibility. In modern CT-based simulation, radiation oncologists apply multiple beams of high-dose radiation from many different angles—all within a 3D plane. 4D planning is increasingly common, taking into account the movement of tissues "intrafraction."

In the 1990s, intensity-modulated radiation therapy (IMRT) was implemented in the clinic. In this technique, thin sliding metal blocks (leaves) enter and exit a field of radiation for varying lengths of time. This can provide superior conformational coverage to the target. The end result is better protection of normal organ tissue and higher doses of finely shaped radiation to cancerous tissue.

The development of exquisitely precise beams and precise localization of the tumor (and patient) in space has given birth to radiosurgery, the application of a high dose of radiation in a limited number of fractions targeted in stereotactic space. Most commonly, radiosurgery is delivered in brain tumors. It again underscores the rapidity of technological development to note that at publication of the last edition of this book, body radiosurgery was quite rare. It is now increasingly becoming a standard practice. Traditional linear accelerators (the standard treatment machines in radiation oncology) can be programed to perform radiosurgery and there are a few dedicated technologies such as Gamma Knife or Cyberknife.

Radiation oncologists also perform brachytherapy, the temporary or permanent placement of radioactive seeds and ribbons (depending on the organ) directly into the patient. Because brachytherapy delivers radiation for a short distance before falling off to negligible amounts in surrounding tissue, oncologists find this method very appealing for primary or adjuvant radiation treatment. It can potentially wipe out tumor without harming the neighboring tissue. Brachytherapy is often performed in the operating room and involves an interdisciplinary team—such as gynecologic oncologists, orthopedic surgeons, neurosurgeons, or urologists—who work alongside the radiation oncologist in performing the procedure.

THE DOCTOR–PATIENT RELATIONSHIP

Although technology and a strong representation in research are appealing features of radiation oncologist for many, it should emphasize that the backbone of a radiation oncologist's practice is clinical care. Very few have a primarily research-oriented practice.

Typically, patients are seen by their radiation oncologist for a short visit once a week during treatment. This on-treatment appointment gives you the opportunity to address the patient's active problems or acute side effects of therapy. Once radiation treatment has ended, follow-up appointments continue, usually on a long-term basis. These follow-up visits are extremely rewarding. You are important to your patients who are keen to recount the many happy events that have occurred in their lives since their last appointment. You become an important personage in many people's lives.

Of course, not all of your patients are cured. Radiation oncology has an important role in the palliation of patients with incurable disease. Approximately 60% of radiation treatment is used with the intent to cure. Temporizing and palliation (in the long or short term) are goals of treatment for about 40% of patients. If you enter this specialty, be prepared to cope with the emotional toll of caring for patients with cancer.

The psychological impact for the treating physician may be more subtle than you imagine, but nonetheless profound. As an outpatient-based service, the practice of radiation oncology is calmer and less dramatic day to day than, for example, the acute setting of inpatient wards. The drama of treating acutely ill patients on the general medicine wards can bring your emotions to the fore. Most of your patients on a radiation oncology service will not be in crisis when you see them. Nevertheless, a sizable percentage of your patients will progress or succumb to disease within a few years. Witnessing this aspect of the human condition can work as insidiously on the physician's psyche as the disease he watches over.

Although emotionally draining at times, caring for these patients and their families is extremely rewarding. As physicians, we want to help people in an important way. As you guide them through rough seas (cancer treatment is not pleasant for anyone), patients want reassurance that they will not be abandoned. Remarkably, it is often this reassurance—more so than any promise of a miracle to cure—that provides patients and their families with solace, comfort, and peace of mind. One impressive oncologist had the ability to convey to every patient that "I'll take you through hell and back to treat your cancer, but every single step of the way, I will be there for you." It was not a comment that had to be made explicit, but the sentiment was there.

Like any physician, radiation oncologists must be willing to accept the ambiguities of medicine and deal with issues that most people generally find discomforting if not plain frightening. Your patients' will to survive and endure intensive treatment—both radiation and chemical therapy—will humble and inspire you every single day. Indeed, this specialty can offer much perspective on life for any busy physician.

RADIATION ONCOLOGY AS A PALLIATIVE MODALITY

Through long-term follow-up with their patients, radiation oncologists assess for clinical stability or signs of recurrence of disease and manage any long-term sequelae of treatment. This is particularly important as these late effects can become manifest weeks to years down the line and may even include iatrogenic (radiation-induced) secondary tumors. Your familiarity with radiation's long-term effects on many organ systems will allow you to identify and medically intervene when necessary.

In light of the potential side effects from radiation treatment, what role does this therapy have for patients who do not have curative disease? Radiation oncologists have an important role maintaining comfort and quality of life for cancer patients by palliating local symptoms. Tumors of all types can be painful or even functionally obstructive. If surgery is not an option to resect a tumor, radiation becomes the preferred (or adjunctive) modality. In particular, radiation oncologists have much success in eliminating the severe pain caused by cancer that has metastasized to bone (particularly lung, breast, or prostate cancer). With just a couple of weeks of therapy, most patients report a partial or complete resolution of tumor-related bone pain. Emergencies in radiation oncology also include spinal cord compression and brain metastasis. Radiation is also used to relieve superior vena cava syndrome, where tumors (usually lung cancer) grow and obstruct the main vessel draining blood from the head and neck into the heart. There is a recent innovative trend toward developing dedicated services for inpatient and palliative care to stand along side more conventional radiation oncology specialties, a wonderful area for a budding radiation oncologist in training to explore and develop.

BEING A PART OF THE MULTIDISCIPLINARY CANCER TEAM

Many medical students, like patients, are under the misconception that therapies for cancer are somehow hierarchical and sequential in their nature that one modality will simply come along and will supplant another (such as radiation therapy) as the modality of choice to treat tumors in the future. This view probably stems from the historical sequence of cancer therapy discovery. For centuries, the only physicians who could treat cancer were the surgeons, who sought to prolong life by cutting out the tumor mass. In the early 1900s, the discovery of x-rays was soon followed by the realization that radiation could be used as a therapeutic modality to destroy cancerous tissue. The promise of chemotherapy caused great excitement a few decades later. Unlike both surgery and radiation, chemotherapy is systemic therapy with the ability to reach cancer cells circulating anywhere in the body. Nearly seven decades later, all oncologists realize that this alone does not typically make for a cure. The literature is rife with attempts to replace discipline's therapy with another's therapy only to find that more often than not, the whole is greater than the sum of its parts. So too, will this likely continue into the foreseeable future.

Today, the focus is on "targeted biological therapy." These drugs (sometimes in combination with radiolabeling) typically seek out particular molecular targets that are preferentially expressed or utilized on cancer cells. Of course, a therapy that is both 100% sensitive and specific to cancer cells—the proverbial "magic bullet"—remains elusive and not likely to be realized in the near future. In fact in concept, modern day "biologics" are not very much distinguishable from cytotoxic chemotherapies, which also optimally sought to target molecular features of cancer cells over normal ones.

Given our greater understanding of the mechanisms of cancer, it seems likely that no single modality—whether surgical, radiation, or chemical—will wipe out malignant disease. A hierarchical model probably is the wrong paradigm through which to understand oncologic therapy. All future oncologists must accept the mantra that "different cancers in different stages respond to different schemes of therapy." These modalities often work best synergistically. Hybrids, such as targeted therapy and chemosensitization to enhance the effects of radiation, are excellent examples of this synergy.

This is why radiation oncologists are integral members of interdisciplinary cancer care teams whose members—across multiple specialties—work together to treat a patient afflicted with cancer. It is important to realize that radiation is just one of three major therapeutic arms in modern cancer treatment. Through conferences known as Tumor Board, the three major types of oncologists come together—along with consultant pathologists and radiologists—to decide on the best course of treatment. For the radiation oncologist then, an awareness of the multidisciplinary approach to cancer is essential. Although surgical oncologists can often resect all gross tumor seen with the naked eye, this approach may not be adequate to achieve a cure. Some cancers are particularly sensitive to radiation (such as prostate cancer), whereas others respond quite well to chemotherapy (such as the type of leukemia often found in kids). Radiation therapy might be used as the primary treatment (instead of surgery) or in conjunction with surgical or chemical therapy. This is especially important because often the appropriate dosage and the timing of radiation treatment depend upon whether or not the patient will go for surgery or certain types of toxic chemotherapy.

LIFESTYLE CONSIDERATIONS AND PRACTICE OPTIONS

The lifestyle of a radiation oncologist is relatively benign compared with that of other specialties, particularly after residency. As physicians practicing in an outpatient setting, they work predictable and humane hours, earn relatively generous salaries, and have low malpractice premiums. Although there are few oncologic-related emergencies that require immediate radiation treatment, oncologists still carry a beeper, typically taking call from home for 1 week several times per year depending upon the kind of practice they are in. As a result, there is ample time (including most weekends off) for radiation oncologists to spend with their families and pursue other interests. Much of your free time, however, is spent in keeping up with fast-evolving medical literature as well as scholarly pursuits if you are academically inclined. Although especially true in residency years, the fluidity of the standards of care in modern cancer treatment requires the attending radiation oncologist to be a lifelong student. The American Board of Radiology makes sure this happens with their 10-year cycle maintenance of certificate program required to keep board certified.

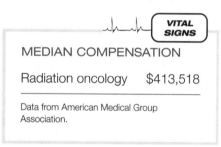

VITAL SIGNS

MEDIAN COMPENSATION

Radiation oncology $413,518

Data from American Medical Group Association.

Radiation oncologists can decide among the three standard choices of practice: academic jobs (often salaried), community/private practice positions, or freestanding/private practice centers. Median income is excellent for radiation oncologists in any of models. In a recent career survey of new physicians, most board-eligible radiation oncologists (50%) favor private practice, while 30% chose an academic setting. The remainder opted for fellowships, locum tenens, military work, or remained undecided.[1] Regardless of choice, the job market for young radiation oncologists coming out of residency remains extremely good. In studies evaluating the trends in the job market for radiation oncologists, program directors viewed the job market strongly.[2,3] Starting salaries are high and rising, and choice academic positions are available. The practice of radiation oncology requires an extensive amount of expensive equipment, supplies, and staff. Because private practice models come in many flavors, fresh residency graduates will need to brush up on their business skills and acumen. This is because private practice models come in many flavors. The typical scenario involves 2- to 5-year tenure as a salaried junior who may eventually become a partner in the practice.

Academic practice tends to be primarily hospital-based work. Since these doctors are frequently paid on salary, the department takes care of money management and spares its frontline physicians from the routine business concerns. Referrals are built-in from the hospital's medical oncologists and surgeons, and the more challenging cases will typically be sent from the community. Many patients self-refer to academic centers to receive what they perceive as the "best" care. Academic radiation oncologists typically have protected time for nonclinical work such as teaching and conducting research, and promotion depends upon success in these areas.

FELLOWSHIPS AND SUBSPECIALTY TRAINING

Perhaps more so than most other specialties, a resident's training experience in radiation oncology can be quite variable program to program. Although there are some uniform ACGME (Accreditation Council for Graduate Medical Education) curricular requirements, techniques and practices between institutions are different enough to make the skills attained by trainees notably broad. For instance, some provide experience with stereotactic radiosurgery and radiolabeled monoclonal antibody therapy; others offer strong brachytherapy programs. Certain areas of radiation oncology—such as pediatric radiation oncology or brachytherapy— are specialized enough to be offered only in select institutions, which does not include all residencies. Furthermore, the technology of this field is not only expensive but also ever evolving. As a result, not every academic medical center can have each type of treatment modality and thus residency experiences differ across the many programs and hospitals.

Because of this varying exposure to techniques and subspecialties in radiation oncology, some residents choose to enter a fellowship program after residency for more in-depth training and subspecialization. Fellowships can provide advanced clinical training in nearly any subspecialty in the field, including head and neck cancer, gynecologic oncology, central nervous system radiation, and pediatrics, among others. They are generally 1 to 2 years long. Typically, you hone your clinical skills, perfect your technique, develop a professional niche, and become an expert at your chosen area of subspecialization. Fellowship is a good place to take advantage of resources to publish in your area of interest and establish an academic foothold.

In this specialty, fellowships can also take the guise of further expertise in a technique rather than traditional sub-specialization in an organ system or population base. Popular fellowships include brachytherapy, IMRT, charged particle therapy, radiosurgery, and hyperthermia. Many people became aware of brachytherapy as a treatment for prostate cancer (in which radioactive seeds are permanently implanted in the intact prostate) after Rudolph Giuliani, the former mayor of New York City, underwent this procedure in 2000. As modern physicians continue to refine this modality, and other equally promising techniques, you will need greater surgical dexterity and skill to attain expertise in this increasingly popular procedure. Some residents opt to take their internship in surgery in anticipation of a career specializing in brachytherapy. Because many medical centers do not offer enough volume to provide adequate training for the interested resident, a fellowship can remedy the situation. Brachytherapy procedures for the head and neck are also common, as is gynecologic brachytherapy. Breast brachytherapy is poised to become another area of demand in remote areas where patients find daily access to a clinic for 6 weeks burdensome.

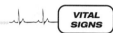

VITAL SIGNS

RADIATION ONCOLOGY 2011 MATCH STATISTICS

- Number of positions available: 171
- 186 US seniors and 39 independent applicants ranked at least one radiation oncology program
- 96.5% of all positions were filled in the initial Match
- The successful applicants: 94% US seniors, 0% foreign-trained physicians, and 0.06% osteopathic graduates
- Mean USMLE Step I score: 240
- Unmatched rate for US seniors applying only to radiation oncology: 14.1%

Data from National Resident Matching Program.

Many radiation oncologists are research-minded folks. If you want to pursue laboratory or clinical research in your medical career, there are many research fellowships available. Some trainees participate in the Leonard Holman Research Pathway, a program offered by the American Board of Radiation Oncology since 1999. This program combines training in clinical radiation oncology (and radiology) with extensive time spent conducting radiation research. Applications are generally accepted during the internship year. Candidates participating in this pathway can still complete their clinical training within the normal length of residency.

RESIDENCY TRAINING

Residency in radiation oncology requires a total of 5 years of postgraduate training. There are currently 80 accredited programs in the United States. The first year of training (PGY-1) consists of a separate internship—preliminary medicine, surgery, or transitional year. PGY 2–5 training is in the specialty of radiation oncology. Radiation oncology is an outpatient-based specialty, so most residents work about 60 hours per week with most weekends off except during call periods in the specialty years. On-call requirements typically last for 1 week at a time, during which the resident takes call from home and only comes to the hospital for an emergency. This can be a busy period particularly in major academic training centers. Despite the relatively benign work hours, residency training in radiation oncology is academically intense. Assignments, case presentations, and participation at conferences are required and frequent. A great deal of outside reading—particularly using the scientific literature—is necessary. To earn board certification after residency, you must pass three components of a written examination (clinical, radiobiology, and physics) as well as an oral examination.

THE INSIDE SCOOP

WHY CONSIDER A CAREER IN RADIATION ONCOLOGY?

Although no medical school requires a clinical rotation in radiation oncology, more and more medical students are deciding on it as their specialty. The number of residency applications for the small number of positions remains at an all-time high, which unfortunately means that many well-qualified candidates may find themselves without a training position in this specialty. Radiation oncologists recognize that it is a great privilege to care for patients suffering from cancer. After all, they provide more than just medical treatment—radiation oncologists are always a source of comfort and hope.

For many aspiring physicians, this specialty has the perfect mix: intimate, one-on-one patient contact; new technology that is continually developing; good working hours and pay; and a high level of intellectual stimulation. Because radiation oncologists interact with physicians, patients, technicians, and other personnel on a daily basis, this specialty requires excellent communication skills. It is a specialty with a singular focus—the cure of cancer through radiation therapy—yet has enough facets to suit a variety of interests, from teaching to research to clinical care.

Although this specialty can be emotionally weighty, particularly when your patients succumb to disease, both the cases of successful treatments and those where you give comfort and care to the patient are some of the most rewarding and satisfying moments of your professional life. Being a radiation oncologist is an exceptionally fulfilling way to practice medicine. You take the latest scientific research and apply its promising discoveries to your patients. You relieve their discomfort, improve their quality of life, and always serve as a beacon of hope.

ABOUT THE CONTRIBUTOR

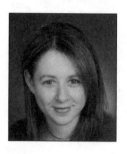 Dr Stephanie E. Weiss completed residency training at Johns Hopkins Sidney Kimmel Cancer Center. She is now an attending physician at Harvard Medical School's Brigham and Women Hospital/Dana Farber Cancer Institute. A native New Yorker, she earned a BA in English and psychology from Franklin and Marshall College and completed postbaccalaureate premedical studies at Columbia University. She then packed her snorkeling gear for medical school at St. George's University School of Medicine in Grenada. Dr Weiss' professional interests include central nervous system disease, stereotactic radiation, and pediatric radiation oncology. She and her husband enjoy skiing, traveling, karate, sailing, and spending time with friends and family. She can be reached by e-mail at stephew03@yahoo.com.

REFERENCES

1. Yasmin, C., Sunshine, J., et al. Radiation oncologists in 2000: Demographic, professional, and practice characteristics. *Int J Radiat Oncol Biol Phys.* 2002;53(3):720–728.

2. Ling, S.M., Flynn, D.F. Results of the 1993 Association of Residents in Radiation Oncology survey. *Int J Radiat Oncol Biol Phys.* 1996;34:221–226.

3. Bushee, G.R., Sunshine, J.H., et al. The status of radiation oncology training programs and their graduates in 1999. *Int J Radiat Oncol Biol Phys.* 2001;49(1):133–138.

31

RADIOLOGY

Derek L. Fimmen

W ith the discovery of the x-ray, the specialty of radiology was born. It has rapidly grown into an advanced, highly cerebral discipline encompassing a variety of high-tech imaging modalities. If you want to serve at the forefront of diagnostic and therapeutic interventions, and be the physician to whom clinicians turn for advice, then take a closer look at radiology.

Radiology is the branch of medicine in which radiologic images are interpreted for the prevention, diagnosis, and treatment of disease. Technological advances in medical imaging—and its growing role in the diagnosis and management of disease—have transformed radiology into one of the premier fields of modern medicine. Many of the greatest achievements in health care have come from radiologists. Now new imaging modalities are being used to pioneer faster, better, and safer procedures. These exciting technological advances, along with the amazing diversity of career opportunities and subspecialties, make it no surprise that radiology has become an increasingly popular and selective specialty.

THE ORIGINS OF RADIOLOGY

Before the discovery of the x-ray, the only way for doctors to peer inside the human body was to open it up through painful surgery or autopsy. Radiology's beginnings, when scientists first obtained a noninvasive glimpse of internal structures, date back to late nineteenth-century Germany. At the University of Wurzburg, Professor Wilhelm Roentgen and his younger colleague, Philip Lenard, were investigating the properties of cathode rays. In these studies, Lenard observed a glow on a fluorescent screen placed near a partially evacuated glass tube. Using his partner's

WHAT MAKES A GOOD RADIOLOGIST?

✓ Likes working with his or her mind.
✓ Enjoys learning about new technology.
✓ Has excellent interpersonal skills.
✓ Is an intellectual and visually oriented problem solver.
✓ Is comfortable with minimal patient contact.

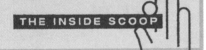

THE INSIDE SCOOP

techniques, Roentgen duplicated this fluorescent phenomenon on his own. By November 1895, he observed that these rays of light could pass through some substances but would leave shadows of others. When he placed his hands in the rays' path, Roentgen discovered that he could see the faint shadow of his bones. He documented that bones, as well as glass made from lead, could stop these rays. Because magnets or prisms could not deflect or refract the light rays, Roentgen excluded the possibility of the rays being either cathode rays or a form of visible light. He concluded that these rays were previously unknown and thus referred to them by the variable x.

The first x-ray ever taken was when Roentgen exposed his wife's hands for 15 minutes to these mysterious x-rays. The result was a photographic plate of Mrs Roentgen's wedding ring floating around her finger. After publishing several radiographs (including this now famous image of his wife's hand) in the journal of the *Physio-Medical Society of Wurzburg*, Roentgen became an instant international celebrity. Within the month, his work was translated into several languages and published in *Science and The New York Times*. Physicians could now "internally" examine patients by looking at x-rays, which was hailed all around the world as a major accomplishment.

The impact of Roentgen's work is still evident today. Those mysterious x-rays became known as roentgen rays, and the *American Journal of Roentgenology* has become one of the specialty's premier journals. When the first Nobel Prize in physics was awarded in 1901, the committee chose only to honor Roentgen. Although Lenard had published research as early as 1895 regarding the fluorescence he observed, Roentgen was the one who further investigated the origin and nature of this fluorescence and was the first to use this phenomenon to create anatomic images. Interestingly, Lenard did receive a Nobel Prize in 1905 for his work with cathode rays, but still furious over previous events, he used this speaking opportunity in Stockholm to denounce the 1901 decision. During his last interview in 1945, Lenard insisted that x-rays were his baby and Roentgen had been only the midwife.

A CLOSER LOOK AT MODERN RADIOLOGY

Today, x-rays are just one of many different kinds of imaging modalities available for the diagnosis of disease. To expose anatomic parts, radiologists are no longer limited to using radiation. One of the other imaging techniques in their arsenal is ultrasound, which is unique in that its origin is in the physics of sound, as opposed to light. The concept of using sound waves to obtain images of covered objects goes back as far as the 1870s. Ultrasound has never been able to provide the same sharpness possible with other forms of imaging. But physicians use ultrasound for a diversity of applications, such as viewing a growing fetus, looking for stones obstructing the gallbladder, and detecting potentially fatal blood clots within the deep veins of the leg.

First demonstrated in London in 1971, computed tomography (CT) scans provide a level of anatomic detail that was previously unimagined. CT scan uses collimated beams of x-rays, which are sent to a series of detectors that in turn transmit signals to a computer for translation into images. Although the technology was initially limited by the data storage capacity of early 1970s computers, this obstacle was quickly overcome. By 1981, there were more than 1300 CT scanners in the United States and their use had gained acceptance by the National Institutes of Health. CT scan has since become one of the most commonly used imaging modalities in modern diagnostic radiology, with which radiologists can examine almost every internal structure. Its diverse applications include diagnosing pathologic processes ranging from colon cancer to hemorrhaging within the brain.

Seeking to improve their ability to look inside a patient's body, radiologists established many of the theoretical and practical aspects of magnetic resonance imaging (MRI) by the 1980s. Drawing from the principles of nuclear magnetic resonance (NMR), which is used in chemistry, MRI uses magnetism—just like x-rays require radiation—to produce images. MRI also benefited greatly from the development of CT, because many mathematical problems involved in translating masses of data into computerized images had already been worked out. MRI rapidly gained widespread acceptance within the medical community. Now radiologists could examine many disease processes in even greater detail. Some examples include herniated intervertebral disks, intracranial lesions, obstructed bile ducts, and ligament tears of the knees and shoulders.

Radiologists in the area of nuclear medicine obtain anatomic images from internal sources of radiation. Many in this field have worked hard to develop positron emission tomography (PET). During radioactive decay, the nucleus emits positrons (the positive antiparticles of electrons) with protons and neutrons. When a source of radiation is placed within the human body, the presence of these particles can be recorded. The development of PET scanning and its applications in monitoring cancer growth is proceeding at an incredibly fast rate. By looking at whether or not cells light up during the study, radiologists can gain insight into the level of metabolic activity within tissue in addition to monitoring gross anatomic changes such as size and shape. This knowledge greatly expands the power of imaging in monitoring the progression of disease as well as its response to treatment.

As you can tell, radiology is the perfect specialty for physicians who want to be at the forefront of medical technology. Radiology makes it possible to diagnose increasing numbers of diseases simply through imaging. When this is not possible, clinicians often turn to more invasive (and painful) means of diagnosis, such as colonoscopy, bronchoscopy, and laparotomy. Even so, radiologists sometimes have to cause discomfort to generate the most accurate imaging study possible, whether it is injecting contrast into a patient for better delineation of anatomic structures, making them drink barium for an upper gastrointestinal swallow study, or giving a barium enema to examine the colon.

Improved imaging techniques, combined with the development of various catheters, have given rise to a field known as interventional radiology. This subspecialty enables radiologists to do much more than just diagnose. These specialists use medical images to help guide small instruments such as catheters through blood vessels or other anatomic pathways in the percutaneous treatment of disease. With these invasive techniques, interventional radiologists are in many ways similar to surgeons. They scrub in, gown up, and perform procedures that are often invasive enough to require general anesthesia. Some examples include draining abscesses, opening blocked areas of the cardiovascular system, creating vascular shunts in the liver, and inserting various devices into patients requiring long-term vascular access (for things such as chemotherapy, antibiotics, or dialysis). As you can see, these radiologists combine the fundamentals of diagnostic radiology with the technical and clinical skills of a surgeon.

Since 1895, when Wilhelm Roentgen first captured an x-ray, the promise of imaging has remained astonishing. Radiology has grown into a multimodality of high-tech imaging using some of the most advanced instrumentation in the world. The remarkable pace of technological advance and the promise it holds for the future have made radiology an incredibly exciting specialty.

THE SCIENCE OF RADIOLOGY

Radiologists must command a great deal of information. In this specialty, there is an increased emphasis on many of the basic sciences. The study of medical physics, for example, is so fundamental to radiology that residents are required to take a physics examination as a part of the board certification process. Radiology, however, is more than just studying magnetic field gradients and trying to understand how the complex technology of x-rays, CTs, MRIs, and PET scans actually works. You have to know many clinical and basic sciences—from pathology to internal medicine—inside and out. This must also be tempered with common sense and practicality. Many doctors agree that radiologists are among the most knowledgeable and academic physicians around.

Of the basic sciences, anatomy and pathology are two of the most crucial disciplines. You will become an expert on the name and location of essentially every single anatomic structure in the human body. You have to be able to identify almost every artery, vein, bone, and muscle that exists. You have to memorize anatomic landmarks such as the ligament of Treitz, the segmental anatomy of the lungs, the structures of the brain, countless normal anatomic variants, and much more. As a radiologist, you will not only know anatomy well but also will be able to visualize and understand anatomic relationships on a spatial, 3D level. When interpreting images, radiologists must be able to draw on their memory to recognize abnormalities (as well as normal variants which can mimic disease), maintain focus on the smallest of details, and be able to extrapolate from radiologic findings into differential diagnoses.

As expert diagnosticians, radiologists must have a detailed understanding of disease processes and be able to formulate differential diagnoses regarding every organ system. They must prepare for consultations by almost every type of subspecialist, such as internists, surgeons, pediatricians, and obstetricians. For example, pulmonologists often request assistance in evaluating lung nodules. If an older man with a long history of smoking receives a chest x-ray that shows a nodule, radiologists first use their knowledge of anatomy (eg, the segments of the lung) to identify the location of the lesion. They then use their knowledge of medicine to come up with a differential diagnosis (malignancy, pneumonia, granuloma, etc) based on the precise nature of the radiologic finding.

This process can be more complex than most people realize. Radiologists first describe the appearance of the lesion in radiologic terms (eg, upper-zone predominant reticulonodular pattern). They then guide the clinician to a more likely diagnosis by combining information from the clinical history, physical examination, and laboratory data with the radiologic findings. Radiologists have to meet the challenge of appropriately labeling states of health, normal anatomic variation, and disease.

BEING A CONSULTANT PHYSICIAN

Radiologists' role as behind-the-scenes consultants with limited patient contact has led to many misconceptions about the specialty. It is wrong to think of it as a field in which one is isolated from others and has no need for good communication skills or bedside manner. The increased invasiveness of radiology means there are opportunities for extensive direct clinical involvement with patients, if you so desire. Radiologists are consulted by almost every type of clinician, so they are in continuous discussions with a variety of colleagues. Because radiology is a referral-based specialty, your success depends on being able to communicate findings, both in writing and orally, in a clear, timely, and helpful manner. Remember that radiologists spend a great deal of time dictating reports, editing preliminary drafts, and discussing cases directly with the clinicians.

It is important to understand what it means to work behind the scenes as a technical consultant. Radiologists often contribute to the diagnosis and management of disease without ever meeting or examining the patient. Except among physicians, their role is one of relative anonymity. In the days after President Ronald Reagan was shot, for example, little attention was paid to the physicians who provided his anesthetic care, the clinicians who appropriately managed his antimicrobial therapy, or the radiologist who helped to locate the bullet. A great deal of press, however, was given to the surgeon displaying the bullet fragment he had removed from the President's chest. Although radiology may lack the glamour of plastic surgery, the drama of emergency medicine, and the personal bonding of family practice, it is a field in which the rewards come from your daily challenges and accomplishments.

As the physician who is consulted by so many other physicians, radiologists have come to be known as "a doctor's doctor." They must be able to assist in the diagnosis and clinical management of a great diversity of pathology. Radiology is thus ideal for those who love to read, explore, and teach. To play this role in the management of disease is a great privilege, but it also requires a great deal of personal sacrifice as well as a commitment to a lifetime of learning. Be prepared for an extensive amount of reading on a daily basis.

Clinicians seek out consultations with radiologists for two reasons: (1) help with a diagnosis (the interpretation of a particular imaging study) and (2) advise on the best and most appropriate imaging study to order. Radiologic imaging gives clinicians additional evidence that will support or weigh against a particular diagnosis. Every physician, therefore, needs the radiologist. Neurologists rely heavily on brain CTs and MRIs to diagnose neurologic disease. Critical care specialists rely on radiologists to evaluate endotracheal tube and central line placement on chest x-ray. If an emergency medicine physician suspects that a patient may have acute appendicitis (because the patient came into the ED with fever and right lower quadrant abdominal pain), he or she may order a CT scan of the abdomen. If the radiologist is able to identify a normal appendix, then this is excellent evidence against the diagnosis of appendicitis. If it were not for radiologic testing, a patient such as this might end up having his abdomen opened in the operating room when it did not necessarily have to be.

A GLIMPSE INTO THE FUTURE: TELERADIOLOGY

The last decade has brought with it substantial growth in the sharing of information among networks of hospitals and clinics. Teleradiology—the ability to read digitized radiologic images from different locations—was developed in the early 1990s and soon became a functional part of the health care industry. Creation of the necessary infrastructure to transmit images reliably with large amounts of data around the world has made this possible. The ability to provide radiologic interpretations from remote locations is becoming more and more common. Teleradiology can allow radiologists who have hospital-based practices to interpret images from home. It also enables full-time practice opportunities that are entirely from home, plus the opportunity to practice in several overseas locations while being employed in the United States. Despite legal, regulatory, and reimbursement policies that have acted to slow down the growth of teleradiology, we have seen telecommunication's role in the delivery of medical care continue to expand. Trends in the current health care system suggest that many "night hawk" teleradiology firms are providing the right service to the right marketplace at the right time.

As networks between hospitals and clinics become easier to set up and maintain, we will continue to see significant growth in the sharing of telemedical resources. Sharing medical technology is a cost-effective way to distribute expertise; it decreases the overall cost to each component in the system. It also, of course, gives a greater number of patients access to physician groups with additional expertise. Small hospitals can access a greater pool of resources by linking themselves with tertiary care facilities, and the larger institutions can increase their population base and volume of interpretations.

The media often spins teleradiology as a low-cost alternative to more traditional methods. This is simply wrong. Teleradiology can decrease the waiting time for radiologic interpretations. There are clinics in which images can be obtained, transmitted to a distant site, and interpreted in a prompt, thorough, and detailed manner by radiologists with established expertise. This cost-effective and efficient technology can provide high-quality radiology services to facilities that may not have sufficient volume to support full-time in-house night coverage. Teleradiology, therefore, has led to a diversity of new career opportunities while also alleviating some of the traditional overnight on-call duties for many practicing radiologists.

LIFESTYLE CONSIDERATIONS AND PRACTICE OPTIONS

Many of today's medical students are seeking careers in specialties that afford them time to raise a family and pursue outside interests. It is no secret that radiology — with its humane and more regular working hours — is often referred to as one of the lifestyle fields. Choosing radiology for this reason alone, however, is a mistake. First of all, many tales of the cushy lives of radiologists are exaggerated. And times are changing. The expanded role of imaging places increased demands on all radiologists. The role of the radiology resident-on-call has become very demanding in many academic institutions. Recent data suggest that, over the last decade, the workloads of radiologists in both private practice and academics have increased dramatically.[1]

After the completion of residency, however, you do have a great deal more control over your lifestyle. Radiology offers opportunities to work full time, or part time, in both private and academic settings. Opinions differ regarding the advantages and disadvantages of private versus academic radiology. While factors such as academic interests, research opportunities, and teaching responsibilities are fundamental considerations in deciding between the two paths, there are important differences. Many radiologists state, as a generalization, that in private practice one has to work three times as hard to make twice as much. One study found that the workload in relative value units for academic radiologists is approximately 35% less than that of their private practice counterparts.[1]

During the early 1990s, amidst misguided forecasts of a surplus of radiologists, applications to diagnostic radiology residency programs decreased dramatically. By the late 1990s, once the flaws in these projections became apparent,

---

~~~~⌐ VITAL SIGNS ⌐

MEDIAN COMPENSATION

Radiology—	
diagnostic	$438,115
Radiology—	
interventional	$478,000
Radiology—	
neurointerventional	$458,187

Data from American Medical Group Association.

radiology again became a highly competitive specialty. Furthermore, most surveys of physician income per specialty show that radiologists are among the highest paid of all physicians. In recent years, the number of applicants, and the percentage of US seniors left unmatched from the specialty, has continued to rise.

ALTERNATIVE PATHWAYS TO BECOMING A RADIOLOGIST

Today, securing a residency position in diagnostic radiology is no easy feat. However, medical students should know that there are alternates to the standard pathway of residency training in radiology. Several programs around the country have experimented with combining radiology training with other specialties, or providing some form of prespecialization during residency. (These alternate pathways are subject to change on a year-to-year basis.)

The combined triple-specialty training program in neurology, radiology, and neuroradiology requires a total of 7 years (see Chapter 7). It leads to board certification in neurology and diagnostic radiology, as well as a certificate of added qualifications in neuroradiology. The goal of these programs is to prepare physicians to serve as leaders in both academic and clinical settings in the image-guided diagnosis and treatment of neurologic disease.

A second alternative for training is the clinical pathway for "vascular and interventional radiology." The American Medical Association officially recognized interventional radiology as a medical specialty in 1992, and today there are more than 5000 interventional radiologists in the United States. This growth prompted the Society of Cardiovascular and Interventional Radiology to address the lack of training options for individuals interested in obtaining broader clinical and research experience. A pathway has been created for trainees interested in the clinical diagnosis and care of patients with diseases commonly treated by interventional radiologists. Six years of training (preferably at a single institution) satisfies the requirements for diagnostic and interventional radiology. Planning for this pathway should occur as a medical student or during the PGY-1 year.

FELLOWSHIPS AND SUBSPECIALTY TRAINING

Newly trained residents in radiology can choose to subspecialize in more narrow areas of radiology. Is this a popular option? A recent study found that although the majority (72%) of diagnostic radiologists are generalists, subspecialization, however, is a growing trend.[2] Subspecialty expertise may be an important factor in providing a higher quality of service while also serving as an important marketing

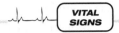

VITAL SIGNS

RADIOLOGY 2011 MATCH STATISTICS

- Number of positions available: 1124
- 948 US seniors and 371 independent applicants ranked at least one radiology program
- 96.4% of all positions were filled in the initial Match
- The successful applicants: 82% US seniors, 6.7% foreign-trained physicians, and 5.7% osteopathic graduates
- Mean USMLE Step I score: 240
- Unmatched rate for US seniors applying only to radiology: 2.1%

Data from National Resident Matching Program.

tool. Among new graduates, more than 70% choose to pursue fellowship training before entering the job market. The following Accreditation Council for Graduate Medical Education (ACGME)-accredited fellowships generally require 1 to 2 additional years of training. In addition, it is important to be aware that fellowship training is available in areas other than those approved by the ACGME. Examples include modality-based fellowships dedicated to further study of CT or MRI.

Abdominal Radiology

This fellowship provides expertise in the application and interpretation of CT, ultrasonography, MRI, and the use of interventional techniques for diseases involving the abdomen and pelvis. Abdominal radiology includes the study of the gastrointestinal tract, hepatobiliary system, genitourinary tract, and intraperitoneal and extraperitoneal abdominal organs.

Cardiothoracic Radiology

This fellowship provides expertise in the application and interpretation of imaging examinations and interventional procedures related to the lungs, pleura, mediastinum, chest wall, heart, pericardium, and the thoracic vascular system. The imaging methods and procedures include plain films, fluoroscopy, CT, MRI, ultrasound, and interventional techniques such as image-guided lung biopsies.

Endovascular Surgical Neuroradiology

This fellowship is generally of 2 to 3 years. You gain expertise in combining catheter-based interventional techniques with various forms of radiologic imaging for the diagnosis and treatment of central nervous system pathophysiology.

Fellowship training provides experience in the clinical management of patients with neurologic disease as well as the technical training to perform endovascular surgical neuroradiology procedures. Examples of these procedures include the treatment of cerebral aneurysms and arteriovenous malformations, as well as the embolization of neoplasms. These rigorous training programs usually contain 1 year of diagnostic neuroradiology and 2 years of neurointerventional training.

Musculoskeletal Radiology

This fellowship is ideal for those who want to learn more about the application and interpretation of imaging examinations and procedures as they relate to the analysis of the musculoskeletal system, including bones, joints, and soft tissues. The imaging methods and procedures include, but are not limited to, plain films, CT, ultrasonography, radionuclide scintigraphy, MRI, arthrography, and image-guided percutaneous biopsy techniques.

Neuroradiology

This fellowship comprises the study of diseases related to the central nervous system as well as diseases of the head and neck. You will gain additional experience in the selection, interpretation, and performance of a diverse set of neuroradiologic examinations and procedures. Fellowship training includes the study and use of imaging modalities such as plain films, CT, MRI, and angiography related to the brain, spine and spinal cord, head, neck, and organs of special sense.

Nuclear Radiology

Nuclear radiology is defined as a clinical subspecialty of radiology involving imaging by external detection of radionuclides in the body for diagnosing disease. Fellowship programs in nuclear radiology provide advanced training in the medical uses of radionuclides for a wide range of in-vivo imaging. Examples of these procedures include studies ranging from bone scans to nuclear cardiology to PET scanning.

Pediatric Radiology

In this fellowship, radiologists become experts in the pediatric applications of imaging techniques. These programs provide experience in all forms of diagnostic imaging as they pertain to the unique clinical and pathophysiologic problems of the newborn, infant, child, and adolescent. You draw on your medical knowledge

Residency in radiology requires 5 years of postgraduate training. There are currently 188 accredited programs. The first year consists of a broad-based clinical internship, usually an internal medicine or transitional program. During the 4 years of radiology training, residents complete monthly rotations in abdominal imaging, neuroimaging, thoracic imaging, pediatric imaging, musculoskeletal imaging, mammography, nuclear medicine, ultrasound, and interventional radiology. Call schedules vary greatly between programs, although most are front loaded, with significantly less call during the last year of training. Many programs have instituted a night float in which residents are on call for 2 to 4 weeks at a time, usually from 7 PM to 7 AM. Resident responsibilities during call hours vary among institutions, but most are responsible for interpreting plain films, CT, MRI, and performing ultrasound. For more complex procedures or cases, there is usually some form of backup provided by a senior resident, fellow, or attending. The process of taking call, and being the only radiologist in the hospital,

(continued)

of growth, development, and congenital disease. This is a highly clinical fellowship that involves close work with the department of pediatrics.

Vascular and Interventional Radiology

The unique clinical and invasive nature of practice in vascular and interventional radiology requires special training and skills. Vascular and interventional procedures are guided by a number of imaging modalities such as fluoroscopy, angiography, CT, and ultrasonography. This fellowship provides experience in the evaluation and management of patients requiring imaging-guided procedures, experience in performing the procedures, and an understanding of the medical and surgical alternatives.

With medical imaging having potential applications in almost every disease process, radiology has become a field of incredible diversity. Diagnostic radiology has come to include modalities like ultrasound, CT, MRI, and PET. Radiology offers many avenues for intellectual curiosity. In this specialty, a physician can still choose to study and specialize in almost any organ system—pediatric or adult. You can also decide to be incredibly invasive procedurally and involved clinically or choose to have little patient contact. Advances in teleradiology have created opportunities for people to work not only from home but also from distant corners of the earth.

The diversity that radiology has acquired over the last century, as well as the growing role of imaging in health care, has made the radiologist indispensable. Technologies such as CT and MRI are relatively recent additions to modern medicine, yet they have revolutionized heath care. One can only imagine what is to come. A great deal of work, for example, is currently being done with molecular imaging. Along with gene targeting, molecular imaging carries the hope of applying imaging to the physiologic processes of disease at the cellular and genetic levels. The incredible pace of technological advance within new and existing imaging modalities, in combination with their seemingly infinite applications to patient care, makes radiology an incredibly exciting field to be a part of.

> puts the resident in the position of being responsible for expertise in all aspects of imaging and being asked to rule out everything from appendicitis to pulmonary emboli.
>
> **THE INSIDE SCOOP**

Deciding on a specialty is an attempt to define both present and future priorities; balance influences from friends, family, and colleagues; and, ultimately, to select a path. But choosing wisely is not easy. Often times, and for countless reasons, residents leave one specialty for another. You can, however, maximize the chances of being happy with the final decision by educating yourself about a variety of specialties and honestly evaluating your priorities. If, after all this, you find yourself attracted to a career in radiology, then definitely work hard and try to gain exposure as early as possible to this exciting specialty.

ABOUT THE CONTRIBUTOR

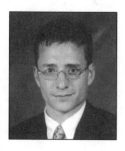

Dr Derek Fimmen is member of Cape Radiology Group, headquartered in Cape Girardeau, Missouri. After growing up in central Illinois, he earned his undergraduate degree in chemistry from Grinnell College. In his free time, he can be found on the golf course or in his sailboat. He also enjoys spending time with his wife, Stephanie, and their three dogs. Dr Fimmen received his medical education from the University of Chicago—Pritzker School of Medicine. Dr Fimmen also completed radiology residency at the University of Chicago. He can be reached by e-mail at dlfimmen@hotmail.com.

REFERENCES

1. Hunter, T.B., Krupinski, E., et al. Academic radiology and doctor discontent: The good news and the bad news. *Acad Rad*. 2001;8:509–511.

2. Crewson, P.E., Sunshine, J.H. Diagnostic radiologists' subspecialization and fields of practice. *Am J Roentgenol*. 2000;174:1203–1209.

32
UROLOGY
Jane M. Lewis

I f you want to operate on patients, urology is one of the best surgical specialties around. Other than hearing jokes about the Viagra phenomenon, most medical students have had little experience with urology. It is a highly focused area of medicine that treats diseases of a more sensitive nature—the urinary and male genital systems—and has rather good treatment outcomes. It is a specialty where you can have long-term relationships with patients (yet not be their primary care physician), where you can perform surgery and procedures (yet still get a decent night's sleep) and truly help improve patients' quality of life.

AN OVERVIEW OF UROLOGY

Urology is a surgical subspecialty focusing on the urinary tract of men and women, as well as the reproductive system of men. A common perception of urologists is that they operate on men's "private parts" and, well, that is about it. Although urologists do in fact operate on the male genitalia (penis, testicles, and scrotum), there is much more to the practice of urology than the penis. They are experts on the diagnosis and management of diseases involving the kidney, ureters, prostate, bladder, urethra, and male genitalia.

Urologists are masters of everything that has to do with the passage of urine, from its production in the kidney to its release through the urethra. They surgically correct problems such as obstructing posterior urethral valves in newborn boys or bladder outlet obstruction caused by benign prostatic hypertrophy (BPH) in elderly men. Urinary tract infections (UTIs), which affect every age group and can be quite destructive, make up a large proportion of cases seen by urologists, especially if it progresses to a worrisome infection of the kidney itself (pyelonephritis).

These UTIs could actually represent serious underlying problems of the urinary system. Urologists, therefore, make use of sophisticated testing (laboratory urine analysis, urodynamic flow studies, cystoscopy) to make diagnoses and begin formulating treatment plans.

In the pediatric population, the focus is on male and female congenital abnormalities. The urinary tract is affected by nonfatal congenital anomalies more than any other organ system. This means undescended testicles (cryptorchidism), ureters poorly implanted into a bladder such that urine refluxes back to the kidneys (vesicoureteral reflux), bladder exstrophy, and the technically difficult arenas of cloacal malformation and disorder of sexual differentiation. Certainly, a general practice urologist will feel comfortable treating some of the more minor conditions, but will likely refer the more complex cases to specialists in pediatric urology.

Kidney stones (nephrolithiasis), which form in both women and men, fall under the expertise of the urologist. Some nephrologists also have an interest in treating patients who form stones, but once a stone is obstructing the urinary system, it is up to the urologist to take it out. Stone surgery dates back to some of the medical writings of Hippocrates. Certainly, a lot has changed since then; with the recent advent of endoscopic technology, minimally invasive techniques can be used to fragment stones and allow passage of the pieces without making an incision. Now urologists use high-tech tools such as rigid and flexible ureteroscopy, percutaneous nephroscopy, and extracorporeal shockwave lithotripsy to treat kidney stones (especially if obstructed and causing infection). For those who like video games, that hand–eye coordination will now come in handy. Open extraction of stones has generally fallen to the wayside.

Incontinence affects the elderly in our population, as well as younger people with neurologic problems or spinal cord injury, regardless of gender, and it can hamper patients' lives terribly. Treating incontinence is one area where a urologist can make a significant impact on a person's quality of life. Imagine being afraid to leave the house because you are worried about wetting yourself. This is crippling to some. Armed with advanced diagnostic techniques such as urodynamic studies, the urologist can assess the underlying cause of the incontinence and offer either medicines or surgery to keep the person dry.

Sexual dysfunction is a significant part of the practice of urology. Historically, the focus has been on male dysfunction but more recently, urologists have also thrown their hat into the complicated world of female sexual dysfunction. In the male world, there are medical treatments for impotence such as Viagra and, if those fail, surgical options such as implantable penile prosthesis. In the female world, medical and surgical interventions are still being investigated. Obviously, this is another area where the urologist can make a huge impact on a patient's quality of life.

Two areas of urology that are somewhat rare but certainly could be areas of focus for the motivated are renal transplantation and traumatic reconstruction. Some urologists take on a role in the world of kidney transplant, either as the primary transplant surgeon or as a member of the transplant team. They often perform the donor nephrectomy, depending on the medical center. Transplant is not a part of all urologists' practices and would need to be sought out as an area of interest. Trauma is another area that is not uniformly experienced in the various training programs. Urologists are key members of the trauma team in the operating room (for patients who have urethral, bladder, or renal damage). They draw on advances in renal tract imaging to evaluate quickly for any trauma to the urinary tract. Urethral reconstructive surgery combines interesting aspects of urologic anatomy and plastic surgery.

Urologists also deal with a significant number of cases of malignant disease in their practices. Unless specifically specialized in another aspect of urology, prostate cancer in men is a urologist's major clinical issue. The search for bladder cancer or kidney cancer brings in many male and female patients when they have blood in their urine. Men are surgically treated for testicular or penile cancer by urologists. Fair assumption—cancer is where the big surgery, both open and robotically assisted laparoscopic approaches, exists in adult urology. Often the urologist is part of a multidisciplinary cancer team, performing the surgical excision and providing the ongoing symptomatic follow-up, while the radiation and medical oncologists provide expertise in areas such as external beam radiation therapy and chemotherapy.

Most students are well aware that urologists are experts on diseases of the prostate. But the prostate is not always affected by cancer; in fact, most older men have BPH—an enlargement of the prostate. Many end up having problems with voiding because of their big prostate, which can be very uncomfortable and can even lead to acute urinary retention. Urologists, once again, offer medical and, if necessary, surgical interventions to ease the passage of urine.

UROLOGY IS BOTH MEDICINE AND SURGERY

Although urology is definitely a surgical subspecialty, it overlaps with many other disciplines. Urology requires some working knowledge of general surgery, gynecology, internal medicine (particularly nephrology and endocrinology), pediatrics, neurology, and radiology.

WHAT MAKES A GOOD UROLOGIST?

✓ Prefers working with his or her hands.

✓ Enjoys being an expert in a very specialized area of medicine.

✓ Is an independent and outgoing thinker.

✓ Likes seeing the immediate results of treatment.

✓ Has excellent manual dexterity and hand–eye coordination.

THE INSIDE SCOOP

Every urologist has been trained in general surgery for at least 1 year. Some urologists even completed full general surgery training and then decided to specialize in urology. The training and knowledge base in general surgery is essential. For starters, surgical interns learn the basic techniques—how to hold the scalpel, how to move the "Bovie" (electrocautery), how to grasp the needle driver, how to tie knots, and where your hands should be and when. Also, a surgical intern learns the concepts of postsurgical inpatient care. For example, these young doctors begin to recognize a postoperative ileus and the proper time to insert a nasogastric tube. Fluid management in the postoperative period can be absolutely critical and requires an understanding of the concepts of third spacing as well as cardiovascular restrictions. Wound care, including managing drains of all kinds, is another important concept for all surgeons—general or specialist—to master.

Gynecology–obstetrics has much overlap with urology, considering the anatomic location. A urologist focusing on female urology shares some of the same patients as a gynecologist subspecializing in urogynecology. Even the general urologist, however, must have a complete understanding of male and female pelvic anatomy. And while a urologist would never perform a cesarean section, they could certainly become involved if the gynecologist or obstetrician inadvertently opened the bladder or transected a ureter.

Internal medicine—particularly nephrology and endocrinology—is important to the urologist given the overlays with adrenal, renal, and testicular disorders. If a patient presents to the hospital in renal failure, the urologist is often consulted to participate in the workup. It may be due to prerenal, intrarenal causes and/or postrenal obstruction. As far as endocrinology is concerned, urologists should have a working sense of male hormones, essential to any infertility workup, as well as the workings of the adrenal glands, given that someone with an adrenal mass may initially present to them for diagnosis.

Knowledge of pediatrics is important if the urologist will be focusing his or her career on children. But certainly during the residency training, unlike a general medicine resident who will spend no time at a children's hospital, a urology resident spends approximately 6 to 8 months taking care of children. Of course, it is specific to urologic care, but taking care of children is different than taking care of adults and these differences must be learned. Fluid management is different, medicine dosing is different, comorbidities are different, and, in general, kids have much higher physiologic reserve and therefore can look well up until the moment they crash.

Neurology is a field that plays into the urology database in that people with spinal cord injuries, congenital or acquired, inevitably have bladder dysfunction. Having a working knowledge of the nervous system, particularly as it relates to the pelvic organs, becomes paramount in treating a neurogenic bladder.

Finally, it is essential for urologists to have an understanding of the radiologic imaging that a urologic patient may undergo. As with any surgical specialty, diagnosis is often predicated completely on what the scan looks like. For example, if a man with testicular pain and no palpable mass is sent for a scrotal ultrasound, and a small testicular mass is noted, he will immediately get a workup for testicular cancer. On the basis of ultrasound findings alone, he may require counseling for surgical excision. Or, for example, a woman who has been in a car accident and whose CT scan shows an incidental, irregular 4-cm renal mass that enhances with intravenous contrast. On the basis of these findings alone, she is diagnosed with probable renal cell carcinoma and offered surgical excision. Renal function for patients with an atrophic-looking kidney can be assessed using nuclear medicine. For example, a dimercaptosuccinic acid scan, a radioisotope that binds to renal parenchyma, gives a sense of how well the kidneys are filtering blood, the left compared with the right.

Medical students considering a career in urology must accept that this specialty is definitely still a surgical field. In some European countries, urology has been divided into two tracts: operative urology and office urology. In the United States, some think that urology is headed toward that same division. In the meanwhile, however, urologists still manage both sides of the operating room. In reality, a community practice urologist may opt to refer all big open cases to an academic center (eg, cystectomy with neobladder construction). This referral pattern has evolved due to the amount of work these bigger cases entail and the poor reimbursement standards. This means that a typical community urologist only performs straightforward open surgery (eg, radical prostatectomy, occasional nephrectomy), minor procedures (eg, vasectomy, circumcision), and endoscopic surgery (eg, cystoscopy, ureteroscopy, transurethral resection of bladder tumor or prostate ablative surgery, lithotripsy).

UROLOGY OUTSIDE THE OPERATING ROOM

There are certainly many nonoperative aspects of urology. A typical clinical day could include any number of patients, such as the following.

Patient 1: A 76-year-old man, complaining of increased urinary frequency and nocturia (nighttime urination) five times a night. His most recent prostate-specific antigen (PSA) level is 0.9. On examination, his prostate feels benign but is large. He empties his bladder and you perform a bladder scan showing 50 mL of urine in his bladder. Diagnosing him with likely BPH, you prescribe a trial of alpha-blockers and ask to see him back in a month to assess improvement in his symptoms.

Patient 2: A 58-year-old man, complaining of inability to maintain an erection during coitus, getting gradually worse over the past year. He is a long-term smoker and type II diabetic patient. His cardiac status is good and he takes only cholesterol and blood-pressure-lowering drugs in addition to metformin (his diabetic medication). Diagnosing him with likely erectile dysfunction due to poor vasculature, you offer him a trial of sildenafil and ask to see him back in 2 months.

Patient 3: A 44-year-old woman, complaining of pelvic pain and urinary frequency, says she has been treated for presumptive urinary tract symptoms by her primary care physician, but there has been no relief. She is otherwise healthy but exasperated by this ongoing pain. You send a urine sample to the lab for urinalysis and culture and to pathology to check for malignancy. You determine that after urinating, she has a postvoid residual of 25 mL, so you schedule her for an in-office flexible cystoscopy, suspecting interstitial cystitis but wanting to rule out any abnormalities.

Patient 4: A 62-year-old man, referred for persistent microhematuria found on routine physical examination urinalysis. He has a 50-pack per year history of tobacco use, controlled hypertension, and no physical complaints. After a physical examination, you send his urine off to the laboratory for a repeat urinalysis and cytologic assessment for malignancy and then schedule him for a CT scan of his kidneys, ureters, bladder to look for lesions, and for an in-office flexible cystoscopy to evaluate his bladder for tumors.

Patient 5: A 53-year-old man whom you have seen previously for an elevated PSA. When his primary care physician checked it 6 months ago, it had risen from 2.5

to 4.1 over the course of a year. You performed ultrasound-guided prostate needle biopsy on him last week and prostate cancer was discovered. Now the patient is here to discuss treatment options. After a lengthy discussion, he decides that he would like to have surgery performed. Because you are nearing retirement and slowing down your surgical practice, you introduce him to the bright young partner in the group who performs at least two prostatectomies a week.

THE DOCTOR–PATIENT RELATIONSHIP

Most surgical specialists are simply consultants who treat an acute surgical problem and then send the patient back to their primary care physicians. Urologists, however, do form long-term relationships with their patients. While patients would never treat their urologist as their primary care physician, if they have bothersome voiding symptoms, sexual dysfunction, or cancer, none of these things are an easy fix. Patients with bladder cancer meet their urologist for a workup after their first episode of gross hematuria, for example, and then potentially go to the operating room for cystoscopy with a follow-up transurethral resection of their bladder tumor. Then, depending on the pathology, they either return to the operating room for a cystectomy or to the clinic for weekly intravesical therapy. This could mean follow-up cystoscopies every 3 to 6 months for a few years then yearly cystoscopy for the rest of his or her life.

If a patient with voiding dysfunction is referred to the urologist for evaluation, he or she could be started on a medicine, sent for urodynamic studies, or treated for UTI. Regardless, the patient needs to come back to talk about the improvement or worsening of symptoms and then another move will be made. Possibly an older man could benefit from an operation on his prostate, but many of these patients do very well on medical therapy and continue to have checkups for years and years. Likewise, women with incontinence may either see the urogynecologist or the female urologist and have an ongoing relationship, assessing the symptoms and tweaking the interventions for years.

The patient with sexual dysfunction requires all the interview finesse and sensitivity a physician has. The urologist must be very comfortable talking about sex and all its accoutrements to make the patient feel comfortable, truly uncover all the symptoms, and get to the best diagnosis and treatment. Once again, this starts with medical therapies and requires ongoing visits. The penile prosthetic devices are currently improving but are still not permanent cures; hence, these patients will continue to require urology services in the future.

Certainly, in the pediatric population, the children with major congenital abnormalities will continue to see their urologist for years; most children will have a surgically correctable problem such as an undescended testicle and their relationships will be short. Children with myelodysplasia will have ongoing relationships, potentially, with a urologist, an orthopedic surgeon, and a neurosurgeon, as well as their primary care pediatrician.

LIFESTYLE CONSIDERATIONS AND PRACTICE OPTIONS

Some refer to urology as "surgery light" because of the highly variable surgical intensity. Of course, there are plenty of academic urologists who would never fall under this description. Many urologists readily admit, however, that urology was attractive to them precisely because it allowed them a lifestyle that they never could have had as a neurosurgeon or general surgeon—but it was still surgery.

The average urologist is not called into the hospital in the middle of the night, given the paucity of true urologic emergencies. One emergency is testicular torsion, a twisting of the testicular blood supply such that the testis, if not operated on and untwisted quickly, will die. This surgery, however, is very brief. Ureteral obstruction from stone disease that has led to urosepsis requires prompt decompression via either cystoscopy with a ureteral stent placement or, more commonly, if someone is acutely ill, interventional radiology placing a percutaneous nephrostomy tube to drain the system from above. Someone with hematuria could develop clot retention, but this can be dealt with via a Foley catheter, manual irrigation of the clots, continuous bladder irrigation, and supportive care.

If you crave more excitement in your urology career, the academic setting would probably be the best fit. Or, if you want to see trauma and be called into the hospital at 2:00 AM for the intraperitoneal bladder rupture after a motor vehicle accident, or the penile reattachment or urethral reconstruction after a knife injury, your choice should be a busy urban academic trauma center. One could even choose a rural trauma center where farm equipment can cause some fairly interesting injuries.

An academic career at a nontrauma hospital might mean having a very interesting surgical practice, where the community urologists refer their difficult cases to you. You could be operating every day, or nearly every day, and doing a wide variety of cases—cystectomy with a range of urinary diversions, prostatectomy, pelvic surgery for a mass that nobody else wants to tackle, repair of ureteric injuries from other surgeons, and revision of a urethral sling because a woman is still bothered by her stress urinary incontinence.

Most urologists with academic careers spend a fair amount of time dedicated to clinical research. Some hold positions in which they mostly see patients in the clinic, operating occasionally, and then spending the rest of their time in research endeavors. These academic urologists generally have established themselves as experts within their research field—for example, male sexual dysfunction, prostate cancer, incontinence—and nearly all the clinical patients they see are there precisely for that reason. Every once in a while, these specialists may go to the operating room, for instance, to place a penile prosthesis, take out a prostate, or do a complex continence repair.

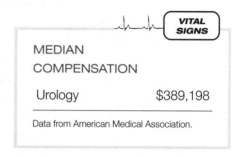

VITAL SIGNS

MEDIAN COMPENSATION

Urology $389,198

Data from American Medical Association.

Most residents, however, choose a career in the private sector. The salaries are higher and the demands are different from the academic world. A group practice will be looking for a junior partner, perhaps because their practice is getting too big for all of them to handle, or perhaps because one of the senior partners is stepping back his patient load with his eye on retiring. Regardless, each group will have different expectations of the junior partner, his or her responsibilities, and how exactly he or she will become a full partner. Some physicians may be partners only in economics and overhead but not in patient care responsibilities. Some practices may be so tight knit that the entire group rounds together every morning at the hospital, seeing whatever inpatients they collectively have, treating all group patients as if they were their individual patient. A urologist desiring a part-time job in a group practice so that he or she can have time for family is not unheard of.

This is a field of professionals who, in general, are nice people, married, the least likely of any surgical specialists to divorce, interested in some hobby outside of medicine, and fairly laid back. Also, given the nature of the anatomy dealt with, most urologists are required to have a pretty good sense of humor.

SPECIAL SPECIALISTS: UROLOGISTS WHO ARE WOMEN

Urology is certainly a specialty that is heavily male dominated—both its area of expertise, patient base and physicians. Given this environment, most women interested in a surgical career may have some hesitation about selecting urology. Patients are often surprised when they encounter a urologist who is a woman. Some may ask you "When did they start letting women do this?" or "Does your mother know you do this?" Despite this, for the most part, men appear to be comfortable with female doctors. Certainly, if the doctor is uncomfortable, the patient will be uncomfortable, regardless of gender.

The demand for women in the field has grown so much recently that women in urology training programs begin fielding job offers well before they are finished with their training. These are inevitably from group practices of urologists, all male, who have had women call asking if they can see a woman doctor. When the answer is no, those women take their business elsewhere if they can.

Of course, the struggle for the general practice woman in adult urology is to see male and female patients. Naturally, women sometimes need a major open surgery such as a nephrectomy or cystectomy, but for the most part, their complaints have to do with voiding dysfunction. This means a woman practicing in general adult urology may end up being a "female urologist," even without doing a year's fellowship training, and maybe without even wanting that focus. Certainly, this is avoidable with awareness and careful planning with the partners.

Being a woman in a surgical field has its own set of personal demands. Men and women, both, are challenged in many ways as residents. Women have some added disadvantages, which obviously have to do with our biologic role with birthing babies. In today's day and age, it is unfortunate that this is still an issue. While any employer is legally required to provide maternity leave, your coworkers are not guaranteed a replacement while you are gone. This could potentially seed resentment if the delivery date is during a particularly stressful time for the department. The same numbers of patients keep coming in, and there may be fewer physicians to take care of them.

Many women have dealt with this challenge by carefully timing the pregnancy during dedicated research time so that your absence hurts only you and your curriculum vitae. Some department heads even find creative ways to support the remainder of the house staff if a female resident was not able to plan the pregnancy perfectly. Still, most female surgical residents do not attempt to have a baby while in residency training.

Another interesting phenomenon is the single female surgical resident. For unclear reasons, there are many super, bright, beautiful, dedicated women who are single. True, nobody has a lot of time for socializing and meeting new people. True, training in surgery is likely a bit threatening to the weaker members of the opposite sex. And true, professional women regardless of career in our culture are staying single longer and longer. It is unclear how or if these truths are related, but they exist.

FELLOWSHIPS AND SUBSPECIALTY TRAINING

Many urologists desire extra training in one particular aspect of the field. This means applying for postresidency fellowship training. They can last anywhere from 1 to 3 years depending on the program.

Endourology and Laparoscopic Surgery

The buzzword in all surgical specialties nowadays is "minimally invasive." In urology, there is a similar effort to develop techniques by which surgeons can operate on the genitourinary system without actually opening the pelvic cavity. Endourology includes advanced training in laparoscopic (including robotically assisted) urologic surgery, percutaneous kidney surgery, and ureteroscopy. Laparoscopy and ureteroscopy have become more commonplace in most urology training programs, so many residents may not feel a need to pursue more of the same training. Many residents, however, would like to perform only minimally invasive procedures in their future practice and seek out intensive training to make that desire a negotiable reality. Most fellowships are 1-year programs integrating both clinical and research experiences.

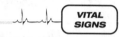
VITAL SIGNS

UROLOGY 2011 MATCH STATISTICS

- Number of positions available: 271
- 339 applicants ranked at least one urology program
- Candidates submitted on an average 48 applications and received 11 interviews
- 98.9% of all positions were filled in the initial Match
- Match rates: US seniors, 86%; US graduates, 62%; women, 82%; foreign-trained physicians, 27%
- Unmatched rate for US seniors applying only to urology: 14%

Data from American Urological Association.

Female Pelvic Medicine and Reconstructive Urology

Remember—women constitute a large portion of the patients seen by urologists. If you are interested in helping women with voiding dysfunction and pelvic prolapse, you should consider this fellowship, which combines both urology and gynecology experience. You will become an expert in all kinds of female reconstructive surgery, such as urethral suspensions, slings, artificial urinary sphincters (for men), and urethroplasty. Women, after all, have their own special set of urologic

Residency in urology requires 5 years of postgraduate training. There are currently 119 accredited programs. The residency begins with 1 year of general surgery training followed by 4 years of clinical urology. In the final year, the resident functions in the capacity of chief resident. Like any surgical specialty, residency in urology is very time consuming and intense. It requires a high level of commitment for excellent patient care, professional development of operative skills and a teamwork mentality, and job responsibilities taking priority over many personal matters. However, call schedules are generally more benign than for other surgical subspecialties. Monthly rotations include general urology and each of its subspecialties (pediatric, oncologic, and renal transplant, among others). Residents also gain a significant amount of outpatient experience in the urology clinic. Upon completion, every new urologist is qualified to perform any operative procedure from minor surgeries such as endoscopy to major reconstructive cases.

THE INSIDE SCOOP

problems, including stress urinary incontinence, urethral diverticuli, and chronic UTIs. In their practice, these subspecialists evaluate patients using diagnostic tools such as cystoscopy and urodynamic studies. The fellowship generally lasts for 2 years (including both clinical and research experience). New therapies for these disorders are constantly refined every year.

Infertility and Sexual Dysfunction

Many men suffer from sexual dysfunction and infertility. Subspecialists in this area become experts in diagnostic techniques, medical therapies, the use of prosthetic devices, and the surgical correction of congenital problems. Because of advances in medical therapy for sexual dysfunction, these urologists develop an in-depth understanding of both endocrinology and reproductive physiology. The area of sexual dysfunction is now expanding from men to also include women. Infertility focuses only on the male side, working in conjunction with the gynecologists who are fellowship trained in infertility. These training programs are of 1 to 2 years depending on the research component.

Pediatric Urology

This fellowship is perfect if you would like to tailor your practice to only children and would like to stay in an academic setting.

Estimates suggest a population of 1 million people is needed to support one pediatric urologist. Hence, the jobs are mostly limited to large referral centers, usually academic hospitals, which are also the centers that train pediatric urologists. Certainly, there are fellowship-trained pediatric urologists who work in private practice as well, particularly in regions of the country, which lack a separate children's hospital. The clinical training is usually 1 year in length. This year is flanked by either 1 or 2 years of research, depending on the program. Obviously, if you are headed into academics, time in research is essential.

Urologic Oncology

If you have a particular interest in cancer, this fellowship provides the opportunity to develop additional expertise in the treatment of cancer in the genitourinary tract. Once again, 1 to 2 years of research precede a clinical training year. This means not only developing laboratory research skills, enhancing one's understanding of the cancer disease process, but also developing prime surgical skills to tackle what usually are the most challenging of urologic surgeries. Of note, most chairmen of academic urology departments have a focus in urologic oncology.

WHY CONSIDER A CAREER IN UROLOGY?

The specialty of urology is constantly changing. Much of this change has been the result of improved technology. Refinements in ureteral and renal endoscopic surgery have already revolutionized the therapy of urinary tract stones and, together with the new generation of extracorporeal lithotriptors, have made many of the traditional surgical and even endoscopic approaches to the problem of renal and ureteral calculi largely obsolete.

The results of other traditional urologic procedures, specifically vasovasostomy and varicocele repair, have improved in selected cases with the use of the surgical microscope. Skill and experience using the surgical microscope will undoubtedly be an important part of urologic practice in the future. Lasers are in their infancy but are already influential in the management of ureteral calculi as well as benign prostatic hyperplasia. Many urologic operations that were done by open surgery in the past can now be performed with a minimally invasive technique. The development of new cancer chemotherapeutic agents has significantly altered therapy for some urologic cancers.

If you enjoy gross anatomy, are a hands-on person, and thrive on interviewing patients about sensitive topics, perhaps urology is for you! These specialists operate (or treat medically), often enacting a cure, and then move on to the next diagnostic problem at hand. You will be joining a field in which the joy of operating can meet the pleasure of some long-term patient relationships in a practice of the intensity you choose. By treating diseases of the urogenital system, as a urologist, you will have the extraordinary privilege of improving your patients' quality of life.

ABOUT THE CONTRIBUTOR

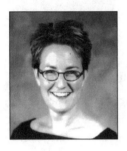 Dr Jane Lewis is currently a pediatric urologist and assistant professor in the Department of Urology at the University of Minnesota in Minneapolis. She completed a pediatric urology fellowship at Children's Memorial Hospital in Chicago. Fellowship was after graduation from the Harvard Urology Residency Program—Longwood area, based at the Brigham and Women's Hospital. Born and raised in Michigan, she earned a BA in sociocultural anthropology at Northwestern University. Over the next 7 years, she worked in Chicago as an anthropology researcher (interviewing elderly Spanish-speaking residents about aging), au pair, substitute teacher, and secretary while taking premedical courses in night school. Dr Lewis then earned her medical degree from the University of Chicago—Pritzker School of Medicine.

APPENDIX: INTERNET RESOURCES GUIDE

Medical Education and Licensing

Accreditation Council on Graduate Medical Education (ACGME) — *www.acgme.org*

American Board of Medical Specialties — *www.abms.org*

American Medical Association — *www.ama-assn.org*

Association of American Medical Colleges — *www.aamc.org*

Council of Medical Specialty Societies — *www.cmss.org*

Federation of State Medical Boards — *www.fsmb.org*

National Board of Medical Examiners — *www.nbme.org*

United States Medical Licensing Exam — *www.usmle.org*

The Match

Educational Commission for Foreign Medical Graduates — *www.ecfmg.org*

Electronic Residency Application Service (ERAS) — *www.myeras.aamc.org*

National Resident Matching Program — *www.nrmp.org*

San Francisco Matching Program — *www.sfmatch.org*

Major Specialty Organizations

American Society of Anesthesiologists — *www.asahq.org*

American Academy of Dermatology — *www.aad.org*

American Academy of Family Physicians — *www.aafp.org*

American Academy of Neurology — *www.aan.com*

American Academy of Ophthalmology — *www.aao.org*

American Academy of Orthopaedic Surgeons — *www.aos.org*

American Academy of Otolaryngology — Head and Neck Surgery — *www.entnet.org*

American Academy of Pediatrics — *www.aap.org*

American Academy of Physical Medicine & Rehabilitation — *www.aapmr.org*

American Association of Neurological Surgeons — *www.aans.org*

American Association of Plastic Surgeons — *www.aapsl921.org*

American College of Emergency Physicians—*www.acep.org*
American College of Obstetricians and Gynecologists—*www.acog.org*
American College of Physicians—American Society of Internal Medicine—
    www.acponline.org
American College of Radiation Oncology—*www.acro.org*
American College of Radiology—*www.acr.org*
American College of Surgeons—*www.facs.org*
American Psychiatric Association—*www.psych.org*
American Society of Clinical Pathologists—*www.ascp.org*
American Urological Association—*www.auanet.org*
College of American Pathologists—*www.cap.org*

Other Useful Web Sites

CareerMD—*www.careermd.com*
Fellowship and Residency Electronic Interactive Database (FREIDA)—
    www.ama-assn.org/go/freida
Internship and Resident Information Site (IRIS)—*www.i-r-i-s.com*
MedCAREERS—*www.aamc.org/medcareers*
Physician's Guide to the Internet—*www.physiciansguide.com*
ResidentWeb—*www.residentweb.com*
Scutwork.com (residency program reviews)—*www.scutwork.com*
The Student-Doctor Network—*www.studentdoctor.net*

INDEX

Page numbers followed by the letter t refer to tabular material.